CLINICAL REASONING IN PHYSICAL DISABILITIES

REBECCA DUTTON, M.S., L/OTR

Assistant Professor
Department of Occupational Therapy
Kean College of New Jersey
Union, New Jersey

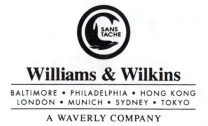

Williams & Wilkins

BALTIMORE • PHILADELPHIA • HONG KONG
LONDON • MUNICH • SYDNEY • TOKYO
A WAVERLY COMPANY

Editor: John P. Butler
Managing Editor: Linda S. Napora
Copy Editor: Judith F. Minkove
Designer: Norman W. Och
Illustration Planner: Ray Lowman
Production Coordinator: Anne Stewart Seitz

Copyright © 1995
Williams & Wilkins
428 East Preston Street
Baltimore, Maryland 21202, USA

Accurate indications, adverse reactions, and dosage schedules for drugs are provided
in this book, but it is possible that they may change. The reader is urged to review
the package information data of the manufacturers of the medications mentioned.

Printed in the United States of America

Library of Congress Cataloging in Publication Data

Dutton, Rebecca.
    Clinical reasoning in physical disabilities / Rebecca Dutton.
        p.   cm.
    Includes bibliographical references and index.
    ISBN 0-683-02740-9
    1. Physically handicapped—Rehabilitation.   2. Physical therapy.
    I. Title.
RM700.D84   1995
617/.03—dc20   94-24714
                                                                    CIP

                            95 96 97 98 99
                    1 2 3 4 5 6 7 8 9 10

To Linda Levy

*who drew me down new pathways and
to the occupational therapy students
at Temple University and Kean College
who sustained me along the way*

PREFACE

Because clinical reasoning is a mental process that cannot be directly observed, students need to hear examples of this type of internal dialogue. It is difficult for experienced therapists to describe the strategies they use to decide what is best for a particular patient; clinical reasoning strategies may be modified many times while working in a wide variety of clinical settings with a wide variety of patients. The strategies and examples presented in *Clinical Reasoning in Physical Disabilities* have been field-tested on more than 450 occupational therapy students and revised over a 9-year period. Many of the ideas presented here are a direct response to the situations that students found confusing. Students will eventually know what to do from experience, but they need concrete strategies to get started. Section I of the text introduces students to clinical reasoning. Early competence in clinical reasoning is especially important inasmuch as students must demonstrate good judgment to pass Fieldwork II evaluations.

FRAMES OF REFERENCE

The biomechanical, neurodevelopmental, and rehabilitation frames of reference are presented in Sections II through IV. This text focuses on the decision tree process, situational thinking, sequencing of treatment, and linking statements. Students will be able to critique tests and select an individualized evaluation package to respond to the time constraints of managed health care. Students will be able to apply theories to unique individuals by seeing *situational thinking* modeled and by being given permission early in their education to use personal judgment about what is best for a given patient. Students will learn in sequencing treatment that it is just as important to know when to implement a treatment technique as how to implement that technique. *Linking statements* document the connection between evaluation results, measurable short-term goals, and functional outcomes. Students will be able to write *linking statements* and understand why they explain occupational therapy to patients and third party payers.

CASE STUDIES

Sections II through IV provide case studies that demonstrate how to apply the biomechanical, neurodevelopmental, and rehabilitation frames of reference. Unlike memorizing concepts fo a multiple-choice examination where there is only one right answer for each question, applying a single frame of reference ensures a successful first experience. Students will also learn how to deal with the discomfort of having to reframe their approach to patient care when they shift to a new frame of reference in the next case study. The result is an eclectic approach to treatment.

Psychosocial, perceptual-cognitive, sensorimotor, and homeostatic concerns are presented in Chapters 14 through 17. These chapters enable students to identify concerns that are ignored when a single physically oriented frame of reference is used. The biomechanical, neurodevelopmental, and rehabilitation frames of reference do not address problems such as pain, infections, and emotional distress. Chapters 14 through 17 enhance awareness of the blind spots in all physically oriented frames of reference.

A final case study (Section VI) suggests strategies for combining frames of reference. Students will develop an eclectic approach by having it modeled for them.

MEMORY AIDS

The memory aids, which cannot be understood without reading the text, are intended to remind the reader of major concepts rather than provide supplemental information as a table does. Using the memory aids during case study exams enables teachers to test judgment rather than memory. The memory aids increase the students' speed of clinical reasoning by chunking information to control the overwhelming flow of information in a case study. Speed is important since they must deal with an entire case in three hours. This 3-hour window is much closer to the "by tomorrow" processing that is expected of students at the beginning of Fieldwork II.

ACKNOWLEDGMENTS

I would like to thank Linda Levy who drew me down new pathways and the occupational therapy students at Temple University and Kean College who sustained me along the way. I would also like to thank my husband, Harley F. Parker, who has encouraged me and brought joy into my life.

CONTENTS

SECTION I

INTRODUCTION

CHAPTER / 1

Clinical Reasoning

The pressure on occupational therapy students to demonstrate good clinical reasoning is very strong. The AOTA fieldwork evaluation form requires students to demonstrate good clinical judgment in addition to technical skill in fieldwork level II (1). This means students will be graded not only on how well a splint actually turns out, but also on how appropriate their thought process was during the evaluation and design phases. Perhaps that is why 49% of over 800 clinicians identified clinical reasoning as the most important skill that *should* be stressed in the education of occupational therapy students (2).

Clinical reasoning is something that experienced clinicians do every day. Yet, it is difficult to describe because experienced therapists know more than they can say (3). In fact, Mattingly and Fleming found that experienced therapists were not aware of making treatment decisions until a researcher asked them to describe their thought process after the treatment session (3). "It wasn't that the therapists didn't think. It was that therapists didn't think about thinking" (4, p. 26). One experienced therapist said, "I never really thought about all of this as much as I have today," when asked to explain why he did something (5, p. 200). If clinical reasoning is an intuitive process that remains a mystery, how can we teach it to the next generation of therapists? How can we evaluate students on clinical judgment during their fieldwork experience? Equally important, how can we empower our clients to participate in the decision-making process if we can't explain what we are doing (5, 6)? The purpose of this book is to demystify the clinical reasoning process and to enable students to demonstrate good clinical judgment very early in their fieldwork II placement.

This chapter introduces you to clinical reasoning by defining basic concepts such as situational thinking, the decision tree process, pattern recognition, knowing-IN-action, frames of reference, reflection-in-action, and the prospective treatment story. This chapter also introduces you to three different tracks of clinical reasoning: the procedural, interactive, and conditional tracks.

CHARACTERISTICS OF CLINICAL REASONING

Clinical reasoning has been called problem solving, clinical judgment, intuition, and critical thinking (2, 3, 5, 7, 8). There are three essential characteristics that define clinical reasoning. Clinical reasoning is:

1. A goal-oriented activity;
2. The practical ability to apply a general theory to a specific patient; and
3. A cognitive process.

First, clinical reasoning is a **goal-oriented activity** (3). Mattingly and Fleming say that the goal of clinical reasoning for occupational therapy is to regain the best possible function for everyday activities (3). This is radically different from the goal of a physician, which is to diagnose physical and mental illness and prescribe treatment. To help a patient regain function, the occupational therapist evaluates functional skills, like dressing, as well as underlying deficits that cause dysfunction, such as loss of range of motion. While early treatment may be aimed at remediating underlying deficits such as abnormal muscle tone, the ultimate goal of clinical reasoning in occupational therapy is to restore the patient to his or her highest level of functional independence.

Second, clinical reasoning is a **practical form of reasoning** that enables you to determine what "the good" is for a particular individual or situation (3). While a theory tells us what to do in the general case, clinical decisions occur in a specific context. Theoretical knowledge is bound to be a crude approximation of what should be done; theory is a starting place rather than a rule book. A particular situation is often more subtle and somewhat different from the complexities of the general case (3). I call this **situational thinking**.

Situational thinking ensures that revision occurs *before* treatment implementation. Situational thinking asks the question, "Are the treatment techniques I've selected appropriate for this specific case?" The therapist mentally tests treatment ideas to see if they are good for this particular patient at this particular time *before* getting feedback.

Experienced clinicians engage in situational thinking by mentally comparing the current patient to treatment stories that have similar components. These clinicians can recall how effective treatment was under similar conditions in the past. However, these treatment stories take time to accumulate. Therefore, the student must initially engage in situational thinking by using common sense to critique treatment ideas before implementing them. For example, pressure applied in the form of Coban Wrap can be used to reduce edema. Yet, Coban Wrap is not always safe. The student needs to reconsider his/her choice if the patient has an open wound. Common sense tells you that Coban Wrap would cut into the unprotected tissues and that other methods to reduce edema, such as elevation, should be used instead.

The situational aspect of clinical reasoning cannot be emphasized enough. Benner said that clinical expertise is embedded in clinical experience (8). When cognitive strategies were taught without practicing them to keep from overwhelming students, improvement in later problem solving did not occur (9). In fact, if students practiced cognitive strategies on logic problems, they did not do well on unfamiliar types of problems, such as visual games (9). Clinical reasoning is a set of domain-specific skills that are acquired through practical experience in specific situations. The types of problems solved in school must be very similar to true clinical problems.

Finally, clinical reasoning is a **cognitive process** that breaks problem-solving down into small steps (3). These steps have traditionally been called evaluation, test interpretation, treatment planning, treatment implementation, and reevaluation. Watts called this series of steps the **decision tree process**, and she defined it as a sequence of decisions involved in problem management that takes into account the uncertainty of events at each step (7). The decisions made at each step influences the decisions made at each subsequent step. For example, how you interpret certain test results will cause your treatment planning to branch off in a particular direction. The final path these decisions make can be drawn in the form of complex flow diagrams. These complex diagrams are very difficult for students to follow on their first attempts at clinical reasoning. That is why I have chosen an outline format in Chapter 2 to describe the decision tree process.

DECISION TREE PROCESS

The steps in the decision tree process are usually identified by the outcomes they produce, like an evalua-

tion report or a treatment plan. However, Elstein found that experienced clinicians created these products by using four mental strategies (10). Elstein observed expert physicians during case simulations to learn what they thought about when trying to arrive at a diagnosis. He discovered that they used:

1. Cue acquisition;
2. Hypothesis generation;
3. Cue interpretation; and
4. Hypothesis evaluation.

Cue acquisition involves recognizing which data are needed in a particular case. Ideally, one doesn't waste time gathering every possible cue; one gathers only the ones that are relevant to the particular case. **Hypothesis generation** initially means creating a list of possible diagnoses, if you are a physician. For therapists, hypothesis generation means creating a list of possible physical and mental deficits and the dysfunction that these deficits cause. **Cue interpretation** means appropriately evaluating which cues are relevant to specific hypotheses under consideration. Elstein reported that a 3-point scale for cue interpretation was used by experts: $+1$ when a cue confirmed a hypothesis, -1 when a cue disconfirmed a hypothesis, and 0 when the cue did not contribute to hypothesis evaluation (10). Elstein found that accuracy in identifying the relevance of cues was strongly related to accurate diagnoses (10). **Hypothesis evaluation** is the final stage, where the expert clinician chooses which hypotheses he/she believes were supported by the evidence.

An expert clinician generates a workable number of hypotheses. Expert physicians generated between 4.2 and 7.0 possible diagnoses for a single case (10). Expert physical therapists generated from one to five possible problems, such as pain and decreased mobility, for a single case (11). The constraints of short-term working memory are seven $\pm$ two pieces of information (10), so extensive lists are not recommended. Experts were able to limit their list of hypotheses to $\pm$ seven hypotheses by (*a*) grouping related hypotheses, such as weakness of the arm and leg, and (*b*) assigning old numbers from hypotheses that were ruled out to new hypotheses as they were generated (10).

An expert clinician generates hypotheses early. Elstein found that expert physicians began generating hypotheses in the first 10% of a diagnostic workup (10). Payton found that nine of 10 expert physical therapists began hypothesis generation very early (11). One therapist began after the chart review. Five therapists began in the first few minutes, while three began within the first third of the evaluation.

However, early generation of hypotheses does not mean premature generation. Elstein's early work found that early hypothesis generation was a critical feature of medical inquiry. Yet, later studies showed that, "As a generalization, that statement is clearly in error" (10, p. 79). Elstein found that expert physicians obtained three to five cues prior to generating their first hypothesis (10). Elstein also compared medical students with high diagnostic accuracy to students with low diagnostic accuracy (10). He found that the more accurate students collected more data before generating a hypothesis (mean number of cues before generation = 4.3) than the less accurate students (mean number of cues before generation = 0.8).

Finally, an expert clinician simultaneously evaluates multiple hypotheses. Physical therapy students who performed most like experts generated multiple hypotheses and then considered cues for several of them at once (12). This ability to consider several possibilities simultaneously is characteristic of the intuitive cognitive style (12). This style is different from the systematic cognitive style, which rules out possibilities sequentially one by one. Systematic reasoning has a weakness. When a correct hypothesis is ruled out too early, subsequent data that support it will not be linked with the proper hypothesis because it no longer exists in the clinician's mind.

STRATEGIES OF EXPERIENCED CLINICIANS

Experienced clinicians don't always go through the decision tree process. Sometimes experts immediately recognize familiar patterns without analyzing the individual behaviors. A clinician will say, "I just know from experience what this patient's problem is." **Pattern recognition** involves comparing the current pattern of clinical cues to previously seen patterns (3). Pattern recognition doesn't always work as well for students. Clinical patterns are more vivid to experienced therapists because they have actually seen patients who exhibit these patterns; students have just read about them in books (3).

Accurate pattern recognition requires a qualitative interpretation of cues that is based on clinical experience. Mattingly and Fleming talked about a psychiatric occupational therapist (OT) who knew that a patient's "slow gait" looked more like the shuffling gait of Parkinson's disease than the slow gait of psychomotor retardation, even though the patient was admitted with a diagnosis of depression (3). Students initially lack a memory file that contains the qualitative aspects of clinical cues to identify similar but subtly different behaviors.

Finally, students don't always understand the value of the signs and symptoms they learn about in their medical conditions courses. For example, dermatomyositis suggests four hypotheses that need to be confirmed or ruled out (13). First, brown pigmentation of the skin may be present, but unlike other skin conditions such as scleroderma, normal elasticity of the skin is maintained. The pigmentation will certainly have emotional consequences, but it usually does not require the student to treat a loss of range of motion. Second, muscular involvement can range from tenderness to atrophy. Treatment and dysfunction will be dramatically different for the two ends of this motor continuum. Third, the disease attacks axial muscles such as neck flexors, laryngeal muscles, and the shoulder and pelvic girdle muscles. The student needs to plan for axial rather than fine motor deficits. Fourth, visceral effusions may affect organs such as the heart and lungs. Students must be prepared for a loss of crucial metabolic support needed for endurance. Students need to turn the medical patterns they learned in school into a plan for action.

After an experienced clinician uses pattern recognition to define a clinical problem, he/she can quickly shift into treatment planning and implementation. A well-formed clinical problem can often be solved with conventional routines. Schön refers to these routine actions as "knowing-IN-action" (14).

Knowing-IN-action refers to the knowledge we reveal through our actions. It includes both observable behaviors like riding a bicycle and internal mental operations like analyzing a balance sheet. Knowing-IN-action gets us through much of our day as clinicians and as people. There are many things we do every day that we don't even have to think about, like starting a car, because we use knowing-IN-action. Knowing-IN-action is both spontaneous and unspoken. If we are asked to say how we do something that is ingrained, we find it hard to describe our actions. Once you've learned how to perform passive range of motion, it is easier to do than to explain.

However, knowing-IN-action has a weakness. Routine actions require a well-defined problem. When you don't have a clearly defined problem, pattern recognition isn't possible, and routine actions do not emerge. As Schön pointed out, [all] "the problems of real-world practice do not present themselves to practitioners as well-formed structures. Indeed, they tend not to present themselves as problems at all, but as messy, indeterminate situations" (14, p. 4).

FRAMES OF REFERENCE

Schön says one way an experienced practitioner clarifies a messy problem is by naming and framing (14). A frame of reference enables you to name a behavior that concerns you, such as weakness. Once you have named the problem, you can then frame this concern within a frame of reference that provides a solution (15). For example, the biomechanical frame of reference suggests several ways to treat weakness.

Frames of reference are an attempt to teach students how to integrate theory and practice strategies. Faculty used to teach theories in school and then assume that their students would figure out how to apply these theories in the clinic. This frequently didn't happen because clinicians felt that theory was disconnected from what they did every day (16). This resulted in differences and inconsistencies in how occupational therapy services were delivered (16).

A **frame of reference** is a set of theoretical concepts that guide clinical practice (16). Frames of reference are practical because they (a) explain human behavior and give these behaviors clearly defined names, (b) suggest specific treatment techniques, and (c) provide rationales that explain why techniques work. Mosey said a frame of reference consists of a theoretical base, function-dysfunction continua, behaviors indicative of function-dysfunction, and postulates regarding intervention (17).

A **theoretical base** produces a set of assumptions about the world that explain and predict events. For instance, the sensory integration (SI) frame of reference assumes that poor motor output is caused by poor central processing of sensory input. This explanation of motor control is different from the one given by sensory reeducation, which says that poor coordination is caused by peripheral conditions that impair sensory input, like deep burns or peripheral nerve injuries.

Function-dysfunction continua identify the specific domains of concern that are addressed by a frame of reference. Function-dysfunction continua are categories of human behavior that can be placed on a continuum, with function on one end and dysfunction on the other end. For example, the SI frame of reference addresses the concern of dyspraxia. Dyspraxia is the inability to perform unfamiliar motor tasks, even though habitually used motor routines are spared. This SI function-dysfunction continuum enables you to "name" the problem as dyspraxia.

Function-dysfunction continua strongly influence what you see when you observe a patient. When staff from different disciplines do a joint evaluation, it is amazing to see how differently each staff person interprets a specific behavior that is simultaneously observed by everyone. The function-dysfunction continua that each discipline brings to the evaluation process create a variety of ways to interpret what we think we see.

Mosey divided function-dysfunction continua into occupational performance and performance components (17). She defined occupational performance as age-appropriate self-care, work, and leisure skills that a person needs to perform his/her roles (17). Occupational performance has also been called performance skills,

and occupational areas. It is more useful to refer to occupational behaviors as **functional outcomes** because third-party payers have shifted approval for reimbursement to improvement of functional limitations (18–20). Clinicians also use the terms function and dysfunction to refer to self-help, work, and leisure skills. **The terms functional outcomes and function/dysfunction will be used in this text**.

Human behavior also consists of performance components. Motor, sensory, cognitive, and psychosocial components form the foundation that make functional outcomes possible. Performance components have been called skill components and performance areas. These "components" are really prerequisite skills. Prerequisite skills are continua with assets at one end and deficits at the other end. **The terms prerequisite skills, assets, and deficits will be used throughout this text**.

A patient is placed on these continua by identifying **behaviors indicative of function-dysfunction**. Specific behaviors can be identified with formal evaluation tools. For example, a child can be placed on the praxis function-dysfunction continuum by reporting his/her score on the Sensory Integration and Praxis Tests. The initial test score tells the therapist whether the patient is closer to the normal or abnormal end of the continuum. Subsequent test scores help the therapist decide if treatment is moving the patient in the desired direction on the continuum.

Finally, clearly defined deficits and dysfunction are "framed" within a particular treatment approach by writing **postulates regarding intervention**. These postulates link goals to specific treatment techniques and explain why the treatment works. For example, scooter board obstacle courses (SI technique) facilitate improved central processing of unfamiliar sensory input (rationale) to produce an adaptive motor response to a changing environment (goal). These linking statements are essential for the patient as well as the therapist. How will the patient know what he/she will gain from actively participating in treatment if a connection between the activity and the goal is not clearly communicated?

REFLECTION-IN-ACTION

Sometimes even a frame of reference won't clear up a "messy" clinical problem. Even the most clearly written postulates regarding intervention may not work as expected. The patient may exhibit surprising responses to familiar techniques because his/her case is unique (14). Schön identified two different ways to respond to this element of surprise (14). We may use **reflection-ON-action**, which consists of thinking back on what we have done. Reflection-ON-action occurs after the event and has no effect on the "action present." Or, we may use **reflection-IN-action**, which consists of on-the-spot inquiry that reshapes what we are doing while we are doing it.

Reflection brings past experience to bear on a unique situation (14, p. 44). Experience enables the practitioner to see the unique situation as both familiar and different. No patient is truly unique in all things, so experience helps us identify what makes this patient similar to past cases. This reduces the burden on the therapist because standard procedures still apply to some of this patient's problems. Experience also helps us recognize which aspects of a case are different from past cases. Sometimes, seeing exactly how a patient is different from other patients suggests a new line of thought.

Reflection results in "**move testing**" (14). The therapist designs an action to produce a desired result. If you get what you want, the action or "move" is confirmed. As Schön says, the key to move testing is to specifically define the result you want. Clinicians do not have the option of using a control group, so we cannot say that our therapy was the only cause for change. However, we can say that the desired outcome was achieved. The patient may demonstrate progress that was not possible until move testing began. Move testing is an excellent way to effect change when familiar strategies are not working.

Finally, Schön says that reflection requires ethical reasoning when there is a value conflict (14). For example, the issue may not be whether we *can* do painful stretching with a patient, but whether we *should* do it. Stretching may not significantly improve the quality of life. Or, the patient may not agree that the discomfort is worth the small gains achieved. Or, hospitals may not be willing to give free therapy to every patient who does not have adequate health insurance.

Schön sums up technical problem-solving as the ability to form clearly defined problems, to appropriately apply theories, to implement routine procedures, called knowing-IN-action, and to use reflection-IN-action when the usual routines fail (14). Individualized, prescriptive problem-solving is embedded in naming the deficit, framing that deficit in an appropriate frame of reference, and reflecting on treatment decisions made before, during, and after treatment implementation.

PROSPECTIVE TREATMENT STORY

The AOTF clinical reasoning project found that experienced therapists embedded their technical problem solving in a **prospective treatment story** (21). Experienced therapists in this project said that treatment goals and techniques were the last ideas they formed about patients (21). First they created a sequence of mental images of the patient. They saw concrete pictures of what patients look like now and what they will look like at discharge. This is a lot like guessing the ending

of a movie as the story moves along. Mattingly calls these images a "prospective treatment story" (21).

This story is not told through explicit storytelling. It is constructed by sharing powerful therapeutic experiences that suggest a particular ending. For example, if a patient regains enough strength to make a fist, both the patient and therapist will begin to think about what valued roles the patient can resume if hand function returns to normal.

Prospective stories are valuable, not because they are completely accurate, but because therapists experience discomfort when there is a conflict between their imagined stories and what really happened (21). Students need to learn that this **mismatch** is good. With the prospective treatment story as a baseline, you can quickly pick up early discrepancies between the expected change and the actual change. Experienced clinicians were quick to recognize this type of mismatch, which led to early revision of the prospective treatment story (21).

These mismatches force us to be aware of the hopes and fears we project to our patients. We all form first impressions of people that we may or may not be aware of. For example, if we have little hope for a patient, our treatment will not be aggressive. Patients try to read our expectations and may jump to wrong conclusions if we don't communicate clearly.

Therapists reported discomfort when there was a conflict between the therapist's and patient's version of the story (21). For example, patients and their families were often more pessimistic about outcomes than the therapists. This can give the impression that the patient and family are "uncooperative" because their version of the story doesn't match the therapist's version. Experienced clinicians were quick to recognize this type of mismatch, which led to renegotiation of the prospective treatment story (21).

Prospective treatment stories are valuable because they act as a catalyst to give patients new pictures of themselves (21). The few weeks we have patients in therapy is not long enough to teach them everything they need to know. All we can do is show them how to generalize gains to a few functional tasks and then turn the story over to them to complete when they go home.

Finally, prospective stories are valuable because they tell therapists to expect change (21). Diagnoses and people are not static. Recovery is a series of stages that enable the patient to progress towards some happy ending. This concept of an ongoing story line prepares experienced therapists for the many changes that occur.

THERAPISTS WITH A THREE-TRACK MIND

Fleming fine-tuned the subplots in the prospective treatment story by studying experienced therapists who participated in the AOTF clinical reasoning project (22). She found that experienced therapists utilized three tracks of clinical thinking. She called them the procedural, interactive, and conditional tracks.

The **procedural track** is the easiest to understand because it is very concrete. It uses frames of reference to identify problems, set goals, and select specific treatment techniques for a specific diagnosis (22). Problems, goals, and techniques for a particular diagnosis have been discussed in print and classrooms for many years. For example, the therapist may identify edema as a problem, a specific circumferential measurement as a goal, and elevation as a treatment technique. When a therapist uses the procedural track, he/she focuses on the treatment of a diagnosis.

The **interactive track** asks the therapist to focus on the patient as a person, instead of as a diagnosis (22). Patients have a life outside of treatment and their own unique personal histories. These personal differences cause different people to react differently to the same disease. While the diagnosis may be the same, the illness experience can vary considerably. Two patients' responses to an injury and their view about the role of therapy can be quite different. Therefore, therapeutic use of self is employed to encourage the patient to reveal the details of his/her illness experience, to engage the patient in treatment, and to monitor the patient's personal response to treatment. The therapist makes "astute observations and fine-tuned adjustments to the moods and motives of the patients" (22). When therapists use the interactive track, they focus on how they should interact with the person.

The third type of clinical reasoning is called the **conditional track** (23). This track creates an image of the patient that is provisional, holistic, and conditional on patient participation. The conditional tract is provisional because it requires the therapist to monitor the patient's physical and psychological responses in order to constantly revise treatment (22). It is very important to stop thinking that a diagnosis and a person are fixed entities. The first question a student should ask is what stage of physical and mental recovery is this patient in right now? If you see a patient in acute care, his/her medical condition and state of mind will be very different from what they might be in an outpatient setting. A lack of awareness about stages of recovery will get a student in trouble very quickly. The conditional track reminds you that conditions change rather than remain static.

The conditional track also creates an image that is **holistic** (22). It integrates impressions into a "whole condition," which includes the medical diagnosis, the person, and the environmental demands. Rather than switching back and forth between the procedural and interactive tracks, the experienced clinician plans treatment and observes responses in both tracks at once. For example, instead of doing 10 minutes of biomechanical treatment and then talking to the patient for 10 minutes, the experienced therapist does both simultaneously. The therapist keeps track of all the details of the whole condition simultaneously.

Finally, successful treatment is conditional on patient participation (3). A successful treatment session is not justified by concrete physical changes alone. Therapists who exhibited thinking in the conditional tract shared a deep-seated value that success also depends on whether the treatment was a meaningful experience for the patient. Treatment is meaningful to the patient only when the patient helps to construct the image of possible outcomes *and then* actively participates in the treatment activities. The patient has to have a stake in his or her own story (21).

PROFESSIONAL GROWTH

No one expects a student to develop all of these clinical reasoning skills at once. Benner described five levels of clinical reasoning in nurses (8).

The "novice" is characterized by the rigid application of rules and principles learned in school. These rules and principles result in a rigid list of procedures that are carried out regardless of what is happening in a specific case. These rules and principles are "context-free" applications of theory.

The "advanced beginner" is characterized by situational thinking. Rules and principles are modified to take into account the specifics of an actual clinical situation. For occupational therapists, situational thinking may mean visualizing how prerequisite goals, like increased endurance, will affect functional tasks for a specific patient with a specific life-style (24). Situational thinking can also mean placing a biomechanical technique like Coban Wrap into the context of a patient's medical precautions and how well he/she tolerates this specific technique. However, the advanced beginner still has difficulty prioritizing concerns. He/she attends only to the behavior that is currently observable because all patient behaviors are equally important to him/her.

The "competent" clinician is able to do both situational thinking and prioritize treatment concerns. This clinician has a broader picture of the patient's illness experience and a more refined understanding of the nuances in a specific case. In addition, daily actions are translated into long-term goals. One nurse said, "I have the whole morning set out and I can go ahead and do things. I am much more organized. I know what I have to do" (8, p. 27). The competent clinician may still lack flexibility which may be expressed by a reluctance to change the initial plan of treatment.

The "proficient" clinician perceives the whole situation rather than isolated parts of the case. Benner described a nurse who thought about treating infants by telling herself a story instead of making a list of things to do. The nurse said, "OK, here's *this* baby, this is where *this* baby is at, and here's where I want *this* baby to be in six weeks. What can I do today to make this baby go along the road to end up being better?" (8, p. 28). Mattingly would call this a prospective treatment story. As the story progresses, the proficient clinician recognizes a familiar pattern from previous experience. Yet when the current pattern deviates from previous cases, the proficient clinician is quick to recognize the mismatch and modify the treatment plan. Proficient clinicians seem to modify treatment plans automatically (24). This flexibility is learned when the student can treat his/her initial plan as a rough draft that has to be fine-tuned as the unique aspects of a case gradually emerge.

Benner calls the fifth level of clinical reasoning the "expert" level. This level is difficult to describe. Experts make clinical decisions in a "truly remarkable way" that is apparent to patients and colleagues. The expert knows what to do because it "just feels right." Benner gives the example of the blind person who no longer feels the pressure of the cane in the palm of his hand, but "simply feels the curb." No text on clinical reasoning will elevate the reader to the level of expert. Hopefully, this book will heighten your awareness of the components of clinical reasoning and clarify the process.

PRELIMINARY CONCLUSIONS

Two studies show that clinical reasoning can be taught. Neistadt exposed occupational therapy students to clinical reasoning strategies (25). Then she compared these students to themselves over four attempts at problem identification. She found that there was a statistically significant increase in percentage of correctly identified problems from their first attempt to their fourth attempt.

Elstein compared independent clinical reasoning practice to clinical reasoning practice plus feedback on how expert physicians performed on the same case studies (10). There was no significant difference among the groups for cue acquisition. However, the groups who received feedback performed significantly better on both hypothesis generation and cue interpretation than the control group, who just practiced on their own. It appears that clinical reasoning can be taught if experience with case simulations is combined with training about clinical reasoning and feedback about how an experienced therapist solved the same case studies.

PREVIEW

Rather than present a summary, I would like to give you a preview of how you will use all the information from this chapter in the rest of the book.

Clinical reasoning has three characteristics. First, for occupational therapists, it is a goal-oriented activity aimed at regaining function. Functional goals will become an automatic part of your clinical reasoning if you know how to create linking statements between treatment procedures and functional outcomes. One of the main goals of this book is to teach you how to write these linking statements. Second, clinical reasoning is the ability to identify the right thing to do in a specific case. Situational reasoning will be discussed in the chapters on biomechanical, neurodevelopmental, and rehabilitation frames of reference. The case study chapters will then guide you through this application process to determine what is "the good" for a particular individual. Third, clinical reasoning is a cognitive process called the decision tree process. All of Chapter 2 is devoted to this complex process. Each case simulation chapter will require you to apply this process to a specific case.

The case simulation chapters will provide practice in applying the four mental stages of medical inquiry. You will learn how to use the four mental stages, which include cue acquisition, hypothesis generation, cue interpretation, and hypothesis evaluation. You will learn how to generate ± 7 hypotheses and evaluate them simultaneously. You will learn how to develop hypotheses early in the decision tree process, but wait to acquire a sufficient number of cues before generating your hypotheses.

Pattern recognition is initially difficult for students. However, your clinical conditions courses will help you generate potential hypotheses for a particular patient with a particular diagnosis. The test results in each case simulation chapter will tell you how accurate your diagnosis based hypotheses were in a specific case.

Frames of reference make up a large portion of this text. You will become very familiar with all the characteristics of a frame of reference. This includes a theoretical base, function-dysfunction continua, behaviors indicative of function-dysfunction, and postulates regarding intervention. To ensure that you know how to apply different frames of reference, you will initially be asked to solve case simulations with one frame of reference.

Reflection-IN-action is a very complex skill that fieldwork supervisors do not expect students to exhibit at the beginning of fieldwork. Supervisors initially expect reflection-ON-action, which takes place after the event. This occurs as a result of both the student's own reflections and the supervisory process. Fieldwork supervisors expect students to recognize their own errors when they occur and seek supervision to correct them before the next session. Reflection-IN-action will develop out of repeated reflection-ON-action.

The procedural, interactive, and conditional tracks are utilized in varying degrees in this text. The procedural track is discussed at length in chapters on frames of reference like the biomechanical frame of reference. These frame of reference chapters are not intended to duplicate the how-to instructions that are fully documented in entry-level texts. The purpose of these chapters is to model situational thinking about assessment planning, sequencing goals, and writing postulates regarding intervention. Case simulations are provided to help you practice clinical reasoning in the procedural track using different frames of reference.

The interactive track can be discussed only in the context of a specific person. Therefore, the case simulation chapters tell the life stories of real people. These case simulations illustrate how the therapist thinks about the interactive track by thinking of psychosocial issues and by using social history to make tentative suggestions about treatment activities. Choosing meaningful activities based on personal history is an initial step in trying to think about the person in addition to the diagnosis. However, the interactive track can be fully experienced only by interacting with a real patient, which is beyond the scope of this book.

Similarly, the richness of the conditional track can be experienced fully only by repeated treatment of the same patient. The provisional aspect of the conditional track is introduced by basing initial treatment plans on the stage-specific causes that produce each deficit. The holistic aspect of the conditional track is modeled in the form of test interpretation that takes into account the "whole condition." Deficits that are not addressed by the primary frame of reference are a part of every case simulation.

I share the legitimate fears about treating from a single frame of reference. By identifying deficits not addressed, you will appreciate that all frames of references have blind spots that leave many problems untreated. The biomechanical, neurodevelopmental, and the rehabilitative frames of reference do not acknowledge or suggest how to treat problems like life-threatening infection, emotional distress, or pain. Yet, problems like these occur with regularity and cannot be ignored. On the other hand, students need to experience success on their first attempts to apply a frame of reference to a specific patient. Applying a frame of reference is not like memorizing concepts for a multiple choice exam. After you become proficient at applying one frame of reference, you will find it easier to use a holistic approach that combines frames of reference. The com-

bined use of several frames of reference is modeled at the end of the book.

The prospective treatment story emerges when the clinician no longer thinks about specific details, but just sees the whole situation. This is the fourth level of professional growth, which Benner calls the "proficient" clinician. This level of thinking requires extended clinical experience. The goal of this book is to make you a "competent" clinician who uses situational thinking to generate and evaluate narrative hypotheses, who can prioritize measurable treatment concerns, and who has some initial flexibility about treatment planning that incorporates the patient's concerns, preferences, and reactions to treatment.

STUDY QUESTIONS

1. What is situational thinking?
2. What are the four stages in the model of medical inquiry?
3. What is pattern recognition? Why is it difficult for students?
4. What are: a frame of reference, a theoretical base, functional outcomes, and prerequisite skills?
5. What do the terms function/dysfunction and assets/deficits refer to in this text?
6. How are reflection-ON-action and reflection-IN-action different?
7. What is a prospective treatment story, and what are the three reasons that it is useful?
8. What are the procedural, interactive, and conditional tracks?

References

1. American Occupational Therapy Association: Occupational Therapy: Directions for the Future. A report of the Entry-Level Study Committee, an ad-hoc committee of the Executive Board of the American Occupational Therapy Association, Inc., Rockville, MD, 1987.
2. Fleming MH, Piedmont RL. The relationship of academic degree and years in practice to occupational therapists' perception of the status of the profession and educational preparation. Occupational Therapy Journal of Research 1989;9:101.
3. Mattingly C, Fleming M. Clinical reasoning: forms of inquiry in therapeutic practice. Philadelphia: FA Davis, 1994.
4. Rogers JC, Masagatani G. Clinical reasoning of occupational therapists during the initial assessment of physically disabled patients. Occupational Therapy Journal of Research 1982;9:200.
5. Greenberg NS. Incorporating critical thinking throughout the curriculum. In: Target 2000—occupational therapy education. Rockville, MD: American Occupation Therapy Association, Inc., 1986:149.
6. Rogers JC. Eleanor Clarke Slagle Lectureship—Clinical Reasoning: the ethics, science, and art. Am J Occup Ther 1983;37:601.
7. Watts NT. Decision analysis: a tool for improving physical therapy practice and education. In: Wolf SL, ed. Clinical decision making in physical therapy. Philadelphia: FA Davis, 1985:7.
8. Benner P. From novice to expert. Menlo Park, CA:Addison-Wesley, 1984.

9. Bruer JT. The mind's journey from novice to expert. American Educator 1993:17:6.

10. Elstein AS, Shulman LS, Sprafka SA. Medical problem solving—an analysis of clinical reasoning. Cambridge, MA: Harvard University Press, 1978.

11. Payton OD. Clinical reasoning process in physical therapy. Phys Ther 1985;65:924.

12. Bork CE. The influence of cognitive style upon clinical evaluation. Unpublished dissertation, State University of New York at Buffalo, 1980.

13. Berkow R, ed. The Merck manual of diagnosis and therapy, 16th ed. Rahway, NJ: Merck & Co., 1992:1323.

14. Schön DA. Educating the reflective practitioner. San Francisco: Jossey-Bass Publishers, 1990.

15. Parham D. Towards professionalism: the reflective therapist. Am J Occup Ther 1987;41:555.

16. Denton PL. Psychiatric occupational therapy: a workbook of practical skills. Boston:Little, Brown & Company, 1987:44.

17. Mosey SC. Occupational therapy: configuration of a profession. New York: Raven Press, 1981.

18. Allen KA, Foto M: Reporting occupational therapy outcomes with the ICIDH codes. Physical Disabilities Special Interest Section Newsletter 1991;14:2–3.

19. Pinson CC. Work programs reimbursement: what is happening across the nation? Physical Disabilities Special Interest Section Newsletter 1991;14:4–5.

20. Dahl M. Money and reimbursement versus OT practice. Philadelphia: Pennsylvania Occupational Therapy Association Workshop, June, 1990.

21. Mattingly C. The narrative nature of clinical reasoning. Am J Occup Ther 1991;45:998.

22. Fleming MH. The therapist with the three track mind. Am J Occup Ther 1991;45:1007.

23. Fleming MH. The therapist with the three track mind. Paper presented at the annual meeting of the Occupational Therapy Association, Baltimore, MD, 1989.

24. Slater DY, Cohn EL. Staff development through analysis of practice. Am J Occup Ther 1991;45:1038.

25. Neistadt MD. Classroom as clinic: a model of teaching clinical reasoning in occupational therapy education. Am J Occup Ther 1987;41:631.

CHAPTER / 2

Decision Tree Process

The decision tree process is a sequence of events that includes assessment planning, problem identification, treatment planning, treatment implementation, and reevaluation. This chapter goes beyond outlining the steps. It applies the clinical reasoning strategies described in Chapter 1 and illustrates each strategy with clinical examples. These strategies are presented in a linear sequence to make learning easier. However, cue acquisition, hypothesis generation, cue interpretation, and hypothesis evaluation are intermingled as appropriate. The decision tree process is not a strict form of linear logic; each mental step is retraced several times to make sure that first impressions do not lead to false conclusions (1, 2).

This branching and retracing of ideas are most accurately conveyed in complex flow diagrams with arrows that point backwards and forwards at the same time. However, these diagrams are overwhelming for students who are trying to learn the decision tree process for the very first time. The nonlinear nature of clinical reasoning can be conveyed more simply in an outline format, which is listed in Memory Aid 2.1. Use this Memory Aid to guide you through this chapter.

CREATING NARRATIVE HYPOTHESES

Clinical hypotheses are not usually stated in the form of statistical predictions. As discussed in Chapter 1, therapists reason in narrative mode in order to construct a prospective treatment story. The first chapter in that story is a set of narrative hypotheses. I call them narrative hypotheses because they take the form of questions about the characters in a story. Will this patient be independent? Will he/she have a loss of range of motion (ROM)?

Narrative hypotheses are lists of potential assets and deficits made *before* evaluation tools are selected by the therapist. Experienced therapists begin cue acquisition and hypothesis generation as they read medical charts

Memory Aid 2.1.
The Decision Tree Process

I. CREATE NARRATIVE HYPOTHESES
1. Generate a Data Collection Schedule
2. Review the chart to generate hypotheses

II. DESIGN AN EVALUATION PACKAGE
1. Formal screening
2. Comprehensive testing
3. Clinical observation
4. Specialty testing

III. INTERPRET TEST RESULTS
1. Generate a Cue Interpretation List
   a. Decide which cues are relevant to which hypotheses
   b. Decide if each cue confirms or disconfirms its hypothesis
2. Evaluate hypotheses
   a. Confirm, revise or disconfirm hypotheses
   b. Resolve discrepancies or plan additional evaluation
   c. Double-check data base for unexpected or new data
3. Write a Problem List

IV. GENERATE TREATMENT GOALS
1. Prioritize prerequisite skills
   a) S–T Goals: are dictated by safety; are functionally significant; have potential for S–T improvement; require direct treatment
   b) Numbers within S–T/L–T: some goals are prerequisites for others
   c) L–T goals may not be WNL, so choose functional outcomes wisely
2. Suggest specific preliminary functional outcomes for every S–T goal
3. Make goals measurable: behavior, criteria, conditions statements

V. DESIGN TREATMENT ACTIVITIES
1. Write postulates regarding change
2. Write postulates regarding intervention
3. Negotiate specific activities

VI. USE THE FEEDBACK LOOP DURING IMPLEMENTATION
1. Modify the activity
2. Revise the short-term goal
3. Change the method
4. Renegotiate functional outcomes
5. Reframe the deficit

and talk to other medical staff. Remember, experts generate multiple hypotheses. For example, does a patient have a loss of range of motion because of pain, contractures, or edema?

Creating a Data Collection Schedule

When students gather data, their knowledge remains fragmented in hundreds of unrelated bits of information, while experienced clinicians organize their data into larger categories called "chunks" (3). **Chunking** is a strategy for organizing data into more manageable, related groups to reduce the anxiety created by overwhelming amounts of information. For example, when doing a 1000-piece jigsaw puzzle, people usually group all of the border pieces together, then group all the pieces of a prominent object in the picture together, and so on, until several piles are formed.

Chunking is a better strategy for handling preassessment data collection than copying everything down verbatim from a chart with no sense of what's important. Memory Aid 2.2 lists the areas of concern associated with different frames of reference used in adult physical disabilities settings. The individual components of each frame of reference are described in detail later in the book. For now, just look at the names of the frames of reference so you can see the wide range of concerns that can generate narrative hypotheses.

Rogers calls a comprehensive list of concerns like Memory Aid 2.2 a "data collection schedule" (4). She believes that it is a valuable memory prompt as long as the list is kept open-ended. Since there is always something that can't be anticipated, it helps to document the unexpected. (See the blank spaces assigned for "other concerns" on Memory Aid 2.2.)

Memory Aid 2.2 is only one example of how to chunk concerns. There are many variations of this list. For example, Neistadt uses the following groups: activities of daily living (ADLs); motor, including active range of motion (AROM), strength, passive range of motion (PROM), muscle tone endurance, and fine-motor coordination); sensation; perception; cognition; equipment; and psychosocial (5). Experienced therapists eventually carry around such a list in their head. This list triggers a thorough and systematic search for data that might otherwise be prematurely excluded because of an incomplete medical chart.

Chunking domains of concern by frame of reference is helpful. Yet it is vital to avoid the assumption that you can use a single frame of reference to treat a single diagnosis. As you will see in subsequent chapters, *every* frame of reference has blind spots. For instance, what if a stroke patient has a swollen hand? A stroke patient is typically treated with the neurodevelopmental approach, but the edema requires a biomechanical treat-

Memory Aid 2.2.
Data Collection Schedule Chunked by Frames of Reference

Rehabilitation Concerns = independence in

1. Self-care skills
2. Work and homecare skills
3. Leisure skills

Homeostatic Concerns

1. Respiratory system
2. Cardiovascular system
3. Integumentary system
4. Immune system
5. Metabolic system
6. Bowel and bladder control
7. Skeletal system
8. Autonomic nervous system

Sensory-Motor Concerns

1. Pain control
2. Somatosensation
3. Coordination

Biomechanical Concerns

1. Structural stability
2. Low-level endurance
3. Edema control
4. Passive range of motion
5. Muscle strength
6. High-level endurance

Neurodevelopmental Concerns

1. Axial control
2. Automatic reactions
3. Limb control (in brain-damaged patient)

Model of Human Occupation

1. Volition: causation, values, and interests
2. Habituation: roles and habits
3. Environment: culture, social groups, objects

Other Psychosocial Concerns

1. Premorbid conditions
2. Sexuality
3. Hospital stressors
4. Stress reactions

Perceptual-Cognitive Concerns

1. Arousal
2. Attention
3. CNS deficits that affect vision/hearing/language
4. Ocular-motor skills
5. Simple visual perception
6. Complex visual perception
7. Motor planning
8. Memory
9. Executive functions

Other Concerns

1.
2.

ment. If you insist on using only one frame of reference, you will leave many deficits untreated. Therapists cannot expect a single theorist to address every single deficit known to the human race. Therapists must use a variety of frames of reference to be holistic.

Many textbooks chunk concerns by listing signs and symptoms associated with each diagnosis. This creates an unwieldy set of lists that grows every time a student learns about a new diagnosis. A compact list like Memory Aid 2.2 is more practical. A comprehensive list of concerns by frame of reference is also conceptually closer to the types of therapeutic decisions therapists have to make (6). For example, a therapist must determine if there is weakness or tightness in order to choose between resistance vs. stretching, regardless of the diagnosis. A deficit list for a specific diagnosis is also frequently incomplete. For example, deficit lists developed for arthritis are classically restricted to biomechanical and rehabilitation issues with no reference to psychosocial or perceptual-cognitive issues (7, 8). Rogers and Masagatani found that once a diagnosis was used to develop an assessment plan, some experienced therapists were resistant to changing that plan, even when there was evidence that a change was needed (9). Chunking deficits by diagnosis may result in a cookbook approach to treatment planning.

Reviewing the Chart to Generate Hypotheses

The medical chart is a common place to begin the search for hypotheses. The chart usually contains an established medical diagnosis for the patient. This enables the therapist to begin forming images of what therapy will be like based on previous experience with similar cases. However, patients with identical diagnoses often have different assets, severity of injury, secondary medical diagnoses, and premorbid influences. These individual differences will influence the narrative hypotheses.

As you read the chart, use Memory Aid 2.2 to make mental pictures. Be as concrete as you can. See if you can write narrative hypotheses for the following patient (10).

CASE HISTORY

He is a right-handed automobile assembly worker with deep second- and third-degree burns over 10% of his body from a car accident. The burned areas include his left shoulder and axilla, the anterior surface of his left arm, and the dorsum of his left hand. He has a wife and two teenage children. He is their sole source of support. Ask yourself what deficits-assets and function-dysfunction you would expect. Gather information about the diagnosis (procedural track) and the person (interactive track).

His unburned right upper extremity should be normal (hypothesis #1). If his dominant right hand is spared, this is very important for future hand function. However, the burn on his left upper extremity (LUE) could be deep enough to have charred the joints, melted soft tissue, and restricted ROM. The dorsum of the hand is especially vulnerable since it has no muscle mass to protect the extensor tendons. You should inquire about structural instability of the extensor tendons (hypothesis #2 = biomechanical). He may not be permitted to stabilize objects with his burned left hand because fist-making could rupture the exposed extensor tendons. This will impede tasks that require two hands, such as cutting meat. Yet, he should be able to perform ADLs one-handed with a few adaptive devices (hypothesis #3 = rehabilitation). You also should get a pre-grafting AROM baseline for finger flexion of individual joints, since the dorsum of the hand was burned, and a baseline for elbow and wrist extension, since the arm was burned on the flexor surface (hypothesis #4 = biomechanical). It is impossible to predict which specific shoulder motions would be limited because you don't know which surfaces of the shoulder and axilla were burned. You

should screen all shoulder motions (#5 hypothesis = biomechanical). Will he experience stress reactions when his wife and sons see how he looks (hypothesis #6 = psychosocial)? Finally, how and when will he return to work to support his family (#7 hypothesis = MOHO)? Don't just read the words in the chart. Turn the words into a prospective story about what the patient will experience!

Narrative hypotheses are immediately useful. First, they facilitate patient-therapist rapport. It helps if you can tell a new patient why you are seeing him/her. This is difficult to do when the referral form reads "OT evaluation." You could at least tell your patient you are going to evaluate his/her range of motion and functional independence. This general introduction creates a meaningful experience during your very first interaction with the patient. Narrative hypotheses also prevent embarrassing situations. Before you talk to a patient for the first time, it's nice to know about such things as cognitive status, ability to cooperate, pending surgery, or imminent discharge (9). Finally, narrative hypotheses ensure the patient's safety because the therapist knows about the necessary medical precautions that should be followed. Watts says that without this ability to "subjectively estimate the likelihood of future occurrences, clinicians would be unable to act" (6, p. 20). Failure to generate narrative hypotheses may explain some of the paralysis that students experience before seeing a patient for the first time.

DESIGNING AN EVALUATION PACKAGE

Every department seems to have its own initial evaluation form. These forms change from facility to facility, unit to unit, and even year to year. This constant change is a response to the changing needs of the patient population. These evaluation forms are helpful because they encourage entry-level therapists to be thorough, but they are often long.

Before diagnosis-related groups (DRG) guidelines restricted lengths of stay, therapists didn't have to worry about the length of their initial evaluations. They could pull out extensive test batteries. Yet, some data in a wastefully broad evaluation may never be used in designing treatment (6). The cost of unused portions of comprehensive evaluations can no longer be justified.

Today, therapists express concern over the inability to complete an evaluation due to repeated preemption of therapy time (9). Shorter lengths of stay require patients to start therapy earlier, while they are less medically stable. Illness and medical tests can result in poor attendance and tardiness. DRGs have forced therapists to complete initial evaluations in a matter of a few hours instead of days without neglecting to gather any essential information. This double bind of time constraints and thoroughness can be resolved only by applying a decision tree process.

The decision tree process means that evaluation data are gathered in stages that include formal screening, comprehensive testing, clinical observation, and specialty testing. For example, the burn patient just described had his dominant hand spared. Since many self-care tasks can be done one-handed, initial evaluation of self-care can probably be *restricted to* screening for two-handed tasks like cutting meat and buttoning. After some healing occurs in his hand, a comprehensive evaluation of his burned hand during self-care, home care, and work tasks would be in order.

Table 2.1 lists a few examples of tests that are used in the different stages of evaluation. With time, you will know the names of all these tests, but for now, you need to be aware that testing occurs in four stages. These stages of testing are the key to developing a good assessment plan. Remember, the point of cue acquisition is to gather data that are needed in a particular case, not every type of data you learned about in school.

Formal Screening

This is the first and most superficial stage of evaluation. Screening has been routinely used by clinicians with unwieldy caseloads, like therapists working in the school system. Yet, screening is more than a case management technique. Screening is also a way to manage your assessment time effectively. Unfortunately, formal screening tests are difficult to identify because they rarely have the word "screening" in the title. Screening tests can be identified by their purpose and length (Table 2.2).

The purpose of screening tests is to quickly detect abnormality. These tests achieve their purpose by:

1. Suggesting appropriate tests when narrative hypotheses are sparse;
2. Quickly ruling out the need for comprehensive testing;
3. Justifying referral to occupational therapy; and
4. Justifying referral to other disciplines.

When you derive little information from reading the chart and talking to other team members, screening will assist you in test selection. A referral for a patient "who was in a car accident" is vague and can make test selection difficult. Does this patient have a closed head injury? The Neurobehavioral Cognitive Status Examination at bedside tells you if you need to do in-depth

---

Table 2.1.

Examples of Evaluation Tools in Different Stages of Testing

Problem Areas	Screening Tests	Comprehensive Tests	Specialty Tests	Clinical Observations
Passive ROM	Eyeball PROM	Formal goniometry	Volumetry	End feels
Muscle Strength	Eyeball AROM Grip/pinch strength	Manual Muscle Test	Muscle Palpation	AROM during ADLs
Endurance	Cardiac Activity Level Activity tolerance in minutes	*Valpar Sample #19: Dynamic Physical Capacities	Duration or # of repetitions during work samples	Fatigue during ADLs
Coordination	*Nine-hole Pegtest	*Jebsen-Taylor Hand Function Test	*Minnesota Rate of Manipulation Test	Write name Buttoning
Somato-sensation	Stereognosis Test	Somatosensory battery	*Moberg Pick-up Test	Spontaneous limb use
Axial Control	Axial movements during handling	Muscle Tone Eval GM Trend I, II, IV	Not available	Sits symmetrically Axial weight shifts
Automatic Reactions	Equilibrium in sitting and standing	Fiorentino's Reflex Testing	Inner ear tests done by the doctor	Sitting balance Rotary righting Protective extension
Limb Control	Brunnstrom Eval: P. 1	Muscle Tone Eval Brunnstrom Eval GM Trend II, III, IV FM Trend I, II, III	Not available	Limb placing and eccentric control LE tone during ADL's Shoulder subluxation
Perception and Cognition	COTE: Part III N.C.S.E.	*LOTCA *Santa Clara	*Motor-Free Visual Perception Test	Need for prompts
Volition and Habituation	COTE: Part I–II	*Occupational History	*Interest Checklist *Life Goals Inventory	Talk to the patient
ADLs and Homemaking	Dressing	*Kenny Self-Care Evaluation	*Routine Task Inventory	Observe a meal

*(Some of these tests are commercially marketed test kits) or copyrighted in the literature

Table 2.2.
Four Stages of Evaluation

Stages	Purpose	Purpose Achieved By	Length
Formal Screening	To quickly detect abnormality	1. Suggesting tests for evaluation when the narrative hypothesis is sparse 2. Ruling out the need for evaluation when deficits are not consistently present 3. Justifying referrals	1. 10–30 mins per test 2. 5–10 items per test or subtest
Comprehensive Testing	To provide a broad database for treatment planning	1. Identifying function/dysfunction 2. Identifying underlying deficits that cause dysfunction 3. Providing a detailed baseline to enable therapist to document small changes	1. 1–10 hours per test 2. 20–30 items per test or subtest
Clinical Observation	To supplement comprehensive tests	1. Quickly documenting assets 2. Providing test results when formal testing is not possible 3. Checking the reliability and validity of formal test results 4. Identifying unanticipated deficits	Variable. This is an on-going process that overlaps other stages of evaluation.
Specialty testing	To focus on specific skills for in-depth evaluation	1. Supplying data that are missing in comprehensive tests 2. Confirming underlying deficits that cause dysfunction	Variable. Frequency of use is a more accurate way to identify these tests.

testing of attention, memory, visual perception, or thinking operations. When your narrative hypotheses are sparse, screening can save time. However, if the chart is rich with presenting problems, you may not need screening tests to help you select specific tests. Make narrative hypotheses work for you, and screen when in doubt.

Formal screening achieves its purpose by quickly ruling out the need for comprehensive testing. Some deficits are inconsistently present. These deficits need to be ruled out case by case without giving lengthy tests. A formal screening test like the Nine-Hole Peg Test can rule out fine-motor incoordination whenever there is a motor impairment. Screening procedures can set your mind at ease with a minimal cost to the patient.

Screening is also useful for obtaining a referral to occupational therapy. A therapist who is sent an order to do self-care may realize that the patient has a cognitive deficit. If the therapist wants the institution to be reimbursed for cognitive assessment or intervention, a second written referral must be obtained. Sometimes the physician will take the therapist's word about the patient's unexpected behavior. Sometimes, however, formal screening results are needed to convince the physician to write that second referral.

Screening tests can also quickly detect deficits that should be treated by other disciplines. This is especially appropriate when other disciplines in your facility do not routinely see certain types of patients or when you must refer a patient to outside agencies. All health care professionals have an ethical responsibility to refer patients to all the appropriate services. Again, sometimes the therapist's observation is sufficient for referral, and sometimes more formal test results are required.

Screening tests can be identified by their relatively short administration time. They can take from 10 to 30 minutes to administer. This range exists because some screening procedures are single tests, while others are screening batteries. A cursory survey of screening tests for adult physical disabilities showed that the number of test items are relatively few. There can be as few as five to 10 items per test (e.g., Nine-Hole Peg Test) or per subtest (e.g., Neurobehavioral Cognitive Status Examination).

Comprehensive Testing

This is the second and most intensive stage of evaluation. These tests should thoroughly evaluate a particular skill, but in practice, they may not truly be comprehensive. Goniometry, for example, does not evaluate the range of motion of the scapula or spine. However, the word "comprehensive" best describes these tests and is used repeatedly in the literature. A comprehensive test can consist of a single test (e.g., the Jebsen-Taylor Hand Function Test) or a battery (e.g., a somatosensory test battery). This is different from a "comprehensive team evaluation," which is an array of tests that are administered by practitioners from several disciplines.

Comprehensive tests are difficult to identify because they rarely have the word comprehensive in the title. They can be identified by their purpose and length

(Table 2.2). The purpose of comprehensive tests is to provide a broad database for treatment planning. They achieve this purpose by:

1. Identifying levels of functional ability;
2. Identifying underlying deficits that cause dysfunction; and
3. Providing a detailed enough baseline to document small changes.

Therapists don't use comprehensive tests to diagnose a patient's illness. Therapists are not licensed to label someone as diabetic, schizophrenic, or mentally retarded. Therapists perform comprehensive testing to identify the patient's level of functional ability and the underlying deficits that cause dysfunction. The exact constellation of deficits and levels of dysfunction can be highly variable, even within a single diagnostic group. For example, some stroke patients can use their affected hand to hold a glass, while others can't. If a stroke patient is unable to drink from a glass, you need to know why. Does the glass slip out of the patient's hand because of low muscle tone? Is the patient unable to open his/her hand to grasp the glass because of spasticity? Is the patient unable to find the glass because of unilateral neglect? Does the patient refuse to use the affected hand because he/she is embarrassed about spilling? It's important to know why a patient exhibits dysfunction before you choose a treatment method. This enables the therapist to provide an individualized treatment plan.

Finally, comprehensive tests achieve their purpose by providing a detailed baseline that the therapist can use as a comparison for future progress. Some patients who are referred for therapy recover slowly, while others are in a particular facility for a short time. Both situations create a problem for clinicians who must justify their services for patients who will not make large gains in a few days. The comprehensive test can provide enough detailed information to permit the therapist to document these small changes.

By definition, comprehensive tests are long. A brief survey of comprehensive tests showed that they can take from 1 to 10 hours to administer. They can have as many as 20 to 30 test items per test (e.g., the Manual Muscle Test) or per subtest in a battery (e.g., the Kenny Self-Care Evaluation).

Clinical Observation

This is really not the third stage of evaluation. Clinical observation is an ongoing process that overlaps the other stages of evaluation. It can be superficial or intensive. The purpose of clinical observation is to supplement formal assessment. It achieves this purpose by:

1. Quickly documenting assets;
2. Providing test data when formal testing is not possible;
3. Checking the reliability and validity of formal test results; and
4. Identifying unanticipated deficits (Table 2.2).

Clinical observation is especially useful for confirming the patient's assets. For example, eyeballing passive range of motion is routinely done to confirm normal joint mobility. Unfortunately, facilities are not reimbursed for extensive testing of normal or above-normal skills, so clinical observation is a cost-effective way to gain this information.

Clinical observation makes a unique contribution to the assessment process when it replaces formal testing. Some patients are unable to follow formal administrative protocols using standard test materials. Some patients cannot physically tolerate a stressful procedure like a complete Manual Muscle Test. The therapist can at least estimate strength by observing active range of motion during dressing changes. These patients would be "untestable" without clinical observations.

Clinical observation is essential for double-checking the reliability of formal test results (see Appendix). Using standardized tests increases test reliability but does not ensure it. Test results may be inaccurate because of the patient's poor motivation, test anxiety, fatigue, or environmental factors such as a noisy test environment. For these patients, a standardized test score is not a reliable indication of what the patient can do. Since the initial evaluation is really only a brief sample of behavior, we need to know if the sample is reliable before we try to predict what will happen.

Clinical observation can also confirm the validity of formal test results. A physiatrist showed me that formal sensory testing is not always a valid way to evaluate somatosensation. She used to listen to my formal sensory test results and then ask my patient to walk down the hallway with a paper under his/her hemiplegic arm. In many cases, the patient dropped the paper immediately and was not aware of it until he/she reached the end of the hallway. The physiatrist was teaching me that sensory discrimination can be present when the patient concentrates exclusively on a impaired limb and still be absent when the patient has to divide his/her attention in a functional context.

Finally, clinical observation achieves its purpose by identifying unanticipated deficits. Students often miss unanticipated deficits because they pay more attention to formal test results, while experienced therapists attend equally to formal test results and informal observations (11). For example, you may have difficulty placing the finger goniometer over the knuckles of a stroke patient because of nodular obstructions. These nodules may be a sign of arthritis. Clinical observation forces you to double-check your preassessment impressions of a patient.

Experienced therapists are particularly adept at using clinical observation to identify unanticipated deficits. However, this skill can be learned only if it is first made explicit. Suppose you are observing a therapist doing a goniometry evaluation. Suddenly the therapist stops and asks the patient to describe how his/her arm was positioned when he/she woke up. The therapist also feels the temperature of the skin and presses on it. This is reflection-IN-action! Try to think about why the therapist would interrupt a formal test procedure. If you're not sure, ask the therapist. You may not notice at first that part of the extremity is red and swollen. The experienced therapist automatically shifts gears from performing formal goniometry to ruling out edema due to poor positioning, a deep vein thrombosis, and an emerging decubitus. The experienced therapist doesn't always share this inner dialogue which causes a sudden change of plans. Don't be shy about asking questions about seemingly unrelated evaluation procedures. Cohn pointed out that "students cannot learn clinical reasoning by watching our actions, because the thought behind the action is not self-evident" (3).

Clinical observation lacks most of the characteristics of formal assessments (see Appendix). It does not have standardized test materials or standardized administrative or scoring protocols. Yet clinical observation can be structured or unstructured. The most structured type involves modifying a formal test, usually by grading down. Any modification should be carefully reported. Once the administrative protocols have been modified, the standardized scores cannot be used. However, the patient's raw score can be used as a comparison when the same modified test procedure is used at discharge. The therapist can also select a specific activity to investigate a specific deficit. Lower extremity dressing is especially good for observing lower extremity muscle tone and sitting balance.

Clinical observation can also be unstructured. The therapist may observe a patient for a specific deficit during an unstructured activity like a party. The therapist doesn't control what happens but still selectively focuses on a specific deficit. The least structured type of clinical observation is truly unplanned, such as the goniometry example just described.

The advantage of structured clinical observation is it can provide guidelines for interpreting patient behavior. Frequency counts and specific descriptions of behavior can be used to compare the patient to him/herself. If the structured observation is repeated later under the same conditions, changes can be compared to the baseline performance. You may note, for example, that a patient initially lacked elongation of the trunk when tilted to the hemiplegic side in sitting. A progress note could then document the gain in trunk elongation following therapy. When the assessment plan is severely disrupted, or no formal test procedures exist, structured clinical observations are an irreplaceable way to complete the assessment process.

Specialty Testing

This stage of testing usually follows screening, comprehensive testing, and clinical observation, but is not always required. Specialty tests can be identified by their purpose and frequency of use. The purpose of specialty testing is to focus on specific skills in more depth than comprehensive tests allow. They achieve this purpose by:

1. Supplying data that are missing in comprehensive tests; and
2. Confirming underlying deficits that cause dysfunction (Table 2.2).

Specialty tests achieve their purpose by supplying data that may be missing from a comprehensive test. For example, goniometry ignores range of motion of the spine. This is crucial information for treating patients with low back pain. Additional test procedures, such as forward bending in standing and vertebral glide, are needed to complete the initial baseline for back-injured patients (12).

Many comprehensive tests have multiple-domain test items. This makes it difficult to identify underlying deficits that cause dysfunction. For example, the Beery-Buktenica Test of Visual-Motor Integration is a test booklet with several pages of geometric designs. The subject is expected to independently copy the designs after complex verbal instructions are given (13). This paper and pencil test requires receptive language, executive functions, memory, complex visual perception, motor planning, and eye-hand coordination. A patient can fail this test for such a wide variety of reasons that the therapist can't pinpoint the specific cause for a below-average test score.

Some specialty tests, on the other hand, are ideal for confirming the underlying deficits that cause dysfunction because they often have minimal-domain test items. The Motor-Free Visual Perception Test eliminates drawing and minimizes the need for language by permitting the subject to point to a response picture or saying the letter underneath a particular response picture (14). All the test materials are manipulated by the examiner and presented in a structured format so that fewer organizational skills are needed than tests like the Beery-Buktenica. Purists say that a truly single domain test item does not exist, and they are right. Even a simple procedure, like testing deep tendon reflexes, assumes that a certain level of arousal is present. Yet, some specialty tests, like the Motor-Free, minimize the need for simultaneous execution of several skills. This enables the therapist to confirm underlying deficits that cause dysfunction with as much accuracy as possible.

Finally, specialty tests can be identified by their frequency of use. They are *not* used routinely for every patient. Muscle palpation and volumetry are examples of specialty tests that are used only with carefully selected patients.

INTERPRETING TEST RESULTS

Test interpretation is traditionally described in the literature as a separate step in the clinical reasoning process. Students, therefore, get the impression that test interpretation begins after test administration ends. When reflection-IN-action occurs, there is no distinct transition from data collection to data analysis. Experienced therapists begin to interpret test results and modify their evaluation plan while they are still collecting the data. Immediate test interpretation guides subsequent assessment decisions. However, for the sake of grouping the clinical reasoning process into manageable chunks, I have kept interpretation separate. Eventually, this line will blur for you as it does for experienced therapists.

Interpretation has to be an ongoing process because assessment is often incomplete at the end of the initial evaluation. Additional testing is often one of the recommendations in an initial evaluation report. However, as Rogers states, "Data collection cannot continue indefinitely" (4, p. 606.). The initial evaluation is complete when the therapist has enough information to begin treatment planning.

How much information is "enough" depends on time constraints imposed by the setting, the diagnosis, and role definition. For example, if you will see a patient for only 5 days, evaluation must be brief. A patient with one mallet finger obviously needs less evaluation than a patient with a spinal cord injury. In some settings, physical therapists do transfer evaluations, and psychologists conduct cognitive screening. In other settings, these domains of concern are defined as occupational therapy's role. How much is "enough" is situation-specific.

Test interpretation includes cue interpretation and hypothesis evaluation. Kari and Kalscheur found that errors are common at this stage of the decision tree process (15). Students suggest solutions before the problem is well defined. Rogers found that experienced therapists spend much more time making sure they have named the problem correctly and have chosen the appropriate frame of reference before they suggest solutions. Students don't distinguish between relevant and irrelevant test results (15). Experienced therapists distinguish between what is observable from what is function-

ally significant. Students see patients as textbook examples of diagnoses, while experienced therapists see a diagnosis as highly variable, depending on the person who has the injury (16). For example, a surgeon with a hand injury has a different set of functional concerns and fine-motor limitations from a truck driver's with a similar injury.

Generating the Cue Interpretation List

Cue interpretation begins by deciding which cues are relevant to which hypotheses. First, write every hypothesis, leaving room underneath to list the actual evaluation results. Second, use that space to list the cues that you believe are relevant to each hypothesis. Third, decide if cues support their hypotheses. Indicate your decision by writing a plus in front of each cue that confirms or a minus that disconfirms a hypothesis (17). Write a ± in front of a cue that partially confirms and partially disconfirms a hypothesis. Write a question mark in front of a cue if its relevance is unclear or if information is not available. Remember, initial evaluation results are often incomplete because treatment must begin quickly. Finally, at the bottom of the list, add new information that is not related to your hypotheses, and precede each item with a capital N. This may sound complicated at first, but it reduces the load on your working memory when you are trying to decide what the test results mean.

Figure 2.1 shows a cue interpretation list for the burn patient (10). Underneath each hypothesis are the cues that are relevant to that particular hypothesis. Remember, the pluses and minuses represent feedback to you on the accuracy of your hypotheses! They *do not* indicate whether the patient has assets or deficits! Remember, too, the conditional track produces a holistic image that includes the diagnosis, the person, and the environmental demands.

Evaluating the Narrative Hypotheses

Hypothesis evaluation is a three-step process. The first step is to confirm, revise, or disconfirm each hypothesis. It is easy to decide when a hypothesis is confirmed or disconfirmed if you have all pluses or all minuses. You have confidence in your impression of the patient based on the preponderance of the evidence. If there are is a mixture of pluses and minuses under one hypothesis, you may have to revise the hypothesis by deleting the part that was not confirmed. In Figure 2.1, the burn patient illustrates how some hypotheses are confirmed (#1, #2, #6) while others have to be revised (#3, #4, #5).

Sometimes, pluses and minuses under one hypothesis propel you to the second step of hypothesis evaluation,

Cue Interpretation List

1. *DOMINANT RUE WILL HAVE NORMAL ROM*
   + RUE has normal ROM
   Confirmed as written

2. *LOSS OF STRUCTURAL STABILITY OF FINGER EXTENSORS*
   + Precaution against active fist-making
   + MP/PIP/DIP joints must be exercised separately
   Confirmed as written

3. *ABLE TO PERFORM ADL'S ONE-HANDED WITH A FEW DEVICES*
   ± Can do ADLs one-handed except for washing/combing hair
   Revision: one-handed techniques insufficient for hair care

4. *LOSS OF LUE AROM FOR ELBOW/WRIST EXTENSION AND FINGER FLEXION*
   − Normal AROM of elbow/wrist
   + Moderate to severe loss of flexion for all 4 fingers
   Revision: loss of AROM for finger flexion

5. *SCREEN FOR LOSS OF AROM OF LEFT SHOULDER*
   ± Mild loss of AROM for shoulder flexion/abduction
   Refined: only shoulder flexion and abduction lost AROM

6. *STRESS REACTIONS WILL BE PRESENT*
   + Withdrawn and depressed
   Confirmed as written

7. *WHEN AND HOW TO RETURN TO MODIFIED WORK?*
   ? Work could not be evaluated due to fist-making precautions

N. Edema of left hand

Figure 2.1. List of cues with two items of new (*N*) information noted at the bottom.

which is to resolve discrepancies. This step requires dialectic reasoning. Rogers says this type of reasoning is like a lawyer pleading a case by presenting facts that support or refute a conclusion (4).

Sometimes, the discrepancy can be explained. Did the patient do poorly on the first day of the evaluation because he/she was nervous and then do better on the second day when he/she was more relaxed? Did you use test procedures that routinely produce different behaviors? For example, stroke patients show more spasticity of leg extensors while standing than sitting. This difference occurs because weightbearing in standing stimulates the extensor muscles, while sitting, which requires leg flexion, inhibits the extension synergy.

Occasionally, the discrepancy can't be explained. A puzzling discrepancy exists in the burn case discussed earlier. Why is this man unable to wash and comb his hair one-handed (hypothesis #3)? A woman would probably have difficulty styling her hair, but a man should be able to handle a short, basic hairstyle easily. Yet, he apparently can cut meat and tie his shoes one-handed. Were adaptive devices provided to make this

possible? Additional information should be gathered to clear up this discrepancy.

The burn case shows how an initial evaluation is often incomplete because certain types of evaluation may be restricted. In the pre-grafting stage, this patient was not allowed to make a fist for fear of rupturing the exposed extensor tendons, so hand strength and coordination could not be evaluated. This leaves hypothesis #7 still unanswered in Figure 2.1.

Hypothesis evaluation is incomplete without the third step. You need to ask yourself if your preconceptions about the diagnosis or the patient may have skewed your thinking. Narrative hypotheses are an excellent strategy for designing an individualized assessment package. Nevertheless, hypotheses produce conceptual biases that encourage us to overlook data that do not support our hypotheses (9). McArthur found that psychologists who held rigidly to applied theories were the poorest judges of personality (18). Elstein found that the most successful clinicians were individuals who repeatedly evaluated the database from different perspectives (24). Therefore, it is crucial to search through the evaluation results objectively to look for data that don't fit your preconceptions. New data, which are marked *N* on the Cue Interpretation List, show that initial hypothesis generation does not anticipate every problem.

Writing a Problem List

Cue interpretation and hypothesis evaluation represent an inner dialogue that is too lengthy to put in a medical chart. A facility wants you to write a Problem List containing general deficits and dysfunction that are limited to brief descriptions. Delete assets and function (e.g., delete burn hypotheses, #1). Keep the number of problems to a minimum by chunking related problems (e.g., chunk burn hypotheses #4 and #5 regarding ROM). Then add all new problems not predicted by your initial hypotheses.

The Problem List for the burn patient discussed in the case study is:

1. Loss of structural stability of extensor tendons;
2. Edema of burned hand;
3. Loss of AROM of finger flexion and shoulder flexion/abduction;
4. Inability to wash and comb hair one-handed;
5. Presence of stress reactions;
6. Need for vocational and leisure potential to be evaluated.

GENERATING TREATMENT GOALS

The problem list helps you focus on the major concerns before writing treatment goals. You must know the difference between two types of treatment goals (19). **Service goals** describe what the therapist will do for a patient, like making a splint. **Outcome goals** state what behaviors the patient will exhibit. For example, the patient will exhibit a functional hand position for writing. Third-party payers will reimburse only for outcome goals.

Outcome goals state what prerequisite skills and functional outcomes the patient will exhibit. Remember, functional outcomes are age-appropriate self-care, work, and leisure activities that a person needs to perform his/her roles. Prerequisite skills seem simple on the surface, but authors don't agree on how to label them. Mosey breaks them down in to sensory-integrative, neuromuscular, cognitive, psychological, and social skills (20). Reed breaks them down into motor, sensory, cognitive, intrapersonal, and interpersonal areas (21). The Uniform Terminology document from the AOTA divides them into sensory-motor, cognitive, and psychosocial areas (22). I followed Mosey's advice and left the naming of prerequisite skills to each frame of reference (20). In this text, prerequisite skills are the skills addressed by the frames of reference listed below the arrow on Memory Aid 2.2.

Prioritizing Prerequisite Skills

When you generate treatment goals, you begin by prioritizing. A patient cannot simultaneously achieve every goal you believe is eventually possible. Your first priority is to regain prerequisite skills so that underlying deficits that cause dysfunction will be permanently corrected. Prerequisite skills are prioritized by dividing them into short-term and long-term goals on the Goal Spreadsheet.

It is difficult to come up with a universal definition of short- and long-term goals. These terms change with the expected length of stay. The length of stay is determined by the number and type of diagnoses. The DRG guidelines, which determine length of stay, are designed to provide a stroke patient with diabetes and a cardiac condition a longer stay than a patient with an uncomplicated stroke. A short-term goal for a 7-day stay is not necessarily short-term goal for a 1-month stay.

In this text, **short-term** is arbitrarily defined as what can be achieved in 5 days of twice-daily treatment. **Long-term** is defined as what you think can be achieved if the patient receives as much therapy as he/she needs. There are numerous intermediate goals, but they are not listed on the Goal Spreadsheet. Listing short- and long-term goals is a practical first step for learning how to prioritize. Once you decide on short- and long-term goals, it is easy to identify intermediate steps when you need them.

Four types of deficits should be given priority in short-term goals:

1. Deficits that must be treated immediately for safety reasons;
2. Deficits that are functionally significant;
3. Deficits that have the potential for short-term improvement; and
4. Deficits that must be treated directly.

First, it may be too dangerous to wait to address a deficit in long-term goals. If joint instability is present, a short-term goal for this deficit must be implemented at the beginning of the first treatment session. Conversely, a deficit may be too dangerous to address in short-term goals because the treatment itself would cause further damage. For example, having the burn patient in the case study squeeze Theraputty could cause his extensor tendons to rupture. Therefore, increasing grip strength was not listed as one of his short-term goals. Short-term goals should include only what is safe; the therapist has an obligation to do no harm!

Second, you need to decide if a deficit is functionally significant. Students tend to think that everything that can be measured has to be treated. Experienced therapists use the question of functional significance to decide if a deficit warrants immediate treatment. With shortened lengths of stay, you will not have time to address every deficit. If you address the most functionally significant deficits in short-term goals, you will make the most important contribution to your patient's recovery before he or she is discharged or moved to another unit.

Formal guidelines for test interpretation do not always help us decide when a deficit is functionally significant. For example, if a patient has 160° out of 180° of shoulder abduction, will this patient be dysfunctional? Whether a loss of 20° of shoulder motion is dysfunctional depends on the patient's roles, height, and remaining assets that substitute for the lost shoulder motion. Therapists use clinical observation to determine if minor deficits interfere with function.

At discharge time in the burn case, mild loss of shoulder range was functionally significant only for activities that required quick movements. He was unable to resume playing golf because the scar tissue in his axilla would not accommodate the quick stretch required during the golf swing.

Third, short-term goals should include deficits that have the potential for short-term improvement. Do you think it is reasonable to achieve a particular short-term goal in the time allotted? Remember, in this text, short-term is arbitrarily defined as 5 hours of treatment spread out over 5 days. Look at the initial evaluation and guess conservatively upwards.

Fourth, short-term goals should include only deficits that must be treated directly. Some goals can be achieved indirectly. For example, the pectoralis major is a prime mover for horizontal adduction, but it is also recruited as an assister during shoulder flexion. If you strengthen the pectoralis major during shoulder horizontal adduction, it is likely that shoulder flexion strength will also improve. It is not necessary to directly treat every functionally significant deficit in the first week.

Long-term goals may indicate that we think some deficits can never be fully remediated. I don't recommend sharing long-term goals with the patient during early treatment! Even experienced therapists can never be sure of what will happen. However, long-term goals can help us let go of guilt so we can to switch to the rehabilitation frame of reference. We would like to be able to solve every problem, but we can't. Denton told a priceless story of a patient who said he wanted to go to occupational therapy, and was told, "But once you start going you have to go for life" (19, p. 93). The only people he knew who had completed treatment were patients who were discharged or dead.

Indicate your priorities within short- and long-term prerequisite skills with numbers (i.e., priority #1 is at the top of each column). The Goal Spreadsheet in Figure 2.2 was written during the pre-grafting stage for the burn patient described earlier. A good strategy for determining what should be treated first is to ask yourself if one particular deficit is a prerequisite for another deficit. For example, in Figure 2.2, it would be difficult to perform ROM testing on a swollen hand, so it makes sense to reduce edema first. On the other hand, there may be

---

BIOMECHANICAL GOAL SPREADSHEET

Short-term Prequisites, Pregrafting stage
1. Prevent all further structural damage to extensor tendons
   FO: for hand opening during independent two-handed eating
2. Reduce edema of hand after baseline evaluation
   FO: for hand closure during *MODIFIED* auto assembly line work
3. Maintain current PROM of
   • shoulder flexion and abduction at 145°
   • MP flexion at 45°, PIP flexion at 30°, DIP flexion at 5°
   FO: to independently reach over head to grasp gardening tools

Long-Term Prerequisites
1. Complete recovery of structural stability of tendons
2. Increase PROM of shoulder to normal limits
3. Increase PROM fingers: 60° PIP flexion, 20° DIP flexion
4. Increase hand strength: 25-lb lateral pinch/30-lb gross grip

---

Figure 2.2. Short- and long-term treatment goals.

---

no compelling reason why one goal should be achieved before another goal. In Figure 2.2, the two parts of long-term goal #3 related to ROM could easily be reversed.

Preliminary Functional Outcomes

Every short-term goal must be paired with a preliminary functional outcome. The relationship must be specific! Stating that every prerequisite goal will improve all functions is untrue. For example, full shoulder ROM is not needed for self-feeding. Functional outcomes should also state what level of independence you think is realistic. Look carefully at your long-term goals before you promise a patient full recovery.

Making Goals Measurable

Now that your prerequisite skills are prioritized, you need to make these goals measurable. The Goal Spreadsheet must list observable behaviors. This permits two or more people to agree that they have seen the same behavior. Goals that are measurable are made up of behavioral, criterion, and conditions statements (19, 20, 24). The **behavioral statement** names what behavior will be achieved. The **criterion statement** states what level of performance the patient has to exhibit to achieve the goal. Level of performance can be described qualitatively, such as with supervision, or listed quantitatively, such as 90°. The **conditions statement** describes where and with what the criterion will be met. "Where" is the environmental context. "With what" is the nonhuman environment, such as built-up handles. Look at the two examples below.

1. The patient will sit symmetrically (behavior = what prerequisite skill) with head erect, shoulders level, and feet flat on the floor (criterion = what level) using a lapboard (condition = with what).
2. The patient will demonstrate 90° (criterion = what level) of active shoulder flexion (behavior = what prerequisite skill).

The first example demonstrates the value of qualitative descriptions. A therapist may want to improve the quality of the performance instead of increasing frequency or duration. In the second example, the condition statement is absent. This omission is common for prerequisite goals. It may be appropriate, but it should be done consciously rather than by default.

It is important to make short-term goals measurable. This is the only way you can quickly detect a mismatch between your intervention and the patient's response. It is not important that the criteria statement be perfectly accurate, as long as it challenges you to reevaluate how treatment is going.

Even experienced therapists can only estimate short-term criteria. In one study, an experienced therapist accurately predicted short-term gains in range of motion and muscle strength 69% of the time *if* accuracy was defined as within 75% of the predicted criteria (25). In another study, experienced therapists accurately predicted the functional level of stroke patients 80% of the time *if* accuracy was defined as within one functional level on a scale of 0 to 7 (26). It's okay to be slightly off, as long as you use the initial criteria to see if you need to modify your treatment.

As a student, you may struggle to generate measurable short-term goals. Your frustration will escalate if you ignore your primary resource. Don't try to pull criteria and conditions out of thin air; they come from the initial evaluation. You can never be totally sure of how much a patient will gain, but it's not unreasonable to hope that the patient will improve a little beyond the initial evaluation. If you are not sure, guess conservatively upwards from the baseline.

It never hurts to be conservative as long as your short-term goals are greater than the measurement error like ±2° for ROM. If you are too conservative:

1. You and your patient will have an immediate success experience; and
2. Your progress note will document predicted improvement.

If your goals are too high:

1. You may treat too aggressively and injure your patient;
2. You and your patient may have an immediate failure experience; and
3. You may have to write a long progress note to explain how the patient has improved even though he/she has not achieved your goals.

It is also important to make long-term goals measurable. First, stating that you will ''maximize'' or ''increase'' an asset or function does little to help you make realistic discharge plans. Second, our beliefs about a patient's long-term potential are very powerful and can become self-fulfilling prophecies. You will treat the patient in a certain way based on what you believe will happen. For example, if your prospective treatment story says that a patient is going to a nursing home, your treatment won't be aggressive. Patients often know what our long-term goals are just by the way we act. Your patient may buy into your story, whether it is true or not. Measurable long-term goals make us more aware of the images we are projecting through our actions.

The uncertainty of long-term predictions is frustrating for students. The only way to learn is to start predicting and then check to see how accurate your prospective treatment stories are. Even experienced therapists are often wrong at the beginning of treatment, so they revise their long-term goals as the patient progresses. It's better to be wrong than to be unaware of your long-term images for your patient.

DESIGNING TREATMENT ACTIVITIES

Once you have a Goal Spreadsheet, you are ready to design treatment activities. Begin by making postulate statements. These statements show the link between deficits, goals, and therapeutic activities (20). The need for linking statements is clear. Rogers and Masagatani reported that even experienced therapists may fail to connect the patient's problems with specific treatment activities (9). In one patient record, an experienced therapist listed making a splint (method) and increasing range of motion (goal) as two separate and unrelated goals. She was able to connect these two goals during recall sessions, but that didn't help third-party payers or her patient make the connection. Perhaps more patients would actively participate in their therapy if they knew what they would gain.

Writing Postulates Regarding Change

The Goal Spreadsheet requires students to make connections between prerequisite goals and functional outcomes. Now new connections need to be added to make your thought process complete. You can learn to make these new connections by learning how to write postulates regarding change. The format for a postulate regarding change is as follows. A *general deficit* due to a *stage-specific cause* will be resolved by achieving a *measurable short-term prerequisite goal,* which results in a *functional outcome.* An example of one postulate regarding change is written *vertically* in the left-hand column of Figure 2.3.

The deficit can be general, like weakness of the arm or poor axial extension, because the short-term goal for that deficit must be specific and measurable. Both could be written in specific form, but this just doubles the paperwork. It is more important to have a specific, measurable goal.

The stage-specific cause is not the diagnosis. The stage-specific cause is the disease process that occurs during a particular stage of recovery. Remember, the conditional track forewarns you that an illness experience is constantly changing. For example, a patient with a severe burn of the dorsum of the hand may initially have a loss of range of motion because of precautions against fist-making. Later on, the loss of range can be due to hypertrophic scarring, which requires aggressive stretching. When the stage-specific cause is identified, treatment can be specific (9).

Deficit/Cause/Goal/FO	Method/Rationale	Specific Modality
Deficit #3: loss of ROM of left shoulder and hand due to	1) *Heat,* which increases the elasticity of soft tissue	*Neutral warmth:* Bioconcepts garments. See Deficit #2 for precautions.
Stage-Specific Cause: hypertrophic scarring in post-grafting stage of burn	2) *Scar remodeling,* which provides stretch pressure to deeper structures	1. *Deep friction massage* to shoulder scar 2. *Tendon-gliding exercises* in the fist and straight fist positions
S-T Biomechanical goal: increase PROM of • shoulder flexion and abduction to 160° • MP flexion to 70° • PIP flexion to 50° • DIP flexion to 15° • Fingertips 1/2″ from distal palmar crease	3) *Passive stretch* beyond the currently available range which elongates collagen fibers in soft tissue	*Distraction approach:* help patient touch objects over head. One hand assists scapula to upwardly rotate, while other hand cradles patient's upper forearm. Then help patient wrap hand around a dowel. Put your index finger over his/her index finger, etc. Stop when firm, white bands appear. Repeat.
Functional Outcome: independently use unadapted gardening and woodworking tools	4) *Positioning/splinting,* which maintain gains from stretching during cool-down/ between Rx	See Deficit # 2 for details
	5) *Role-related activities* through the increased range which ensure that gains will be generalized to daily routines	*Wooden flower pot:* have patient get woodworking tools from overhead cabinet with moderate assistance while sitting on a tall stool. Build up diameter of handles on tools so fingertips are 3/8″ from distal crease. Turn patient sideways to return tools to cabinet.

Figure 2.3. Biomechanical postulates. One postulate regarding change is written *VERTICALLY* in the left-hand column. Five postulates regarding intervention are written *HORIZONTALLY.*

While each short-term goal must be measurable, don't turn each goal into its own postulate, such as three separate postulates for increased MP, PIP, and DIP flexion. This can create an unwieldy list of 30 or more postulates, and that can overwhelm you if you think about treating them all at once. There is often some practical way to chunk closely related goals into one major goal. One way is to chunk goals together that share the same methods. In Figure 2.3, the MP, PIP, and DIP joints will all receive heat and stretch, so why list them separately?

However, you have to double-check this chunking-by-shared-methods strategy when you design the specific treatment activity. Sometimes it is too difficult to make one activity achieve every part of a large goal. For example, if the activity chosen for the ROM goal in Figure 2.3 was rolling out cookie dough, it would be difficult for the patient to see the dough above head height to stretch the shoulder. Check to see if the activity meets all the goals you intended. It might be more realistic to subdivide the ROM goal into 3a and 3b to indicate that two different activities will be used for the shoulder and hand.

Finally, functional outcomes are an essential part of postulates regarding change. Improvement in prerequisite skills will not be reimbursed by Medicare, workers' compensation, and Medicaid unless they result in func-

tional gains (27–29). When prerequisite skills are not linked to functional outcomes, third-party reviewers must make a "leap of faith" that the therapy was really useful to the patient (30).

However, functional outcomes are more than just a strategy in the documentation game. They also help patients become invested in their therapy program. I learned this while undergoing knee surgery. While I found the details of how the surgeon restored the smooth contour of my kneecap interesting, I was primarily concerned about whether or not I could resume downhill skiing. Once I found out I could resume a valued activity, the painful, repetitive exercises became my therapy plan, not the doctor's.

A therapist is trained to identify which functional outcomes are possible once certain prerequisite skills are achieved. Yet only the patient can determine what functional outcomes *should* be achieved (4). Therapists have an ethical responsibility to take the patient's valued goals seriously. It is particularly easy to encourage patients to select functional outcomes because they readily understand them. A functional outcome, like driving a car, makes sense to a patient.

However, therapists and patients do not always value the same functional outcomes. When there is a major discrepancy between what the therapist and patient thinks is important, you don't have to wait for the patient to go home to see mismatches. A patient can work toward a functional outcome with the therapist and fail to implement it outside the therapy department with little cognitive dissonance. One patient felt that the least his family members could do is feed him after he worked all his life to put food on the table. If the patient does not value a particular functional outcome, like independence in feeding, the therapist is likely to find a family member feeding this patient in the patient's room.

A therapist may not like a particular patient's choices, but imposing functional outcomes on the patient only allows the therapist to save face. Patients may choose functional outcomes that are below or above their potential. However, the therapist should negotiate rather than impose what he/she believes is a more realistic choice. Of course, the therapist cannot let the patient do anything that is dangerous, but this is different from telling the patient that his/her functional goals aren't important. Remember, the conditional tract says that successful treatment is conditional upon the patient's active participation. This means giving the patient a say when functional outcomes are chosen.

A postulate regarding change is overly simplistic because it only has one functional outcome. For example, normal strength finger flexors would give a truck driver adequate grip strength for controlling the steering wheel. However, grip strength probably has an impact on several other functional outcomes. Yet, making a long, academically complete list of functional outcomes for each prerequisite skill is not important. Even dividing functional outcomes into short-term and long-term is not important. What is really important is making the connection between your prerequisite skills and functional outcomes that the patient cares about!

Writing Postulates Regarding Intervention

Once the postulates regarding change are written, you are ready to write postulates regarding intervention. Students often want to select a therapeutic activity *before* the goal is clearly stated. It is the goal that must come first! The format for a postulate regarding intervention is as follows. A *short-term prerequisite goal* or *functional outcome* will be achieved by using a *general method* that has a *rationale* that guides selection of a *specific modality*. Five postulates regarding intervention are written *horizontally* in Figure 2.3.

In Figure 2.3, all five postulates start with a short-term prerequisite goal. However, there are many times when no change can be expected in a prerequisite skill. A patient with a spinal cord injury will not get any motor return below the level of the injury. When this happens, the therapist must shift gears from remediation to compensation training; prerequisite goals are omitted,

and the methods used come from the Rehabilitation frame of reference (e.g., adaptive devices).

The **method** is a general category of treatment techniques. For example, in Figure 2.3, heat is the general category from which neutral warmth was selected. Selecting the general category first is not an academic nicety for three reasons.

First, the general method is a good way to develop self-cuing. The method column cues students to recall what they have memorized about the methods of a particular frame of reference before they select specific treatment techniques. It is easier to think about which specific type of heat you want to use after you have recalled that heat is a general method to increase ROM.

Second, the general method is a practical strategy for narrowing down your choices. This reduces anxiety during activity selection. For example, the method of active stretch provides clues for eliminating certain types of activities. Since you want maximal excursion during stretch, you don't want to confuse the patient by asking for a maximal contraction. This eliminates highly resistive activities, like lifting heavy boxes when you want full shoulder flexion. Stretching also means finding an activity that goes beyond the patient's current range. If your patient needs full finger flexion, you can eliminate activities that require minimal finger extension, like knitting. The process of elimination helps reduce anxiety and improve selection when there are too many options (e.g., buying a car).

Third, starting with the general method first also reminds you to keep your mind open to a variety of different therapeutic approaches. Methods often evolve out of treatment for a specific diagnosis, but they should be generalized to other types of patients. For example, work simplification was first used during homemaking for the arthritic patient, but it is just as important for a patient with quadriplegia to gather all of his/her clothes before dressing on the bed. By systematically arguing for and against each method, the student can rediscover old friends and investigate new allies.

Negotiating Specific Activities

While there are only a few methods for each goal, there are endless numbers of therapeutic activities. Students believe they must discover the one right treatment activity for each problem (3, 5). Experienced therapists assume that it is possible to have several correct solutions to a problem. This provisional aspect of the conditional tract makes experienced therapists quicker to change strategies when things don't go as planned. Supervisors initially make students write up treatment activities to give the student an emotional safety net. With experience, a student will learn to bring a list of treatment activities to the first treatment session and let the patient try several activities until the best one is found (1). Students who use the interactive and conditional tracts attend to the person's preferences and reactions before making a final choice about specific activities for a diagnosis.

It is crucial for the therapist to collaborate with the patient on activity selection. First, while occupational therapists are well trained in activity analysis, they can't know every modality. Patients can frequently supply the how-to information that the therapist then modifies to meet the goal. The therapist doesn't have to know the details of fly casting to modify this activity to facilitate axial weight shifts. Collaboration also acknowledges the importance of the patient's preferences. Patients are more likely to be compliant if they select something enjoyable or valuable to them.

With a few simple explanations, it is amazing to see how easily patients or family members can participate in activity selection and modification. Sometimes patient participation involves positive suggestions. A patient can often sense more accurately than the therapist that craft material should be moved slightly. Sometimes participation takes the form of negative reactions. Even cognitively impaired patients know they don't like spinach.

My favorite example of negotiating a specific activity with a nonverbal client appeared in *Smithsonian Magazine*. Bernstein told the story of how Charles Kettering perfected the diesel locomotive (31). "We didn't design it," Kettering said. "All we did was run errands for it. We said to the engine: now here are a half dozen pistons; tell us which one you like. And here's half a dozen valves; try 'em out. We let the engine evaluate things for four or five years, and finally we put it together." I said, "If that engine doesn't work, it's not our fault."

Activity descriptions don't have to be compulsively complete (Fig. 2.3). It is not necessary to list every step needed to make a pinch pot or to write down all the rules of checkers. The most important information is (*a*) how the patient and materials are to be set up and (*b*) exactly what the therapist will do once the activity begins. This information has to be specific. Stating that the game will be somewhere on the table or the therapist will inhibit tone is too vague. Double-check to see if the description is specific enough to determine if the activity has addressed all the goals and is safely graded to the patient's current level of function.

Figure 2.3 employs cross-references to other activities that are not listed. This is a valuable strategy because it encourages students to use activities for several goals instead of designing a different activity for every goal. Making a flower pot can also achieve a socialization goal by doing it in a group. Once an activity is described, subsequent references only have to list the modifications

that are needed to achieve each additional goal. Repeated use of one activity cuts down on the time needed to negotiate with the patient, set up the activity, teach the patient how to do the activity therapeutically, and clean up.

Finding one activity for multiple goals involves a certain amount of serendipity. A goal may jump out at you for one particular activity. Then, later, you see that the same activity can serve other goals. Or you may find that you still have goals left over, so you have to use a second activity. It doesn't really matter if your starting point produces a different constellation of activities from the therapist next to you, as long as your activities are appropriate.

FEEDBACK LOOP DURING IMPLEMENTATION

Formal reevaluation is a periodic event in every patient's program, but an informal feedback loop runs continuously throughout the implementation phase. The feedback loop is a general systems theory concept (32) that assumes that human behavior is dynamic and interactive. The patient's behavior constantly changes in response to a changing environment. The therapist constantly monitors the patient's output and modifies the input to achieve maximal effectiveness.

Sometimes the feedback is negative. Therapists may feel they have lost control of the prospective treatment story when the patient doesn't respond as expected. There are a number of strategies that a therapist can use to "fix" the treatment story. These strategies include modifying the activity, revising the short-term prerequisite goal, changing the method, renegotiating functional outcomes, and reframing the deficit. These strategies are listed in ascending order of the therapist's resistance to change. This sequence approximates the order most commonly used, but it is not necessarily correct for every situation.

Modifying the activity is the easiest way to revise treatment. Even an experienced therapist has to modify an activity when setting it up for a new patient. Each patient is a little bit different, so there is always some trial and error required. Since the therapist has already tinkered once with the activity, it's easy to redesign it again. The patient may not even be able to tell where the first version of an activity ends and its modified version begins.

Revising the short-term goal is another strategy that comes easily. Goals are only predictions, so they are often a little too difficult or too easy for the patient's current level of function. Even if your first short-term goal is correct, you often must write subsequent interim goals before finally achieving a long-term goal. Therapists expect to revise goals.

Changing the method requires overcoming some resistance in the therapist. Certain methods are routinely used with certain deficits. Shopping for a new method may require the therapist to change treatment routines. Instead of using an adaptive device, maybe the therapist should modify the environment. Sometimes a method isn't fully effective until it is combined with other methods. These combinations require reflection and open-mindedness.

Renegotiating functional outcomes may also produce therapist resistance. It's natural to believe that patients want what we want (4). Because therapists are required to value life-long learning and independence, it's easy to project these values on our patients. It's hard to accept that a patient doesn't want to learn a new way to dress him/herself or that family members feel they must do everything for a disabled patient. It's hard to accept that some patients do not have the financial and social resources to implement functional outcomes that they value. It's hard to accept that a patient cannot return to work because of perceptual deficits that can't be remediated. Functional outcomes are painful to renegotiate.

Reframing the deficit generates the most resistance because the therapist essentially has to start over again. It may require a change to a new frame of reference. Once the therapist recognizes that a deficit is not being addressed by the current frame of reference, he/she must be willing to make new assumptions and use totally different treatment techniques. For the therapist who wants to hold onto one frame of reference, this can create a personal crisis (33).

I will not discuss the feedback loop in the case simulation chapters. It takes both a therapist and a patient to produce a feedback loop. While I can write my side of the prospective treatment story, I would need repeated interaction with a real patient to tell his/her side of it. To write both sides of the story would be an unacceptable fabrication. The feedback loop is best left to fieldwork level II, where students are present on a daily basis for repeated observations of the same patients.

SUMMARY

Since the sequence of events from assessment to treatment planning is so complex, it is difficult to condense it into a few paragraphs. Instead, look at Memory Aid 2.1. Then scan ahead to see how this Memory Aid creates a template for all the case simulations.

STUDY QUESTIONS

1. What are the advantages to chunking the "data collection schedule" by frames of reference instead of diagnoses?

2. How would the narrative hypotheses for the burn patient change if he had burns on both upper extremities?
3. What is the relationship of narrative hypotheses to screening tests?
4. What is the purpose in selecting comprehensive vs. specialty tests?
5. How does clinical observation achieve the purpose of supplementing formal assessment?
6. Cue interpretation begins when you do what?
7. On the Cue Interpretation List, what do the pluses, minuses, and question marks signify?
8. When is it difficult to confirm or disconfirm a hypothesis?
9. What is the difference between a service and an outcome goal?
10. In this text, how is a short-term goal arbitrarily defined?
11. What four types of deficits should be given a priority in short-term goals?
12. What three types of statements are needed to make a goal measurable?
13. Why is it helpful to make long-term goals measurable?
14. What is the format for a postulate regarding change?
15. Why should you identify the stage-specific disease process instead of the diagnosis in a postulate regarding change?
16. Why are functional outcomes important to the therapist and to the patient?
17. What is the format for a postulate regarding intervention?
18. What is the advantage to identifying a general treatment method before selecting a specific treatment modality?
19. Who selects the specific treatment activity for a patient?
20. How specific do activity descriptions need to be when you submit a written treatment plan to a supervisor?
21. What are the advantages of using one activity to achieve more than one goal?
22. What is the sequence of strategies used to modify treatment in the feedback loop?
23. Which of these strategies in the feedback loop are therapists most resistant to use and why?

References

1. Fleming MH. The therapist with the three track mind. Am J Occup Ther 1991;45:1007.
2. Payton OD. Clinical reasoning process in physical therapy. Phys Ther 1985;65:924.
3. Cohn ES. Fieldwork education: shaping a foundation for clinical reasoning. Am J Occup Ther 1988;43:243.
4. Rogers JC. Eleanor Clarke Slagle lectureship—Clinical reasoning: the ethics, science, and art. Am J Occup Ther 1983;37:601, 606.
5. Neistadt ME. From classroom to clinic: anticipation of the patient's need. Paper presented at the annual meeting of the American Occupational Therapy Association, Baltimore, 1989.

6. Watts NT. Decision analysis: a tool for improving physical therapy practice and education. In: Wolf SL, ed. Clinical decision making in physical therapy. Philadelphia: FA Davis, 1985:7, 20.

7. Spencer EA. Functional restoration: neurologic, orthopedic, and arthritic conditions. In: Hopkins HL, Smith HD, eds., Willard and Spackman's occupational therapy. 7th ed. Philadelphia: JB Lippincott, 1988:503.

8. Trombly CA. Arthritis. In: Trombly CA, ed. Occupational therapy for physical dysfunction. 3rd ed. Baltimore: Williams & Wilkins, 1989:543.

9. Rogers JC, Masagatani G. Clinical reasoning of occupational therapists during the initial assessment of physically disabled patients. Occupational Therapy Journal of Research 1982;9:195.

10. Chan SW, Pedretti LW. Burns. In: Pedretti LW, Zoltan B, eds. Occupational therapy practice skills for physical dysfunction. 3rd ed. CV Mosby, Princeton, 1985:116.

11. Cohn ES. Fieldwork education: strategies for providing a foundation in clinical reasoning. Paper presented at the annual meeting of the American Occupational Therapy Association, Baltimore, 1989.

12. Wadsworth CT. Manual examination and treatment of the spine and extremities. Baltimore: Williams & Wilkins, 1988:28.

13. Beery KE, Buktenica NA. Developmental test of visual-motor integration. Chicago:Follett Publishing, 1967.

14. Colarusso RP, Hammill DD. The motor-free visual perception test. Philadelphia:Academic Therapy Publications, 1972.

15. Kari N, Kalscheur J. Clinical decision making: an educational model. Paper presented at the annual meeting of the American Occupational Therapy Association, Baltimore, 1989.

16. Neistadt ME. Classroom as clinic: a model for teaching clinical reasoning in occupational therapy education. Am J Occup Ther 1987;41:631.

17. Elstein AS, Shulman LS, Sprafka SA. Medical problem solving—an analysis of clinical reasoning. Cambridge, MA: Harvard University Press, 1978.

18. McArthur C. Analyzing the clinical process. J Coun Psych 1964;1:203.

19. Denton PL. Psychiatric occupational therapy: a workbook of practical skills. Boston:Little, Brown & Co., 1987:93.

20. Mosey AC. Occupational therapy: configuration of a profession. New York:Raven Press, 1981.

21. Reed KL. Occupational therapy models: organization and taxonomy. In: Reed KL, ed. Models of practice in occupational therapy. Baltimore: Williams & Wilkins, 1984: 81.

22. American Occupational Therapy Association. Uniform terminology. 2nd ed. Rockville, MD: AOTA, 1987.

23. Clark PN. Occupational therapy in pediatrics. In: Clark PN, Allen AS, eds. Occupational therapy for children. CV Mosby, Princeton, 1985:116.

24. Pedretti LW. Treatment planning. In: Pedretti LW, Zoltan B, eds. Occupational therapy practice skills for physical dysfunction. 3rd ed. CV Mosby, Princeton, 1990:22.

25. Kwasniewski RT. A study of the accuracy of outcome projections in occupational therapy. Master's thesis, Temple University, May 1990.

26. Korner-Bitensky N, Mayo NE, Poznanski SG. Occupational therapist's accuracy in predicting sensation, perception-cognition, and functional recovery post-stroke. Occupational Therapy Journal of Research 1990;10:237.

27. Gillard M. Money and reimbursement versus OT practice. Pennsylvania Occupational Therapy Association workshop. Philadelphia, 1990.

28. Pinson CC. Work programs reimbursement: what is happening across the nation? Physical Disabilities Special Interest Section Newsletter 1991;4:2.

29. Marmer LA. How to set up a group. Advance for Occupational Therapy 1992;8:11.

30. Dahl M. Money and reimbursement versus OT practice. Pennsylvania Occupational Therapy Association workshop. Philadelphia, 1990.

31. Bernstein M. A self-starter who gave us the self-starter. Smithsonian Magazine 1988;July:125.

32. Von Bertalanffy VL. General Systems Theory. New York: George Braziller, 1962.

31. Mattingly M. The narrative nature of clinical reasoning. Paper presented at the annual meeting of the American Occupational Therapy Association, Baltimore, 1989.

SECTION II

BIOMECHANICAL FRAME OF REFERENCE

CHAPTER 3

Introduction to Biomechanical Frame of Reference

The biomechanical frame of reference has been in use since the end of World War I. In 1918, Baldwin started an OT department at Walter Reed General Hospital for physically injured soldiers. He was the first person to analyze the use of joints and muscles during purposeful activity (1). Prior to Baldwin, purposeful activities were used for diversional purposes only. He developed methods for measuring range of motion (ROM) and strength to prove that purposeful activities were achieving their goal. Taylor expanded on Baldwin's ideas by coining the terms passive range of motion (PROM), active assistive range of motion (AROM), and resistive exercise (1). She also defined muscle reeducation as the localized action of specific muscle groups without recruiting other muscles whose action is not desirable. Dr. Licht added the goal of increased work tolerance, which we now call endurance, and further refined the concept of strengthening (1). He divided muscle activity into static, shortening, and stretching types of contraction. Today, we call these contractions isometric, concentric, and eccentric.

Presently, the theoretical bases for the biomechanical frame of reference are taught in anatomy, physiology, and kinesiology courses. These scientific bases have added many new facts to our knowledge about this frame of reference since the first theorists showed the medical profession the value of prescriptive purposeful activity.

ASSUMPTIONS

The first assumption of the biomechanical frame of reference is the belief that purposeful activities can be prescribed to remediate loss of ROM, strength, and endurance. This replaces the pre-World War I assumption that purposeful activity was simply diversional.

The second assumption states that if ROM, strength, and endurance are regained, the patient will automatically use these prerequisite skills to regain functional skills. Although this is a strongly held assumption, an exhaustive literature search turned up only two studies that examine the relationship of biomechanical gains to functional outcomes. Glynn and Morgan found a correlation of only .32 between an ADL score and the Jebsen Hand Function Test score in 20 physically dysfunctional adults (2). How can skills such as manual dexterity and strength have such a low correlation with ADLs?

One difficulty with this type of global study is the faulty assumption that *every* physical gain will affect *every* functional outcome. In one study, no more than 45° of shoulder motion were needed to perform three feeding tasks (5). Therefore, there is no correlation between gains in feeding and gains of more than 45° of shoulder ROM. A few weak correlations like this will cancel out high correlations and make the overall association between biomechanical skills and a composite ADL score look quite low.

The relationship of biomechanical to functional gains is very important. Workers' compensation, Medicare, and Medicaid will no longer reimburse for treatment of biomechanical deficits unless there is a proven functional gain (4–6). As more third-party payers reimburse for functional rather than biomechanical gains, this second assumption will no longer be taken on faith.

The third assumption is the principle of rest and stress. First, the body needs rest to heal itself. Then, the therapist can gradually stress the bones, muscles, soft tissues, and cardiorespiratory system to regain normal function. Without a reasonable amount of stress, these structures quickly lose their ability to function. That is why NASA takes valuable time out of every mission to make sure that the astronauts exercise. Even though the astronauts start each mission in peak physical condition, they cannot remain healthy in a gravity-free environment without physical stress.

The fourth assumption states that a patient must have an intact brain that can produce isolated, coordinated movements (7). However, many peripheral conditions produce faulty sensory feedback that can cause an intact brain to produce uncoordinated movements. You may have experienced temporary impairment of oral coordination after receiving novocaine. In our patients, the intact brain may receive tactile paresthesias from scar tissue and regenerating peripheral nerves or impaired proprioceptive from sutured tendons and painful muscles. The intact brain needs more than the sensory input given by hot packs and manual stretch. The brain must learn how to interpret complex sensory input from the body's interaction with unpredictable people and uncooperative objects. The intact brain must coordinate more than the predictable motions used to lift weights and perform repetitions. The brain needs to practice modifying motor output in response to complex, changing environmental demands. If a medical condition violates this fourth assumption of normal peripheral sensation, the biomechanical frame of reference is not the best choice for sensory and coordination retraining.

DEFICITS ADDRESSED

The eight function-dysfunction continua that are addressed by the biomechanical frame of reference are:

1. Structural stability;
2. Low-level endurance;
3. Edema;
4. Maintaining ROM;
5. Increasing ROM;
6. Maintaining strength;
7. Increasing strength; and
8. High-level endurance.

Because of changes in the health care system, structural stability and low-level endurance have been added to the concerns identified by the early biomechanical theorists.

Structural stability is traditionally included under homeostatic issues. Changes in the health care delivery system have made it necessary to include structural stability in the biomechanical frame of reference. In the past, therapists were able to assume that structural stability of bones, muscles, ligaments, skin, and other soft tissues were present before therapy began. Today, shortened lengths of stay require therapists to mobilize patients at such early stages of recovery that structural

stability is often incomplete. Therapists may have to balance the need for rest with the need for early mobilization within a single treatment session. Therefore, it is dangerous to separate biomechanical and structural stability issues in your mind when you write treatment goals.

Endurance is traditionally placed much later in the biomechanical sequence. The rationale for also including it early has to do with another old assumption of the biomechanical frame of reference. This old assumption states that cardiovascular and respiratory function will be stable before mobility training is initiated. Patients used to come to therapy well rested and able to start on sedentary activities. Shortened lengths of stay make this assumption obsolete in acute care and even in rehabilitation programs. Today, patients may be so ill that they cannot even tolerate sitting up when treatment begins.

Edema is traditionally included under ROM because edema restricts ROM. I have separated edema from PROM because dozens of techniques have evolved to treat this specific problem, and the dangers of edema require a strong emphasis on this special problem. In the early stages, the signs of edema are visible puffiness, heat due to local inflammation, and a mushy end-feel during PROM. Advanced edema is characterized by massive swelling, decreased skin temperature due to impaired circulation, impaired PROM, and severe pain. The prognosis for untreated edema is devastating: permanent loss of ROM from stagnant fluids that have become fibrotic, loss of sensation and active movement due to nerve compression, and compromised nutrition of distal body parts, which may lead to amputation.

Chapter 4 discusses increasing ROM and maintaining current ROM. Maintenance is a benign term for a very destructive process. Loss of ROM gradually creates a bedridden patient who needs expensive nursing care. In long-term care settings, maintenance of ROM reduces pain and deformity, which makes it easier to handle the patient. Prevention in long-term care settings is not only more humane, it is also more cost-effective.

Even ambulatory outpatients can experience a devastating loss of function if ROM is not maintained. For example, peripheral nerve injuries leave muscle groups unopposed. If untreated, the muscles that are left intact during the prolonged period of nerve regeneration can produce contractures that require expensive surgery. Similarly, grafted skin in burn patients can form massive scars that require repeated surgery to regain ROM and to enhance a cosmetic appearance. Maintenance is far too insipid a word for these serious problems.

Muscle strength is also divided into maintaining vs. increasing strength in Chapter 4 on biomechanical postulates regarding intervention. Loss of strength is a common problem in the early stages of recovery because normal activity is often restricted in acutely ill patients. Loss of strength can appear in even undamaged muscles after only 6 to 10 days of bedrest (8). Any period of restricted activity should trigger a search for muscle weakness. If weakness can be prevented, less strength has to be regained. We don't want to create an unnecessary need for our services when prevention is such an easy thing to do.

EVALUATION CRITIQUED

The administrative protocols and scoring procedures for biomechanical evaluation like goniometry and manual muscle testing are well documented (9). In addition to developing the technical ability to perform these evaluation procedures, you need to develop critical thinking skills. You need to be aware of test reliability, validity, and sensitivity. Unfortunately, only a few of the commonly used biomechanical evaluation tools have been critiqued in depth.

Goniometry

Inter-rater reliability for goniometric measurements made by two or more therapists sometimes fell below .70, which is the lowest acceptable correlation for the clinic (see Appendix). Inter-rater reliability coefficients for elbow motions and knee flexion were between .88 and .97, but were only .63 to .70 for knee extension (10) and .66 to .86 for wrist movements (11).

Baseline and follow-up evaluations were most reliable when all the tests were performed by the same therapist using the same type of goniometer. Intra-rater reliability, which compares a therapist to himself, was better than inter-rater reliability in three studies. Rothstein et al. found that intra-rater reliability for elbow and knee goniometry was .91 to .99, which is exceptional (10). Horger found that intra-rater reliability for PROM of the wrist was .91 to .96. (11). A therapist can be so reliable that averaging repeated measurements is not more reliable than a single measurement (12).

PROM goniometry requires the therapist to move and hold the limb while measurements are made. Under these conditions, the margin for therapist-related error is generally considered to be ±2° (i.e., you may be off by 2° in either direction). Environmental factors that can affect test reliability should be avoided when possible. They include:

1. Testing at different times of day (e.g., patient may be stiffer in the morning);
2. Changing the OT clinic (e.g., air conditioning makes the patient stiffer); and
3. Providing different activities prior to testing (e.g., relaxing hot packs vs. painful stretching exercises).

If it is not possible to control these factors, make a note that they may be affecting test reliability on the recording sheet.

PROM goniometry provides the therapist with "end-feels" that can help identify underlying causes of joint restriction (13). Types of end-feels include:

1. Bony block: abrupt stop; no "giving in" with pressure;
2. Fixation devices (e.g., pins/casts): same as bony block;
3. Spasticity: "catching sensation" followed by a mild rebounding effect or slow release with maintained stretch;
4. Pain/fear of pain: no tissue resistance; patient stops the motion anywhere in the range;
5. Hypertrophic scarring: firm resistance as scar tissue visibly tightens; white bands may appear;
6. Excessive fat/muscle bulk: visually obvious; soft compression as two body parts come together;
7. Edema: soft, "mushy," "boggy" resistance; and
8. Capsular tightness: firm limitation that occurs prematurely in the range; feels resilient with maintained stretch.

An alternative to passive ROM goniometry is active range of motion (AROM) goniometry. AROM goniometry requires the patient to move his/her limb and then hold it up while the therapist takes a measurement. It does not provide the end-feels that help the therapist determine the underlying cause of the loss of range.

AROM goniometry is interpreted correctly *only* if you have first done PROM goniometry to rule out bony blocks and other causes of joint restriction. If PROM equals AROM, you know that the patient has full movement through the currently available range. On the other hand, when PROM is greater than AROM, you know the patient is weak or reluctant to move.

AROM goniometry is helpful under two conditions. One is when weakness produces such limited AROM that the patient moves only a few degrees into the available range (e.g., only 10° out of 180°). This patient may not show improvement in strength by graduating from a Fair minus to a Fair grade within a few days. An increase in degrees of AROM (e.g., from 10° to 30°) permits you to document immediate short-term progress. This enables you to justify the need for therapy even when the muscle grade does not change during the early stages of treatment. Second, AROM goniometry is also a necessary alternative to manual muscle testing when resistance is contraindicated (e.g., during an acute flare-up of rheumatoid arthritis).

Goniometry has good face validity. It appears to measure joint range of motion. However, the use of ROM norms to interpret a patient's ROM scores is questionable. Range of motion is not a construct that remains constant in the general population. A survey of ROM norms shows considerable disagreement about the accepted degrees of motion for a single joint (12). This variability may be due to the influence of occupation on ROM. Clearly, sex and age have a strong influence on ROM. One study showed that women have greater flexibility than men at all ages (12). Another study found that ROM deteriorated with age (13). There was a decline between 20 to 30 years of age, followed by a plateau from 31 to 60 years of age, followed by a second decline in people ages 60 and over.

Even if separate ROM norms are developed to reflect age, sex, and occupational differences, these norms may not be valid for our patients. "They may even lead to unrealistic expectations and inappropriate treatment" (12, p. 108). A patient may need less or even more than average ROM to make use of compensatory movement strategies. An individual with a high spinal cord injury is a good example. This individual needs tight finger flexors to rake up an object with a claw hand and then hold it with tenodesis action. Conversely, a quadriplegic patient needs excessive hip flexibility to permit long-leg sitting while dressing in bed.

The clinician needs to determine what functional activities the patient cannot perform and then estimate how many degrees of ROM are needed. For example, can a patient who has 80° of shoulder flexion and abduction comb his/her hair? It depends on the length of the patient's arm and the number of compensatory movements and adaptive devices that he/she uses. Appropriate ROM goals can be made only through clinical observation of functional activities.

However, the statement that ROM is within functional limits (WFL) is meaningless unless the functional activities are specifically listed. Is the range functional for feeding, which requires very little shoulder motion, or is the range functional for return to work as an auto mechanic, which requires considerable reaching over the head? Is the range functional for writing, which requires considerable finger flexion, or is the range functional for bathing with an open hand? The statement "ROM is WFL" always requires an appropriate condition statement (e.g., for all ADLs or for return to work as an typist).

Occupational therapists have a special responsibility for assessing the functional limitations of PROM in the lower extremity. The ROM needed for gait is far less than full ROM. The ROM for gait is also far less than what the occupational therapist needs for lower extremity dressing and bathing. The list below shows what is needed for walking on a flat surface (14). These ranges are much lower than those needed for many ADL activities. For example, you need far greater hip, knee, and

ankle motion when you lift your foot to tie your shoelaces. Analyze the lower extremity ROM needed to tie your shoes and write your answers below.

Needed for Gait	Full Range	Needed to Tie Shoes
Hip flexion = 60°	0°–120°	Hip flexion = ____°
Hip abduction = 5°	0°–45°	Hip abduction = ____°
Hip rotation = 5°	0–45°	Hip rotation = ____°
Knee flexion = 60°	0–125°	Knee flexion = ____°
Plantar flexion = 25°	0–45°	Plantar flexion = ____°
Ankle inversion = 5°	0–30°	Inversion = ____°

Finally, goniometry is very sensitive to small changes at both ends of the range. However, norms for unusually flexible individuals such as Olympic athletes are not available, so goniometry has a good basement (where zero is), but a poor ceiling (see Appendix).

Specialty Tests of Range of Motion

The goal of PROM goniometry is to measure *joint* movement, not tendon excursion. Standardized ROM protocols ensure that *joint* range will not be restricted by passive insufficiency of soft tissue. **Passive insufficiency** occurs when a muscle and its tendon have been passively stretched to their maximum length (13). For example, if you fully extend all three joints of a finger simultaneously, MP *joint* extension will look restricted because the slack is taken out of the long flexor tendons before the MP *joint* fully extends. You must flex the PIP and DIP joints to keep some slack in the long finger flexors when you evaluate the degrees of MP *joint* extension.

Because ROM protocols ensure that passive insufficiency will be eliminated by not stretching tendons over several joints at once, early tendon tightness may go undetected in the hand by ROM evaluations. Tests for tightness fill this gap. Make sure you thoroughly understand the Test for Intrinsic Tightness, the Test for Extrinsic Tightness, and the Test for Landsmeer's Tightness described in Hopkins and Smith (15).

Another strategy for evaluating finger tendon excursion is Total Action Motion (TAM) (16). TAM requires the patient to actively flex all three finger joints simultaneously to assess total tendon excursion over all the joints that the flexor tendons cross. Normal TAM for one finger is considered to be 260° (Fig. 3.1). Abnormal TAM is computed by adding the degrees of MP/PIP/DIP flexion and then subtracting the degrees of MP/

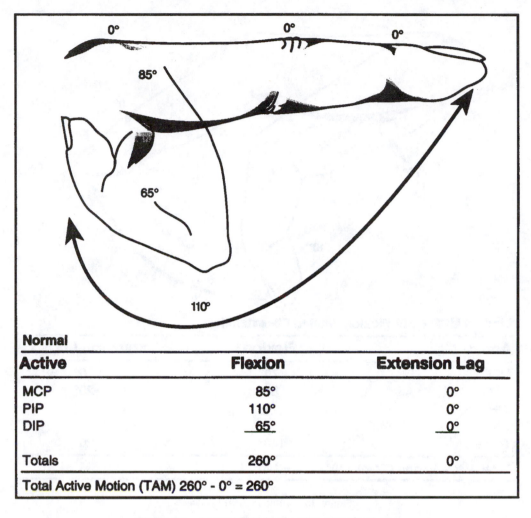

Normal

Active	Flexion	Extension Lag
MCP	85°	0°
PIP	110°	0°
DIP	65°	0°
Totals	260°	0°

Total Active Motion (TAM) 260° - 0° = 260°

Figure 3.1.   Normal TAM (total active motion) values.

PIP/DIP extension that are lacking (Fig. 3.2). When TAM is less than the total PROM for each individual joint, limited tendon glide is suggested (16). TAM is important whenever the disease process suggests that hand function will be restricted by inadequate tendon excursion much earlier than joint restriction.

Other specialty tests for ROM can supplement goniometry. Loss of ROM for hand closure can be documented by measuring how many centimeters the tips of the fingers are from the distal palmer crease. The goal for therapy is to get the centimeters to zero so that the fingers finally touch the distal palmar crease. This evaluation strategy is also used to document how many centimeters the tip of the thumb is to the tip of each finger during opposition. For very unusual hand deformities, the therapist can repeatedly take instant-developing (Polaroid) pictures or even photocopy (Xerox) the hand. These richly detailed pictures can document the gradual recovery of a normal hand shape.

Finally, loss of ROM in the hand can be caused by edema. Edema can be measured by specialty tests such as circumferential measurements of individual digits or by volumetry for the whole hand when skin closure is present. The measurement error for volumetry is considered to be 10 ml of water displacement (16). However, this reliability holds true only if precisely the same test conditions are used each time. For example, the volumeter must be in exactly the same place on the table, the patient must have his/her feet in exactly the same place on the floor, and the patient must submerge his/her hand until the web space between and third and fourth digits rests on the dowel inside the volumeter.

Manual Muscle Testing

Manual Muscle Test (MMT) baselines and follow-up evaluations *must* be performed by the same therapist in order to be reliable. Therapists of different body build

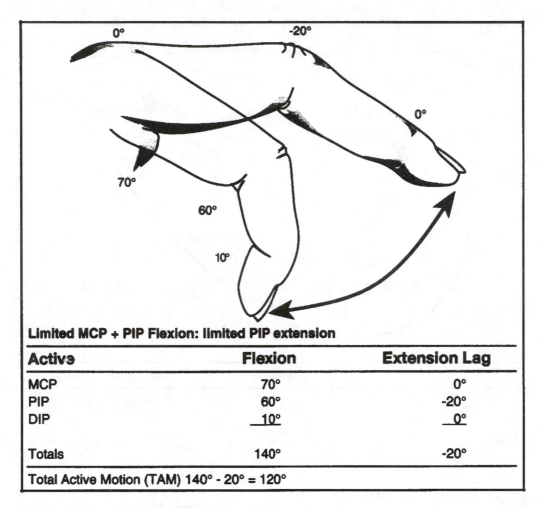

Limited MCP + PIP Flexion: limited PIP extension

Active	Flexion	Extension Lag
MCP	70°	0°
PIP	60°	-20°
DIP	10°	0°
Totals	140°	-20°

Total Active Motion (TAM) 140° - 20° = 120°

Figure 3.2.   Abnormal TAM values.

and strength do not always award identical muscle grades to the same patient. It is not unusual for two therapists to consistently disagree by one muscle grade (e.g., Good minus vs. Fair plus). In one study, three physical therapists agreed within ±one muscle grade 97% of the time, but gave the exact same muscle grade only 67% of the time (17). Record any factors that could affect the reliability of your MMT. These factors include pain, fear, fatigue, and various medical conditions like cardiac or respiratory problems.

Since muscle grades are more subjective than degrees of ROM, the clinician needs to use clinical observation to determine what functional activities the patient can perform with his current level of strength. For example, a frail, elderly woman may only need to overcome minimum resistance (Fair plus) to be functional in her daily life. Using clinical observations to determine whether a given muscle grade is functional makes more sense than constantly changing what is meant by ''maximum''

resistance. To have a different definition of ''maximum'' resistance for an athletic young person vs. a sedentary middle-aged person vs. a wheelchair-bound elderly person would make test-retest reliability questionable.

The MMT has good face validity. It appears to measure static strength. However, is it a valid test of strength for all types of contractions that muscles need to make (17)? What about eccentric contractions? What about strength when explosive movements or coordination are required? Speed and coordination are real problems for patients with neurological impairments. Speed and coordination are also very important for an athlete who must make explosive, complex movements under variable conditions. Are we assessing all types of strength accurately by using a test of static strength?

The MMT is a more sensitive test of weakness than strength. It has many more scores at the low end of the scale, but only two scores at the high end of the scale (i.e., Good and Normal). The MMT does not differentiate well among above-average individuals such as world class athletes. Therefore, the MMT has a good basement but a poor ceiling.

Decision Tree Process

The decision tree process cuts down the length of an evaluation. It is necessary to reduce the time needed to evaluate a patient when that patient has a shortened length of stay or fatigues easily due to an acute illness. Making a conscious decision about what to cut relieves guilt about what was not fully evaluated due to time constraints. You will manage your evaluation time wisely with the decision tree process.

Evaluation should begin with screening for assets. In the biomechanical frame of reference, you start by eyeballing PROM. You move every joint through its full range and visually estimate whether or not full range is present. If you are satisfied that range is within normal limits (WNL), you do not pick up a goniometer to confirm it. If a patient obviously turns his/her hand completely palm-up with no substitutions, you simply record supination as WNL.

If you see an obvious restriction or even suspect that a restriction exists, you go to the second step, which is PROM goniometry. This rules out joint restriction *before* the MMT.

If end-feels during PROM goniometry or the diagnosis of a hand injury leads you to suspect the presence of finger tendon tightness, you proceed to the third step. This is administration of the Tests for Tightness or Total Active Motion of the fingers.

The fourth step in the decision tree process is to screen for strength. You may have no reason to believe that your patient has weakness based on the presenting problem or diagnosis. Assets in hand strength can be documented quickly by testing grip and pinch strength. Upper extremity strength can be screened using AROM. Therapists often ask patients to (*a*) touch their hands together behind the head and behind the back; (*b*) extend the elbows; (*c*) pronate and then extend the wrists; (*d*) protract and retract the scapula while the arms are extended in front of the body; (*e*) supinate and then flex the wrist; (*f*) squeeze the therapist's hand; and (*g*) hold the fingers extended and abducted while the therapist tries to adduct them and then flex them. If the patient does not exhibit full AROM for certain motions, you can select the appropriate muscles for MMT.

If you are sure or even suspect that a patient is weak, the fifth step is MMT. Testing begins in the position that the patient arrives in. For example, if the patient comes to you in sitting, do as many MMT procedures in sitting as you can before repositioning the patient. Weak patients cannot tolerate frequent repositioning and may not be able to complete the MMT if fatigued early in the test session.

The majority of upper extremity motions can be fully tested against gravity in sitting except for five shoulder girdle motions. These five motions are: scapular protraction and retraction, shoulder horizontal adduction and abduction, and shoulder internal rotation. These five motions are gravity-eliminated or -assisted in sitting. Sitting only gives the patient credit for Poor level strength. Yet, these five muscle groups may actually have Fair level strength or above. Your patient wants to receive the highest muscle grade to which he/she is entitled. To correctly award a muscle grade, you must test these five motions in supine or prone, where they are gravity resisted.

Two shoulder motions can never be tested in a gravity-resisted position. These motions are scapular depression and shoulder adduction. When resistance taken is moderate or maximal, it is customary to award a grade of Good or Normal even if they are tested in gravity assisted planes. When resistance taken is minimal or absent, the muscle grade awarded is determined by clinical observation of functional activities like wheelchair push-ups.

If the patient demonstrates very limited degrees of active movement, the sixth step in the decision tree process is to perform AROM goniometry. However, this procedure is used *selectively* only when manual resistance is contraindicated or early progress in strength must be documented by very small increases in degrees of AROM.

Certain conditions, such as peripheral nerve and spinal cord injury, may require the seventh step in the decision tree process. This step is a strength test for individual muscles. Special test positions provide an optimum line of pull for individual muscles. For example, flexing the elbow with the forearm supinated favors the biceps over other elbow flexors. Yet, as soon as increased load (resistance) or speed is applied, the brachioradialis and brachialis are recruited (14). Therefore, to say that the biceps have Good strength against moderate resistance is not a valid statement. You are not testing what you say you are testing. You don't know how much of the resistance was provided by the biceps and how much by other elbow flexors. However, slow, unresisted movement through full range in a special test position does tell you that an individual muscle has at least Fair or Poor grade strength. Within this restriction of no speed and no resistance, individual muscle testing is valid.

The eighth and final step is muscle palpation. This is done when there is no visible movement or if the diagnosis suggests paralysis of individual muscles such as in spinal cord or peripheral nerve injuries.

The decision tree process for joint mobility and strength ensures that successively larger amounts of data will be collected on a selective basis. The steps in this process are:

1. Screen for joint restrictions by eyeballing PROM;
2. PROM goniometry only for restricted joints;
3. Specialty tests of hand ROM for tendon tightness/ edema;
4. Screen for weakness by eyeballing AROM;
5. MMT to test strength of muscles that are known to be weak;
6. Use AROM goniometry to evaluate strength when active range is very limited movement (e.g., only a few degrees of total) or when resistance is contraindicated (e.g., acute arthritis);
7. Test strength of individual muscles with unresisted, slow, AROM in special test positions with optimum lines of pull; and
8. Muscle palpation when no visible motion occurs.

Evaluation of Endurance

Doctors and therapists use activities to establish an endurance baseline and then compare the patient to him/herself on later activities. Endurance data can be collected in the form of metabolic requirements of activities, a particular step on an cardiac activity chart, the level of intensity during activities, the onset of signs and symptoms during monitored activities, the duration of an activity, and the number of repetitions performed during a particular activity.

The metabolic requirements of various activities have been computed using Metabolic Equivalent units (METs). One MET represents the amount of energy it takes to rest while sitting in a semi-reclining position (18). The MET values for different activities are shown in Table 3.1. These MET values can only be used as a guideline because the data were collected on normal individuals. A patient with a spinal cord injury will probably use more energy to perform an activity than is listed on an MET chart because he has fewer intact muscles to do the same job. However, the MET charts provide valuable information about sequencing the level of metabolic demands made by different activities. If a patient is struggling with level 3 MET activities, you should wait to introduce level 4 MET activities.

Cardiac activity charts break the least demanding activities down into much smaller steps than MET charts (18). For example, a patient may be ordered to feed him/ herself while sitting propped up in bed before he/she is allowed to sit upright in a bedside chair to eat (Table 3.2). This baseline endurance information is easily obtained from the nursing staff, who routinely receive orders regarding the patient's "a.m. privileges." While these charts were initially developed for cardiac patients, they can be used with any patient who has very low endurance abilities, such as acutely ill patients who must be treated at bedside.

Another practical method for evaluating endurance comes from the cardiac literature, but it is useful for all diagnoses. This is the method of recording the intensity of effort during activities. Guidelines for recording intensity include event targets and target heart rates.

Event targets are selected by recording how many minutes it takes to complete an activity. From this baseline, you gradually increase the number of events performed within a set time or reduce the amount of time allowed. Dressing in 10 fewer minutes than baseline is an example of an event target that increases intensity.

Target heart rates are another way to evaluate intensity. The doctor may specify a maximum allowable heart rate, such as 140 beats per minute (bpm), based on clinical judgment. The doctor may specify a training heart rate based on a percentage of the maximum heart rate that is safe for a person's age (19). For example, 220 minus the age of 70 equals 150, which is then multiplied by a 75% intensity level (set by the doctor). This equals a maximum training heart rate of 112 bpm (i.e., $220 - 70 = 150 \times 75\% = 112$). The patient must maintain this target heart rate for at least 20 minutes to achieve cardiac reconditioning. Finally, the doctor can determine a safe target heart rate by administering a treadmill test (20). Unfortunately, many acutely ill patients cannot tolerate the treadmill test, so the physician often has to rely on clinical judgment or age-related formulas.

When the physician doesn't provide a target heart rate, the therapist can evaluate the patient's initial endurance level with a monitored activity (21). The first step in a monitored activity is to take vital signs while at rest. An adult's resting pulse is normally between 60 and 100 bpm. An adult's blood pressure (bp) is usually 120 over 80. An adult's breathing rate is usually 15 to 20 breaths per minute (bpm). The second step is to have the patient perform an activity while the therapist watches for signs and symptoms. The third step is to take the vital signs as soon as activity stops. Pulse rate should be taken first since this drops off dramatically as soon as the patient becomes still. The fourth step is to let the patient rest for 5 minutes and then retake vital signs.

During the monitored activity, you need to watch for obvious signs of distress such as confusion, shortness of breath (**dyspnea**), profuse sweating in association with cold, clammy skin (**diaphoresis**), and straining while holding one's breath (the **Valsalva maneuver**). The Valsalva maneuver is especially dangerous for patients with heart disease because it raises blood pressure. You also need to give serious attention to the patient's report of symptoms such as fatigue, chest pain, nausea, and lightheadedness (**syncope**). Try to find out exactly where the chest pain is located (e.g., over the sternum), what type of pain it is (e.g., burning), when it began, and what the patient's subjective estimate of how much

Table 3.1.
MET Levels for ADL, Work and Leisure Activities

1 MET		2 METs		3 METs	
DAILY LIVING					
Resting supine	1	Walking 1 mph	2	Walking 2 mph	3
Sitting in armchair semi-reclined 45°	1	Walking 1.5 mph	2.5	Using bedside commode	3
Sitting unsupported on edge of bed	1.3	Wheelchair propulsion 1.2 mph	2	Lukewarm shower	3.5
Self-feeding: sitting supported	1.2	Driving a car	2	Stairs: slowly at 24 ft/min	3.5
Standing relaxed	1.5	Washes hands, face and brushes hair	2	Bowel movement: on toilet	3.6
Transfer from bed to chair	1.7	Dress, undress	2.5		
		Washing, dressing, and undressing	2.7		
HOMEMAKING					
Hand sewing	1	Polishing furniture	2	Preparing meals	3
Machine sewing	1.5	Dusting	2.5	Waxing floor	3.4
Sweeping floor	1.5	Scrubbing: standing	2.5	Ironing: standing	3.5
		Peeling potatoes	2.5	Mopping	3.5
		Kneading dough	2.5	Hanging wash	3.5
		Wash small clothes	2.5	Wringing by hand	3.5
		Electric vacuum	2.6	Light bed-making	3.9
		Manual vacuum	2.9	Cleaning windows	3–4
		Misc. carrying	2.9		
CLERICAL TASKS		**TRADESMEN**			
Manual typing	1.1	Shoe repair	2.2	Auto repair	3
Electric typing	1.2	Tailoring: cutting	2.2	Light janitorial work	3
Desk work	1.8–2.2	Industrial sewing machine	2.5	Bartending	3
Operating electric		Radio, bench assembly	2.5	Locksmith	3
office machines	2.2			Tractor plowing	3.5
				Tailor: pressing	3.6
ENGINEERING		**BUILDING**			
Watch repair	1.5	Metal work (hammering)	2.1		
Light assembly line	1.5	Hacksawing: standing	2.5		
Draftsman	1.5	Light brick work	2.7		
Setting type: stand	1.6	Measuring, sawing	2.8		
Printing	1.8				
RECREATIONAL TASKS					
Watching TV	1	Playing piano	2	Golf: power cart	3
Knit, crochet	1	Bimanual sanding: 50 strokes/min	2	Cycling: 5 mph on level ground	3
Rug-hooking	1.1	Flying	2	Powerboat: drive	3
Leather tooling: sitting	1.4	Motorcycling: 2.5 mph	2	Billiards	3
Painting: sitting	1.5	Canoeing: 2.5 mph	2.5	Shuffleboard	3
Playing cards: sitting	1.5	Horseback ride: slow walk	2.5	Playing most musical instruments	3
Writing: sitting	1.6	Weightlifting: 10 lb 15/45 min	2.8	Bowling	3.5
Weaving floor loom	1.6			Playing with children	3.5
Carving	1.7				
Drawing: standing	1.9				

pain is present on a scale of 0 to 10 (21). The doctor will want to know all this subtle information when you call him/her about precautions.

These warning signs and symptoms may appear during step 2 of the monitored activity before the therapist has a chance to take the vital signs at the end of the activity. The therapist should *stop* the activity and call the doctor for instructions if the following occur: (*a*) patient reports of symptoms such as chest pain or syncope, (*b*) confusion, (*c*) diaphoresis, or (*d*) level 2 dyspnea. Dyspnea can be assessed by having the patient count out loud to 15 (22). If a patient can count to 15 in one breath, there is no dyspnea (a grade of zero). If a

patient needs two breaths to count to 15, he/she has level 1 dyspnea. If a patient needs three breaths, he/she has level 2 dyspnea, and the activity should be stopped immediately.

Once the baseline data suggest a particular level of endurance training, the therapist still needs to carefully monitor the patient during every treatment session. Activity endurance can change from day to day, especially if the patient is not medically stable or has a change in schedule. During endurance training, watch for subtle signs of distress as fatigue sets in, such as escalating frustration, gradually slowing down the work pace, hurrying to finish, progressively moving through less and

Table 3.1 (continued)
MET Levels for ADL, Work and Leisure Activities

4 METs		5 METs		6 METs	
DAILY LIVING					
Hot shower	4.2	Marital sex	5	Walk with braces and crutches	6.5
Walk down stairs	4.5	Up/down stairs:			
Bowel movement: on bedpan	4.7	30 ft/min	5		
		36 ft/min	5.5		
		Walking 3 mph	5.5		
HOMEMAKING					
Push power mower	3–4	Carrying groceries	4–5	Shoveling light earth, digging garden	5–6
Polishing floor	4.1	Raking leaves	4–5	Mowing lawn: manual mower	6.5
Washing floor: kneeling	4.3			Splitting wood	6.5
Bed-making: stripping	4.4				
TRADESMEN					
Welding: mod. load	3–4	Light carpentry	4–5	Shoveling light earth	5–6
Wheelbarrow:		Paper hanging	4–5	Planing soft wood	6.1
115 lb/2.5 mph	4	Painting	4–5	Planing hard wood	6.6
Chiseling	4.6	Horse ploughing	5		
		Sawing soft wood	5.1		
		Drilling hard wood	5.7		
		Sawing hard wood	5.9		
		Haying	5.9		
RECREATIONAL TASKS					
Energetic musician	3–4	Many calisthenics	4–5	Stream-fishing: walk in light current	5–6
Archery	3–4	Dancing: Foxtrot	4–5	Canoeing 4 mph	5–6
Sailing small boat	3–4	Table tennis	4–5	Cycling 10 mph	5–6
Fly-fishing: standing in water	3–4	Tennis: doubles	4–5	Push-ups	6.5
Horseshoe pitching	3–4	Badminton: singles	4–5	Weightlifting: 10–20 lb lifted	
Volleyball: 6 men noncompetitive	3–4	Golf: carry clubs	4–5	36 times/15 min	6.5
Badminton: social doubles	3–4	Cycling: 8 mph	4–5	Horseback riding: trotting	6.5
Golf: pull bagcart	4	Rollerskating: 9 mph	5		
Swimming 20 yd/min	4	Ice skating: 9 mph	5		
Gardening: raking, hoeing, weeding	4.5	Deep knee bends	5.5		

7 METs		8 METs		9+ METs	
DAILY LIVING					
Ascending stairs with 17-lb load				Ascending stairs with 25-lb load	
at 27 ft/min	7.5			at 54 ft/min	13.5
HOMEMAKING					
		Tending furnace	8.5		
TRADESMEN					
Shoveling 10 lb for 10 min	6–7	Digging ditches	7–8	Shoveling 14 lb for 10 min	8–9
Heavy hammering	7.4	Carrying 30 lbs	7–8		
RECREATIONAL TASKS					
Waterskiing	6–7	Jogging: 5 mph	7–8	Cycling: 13 mph	8–9
Dancing: folk and square dancing	6–7	Cycling: 12 mph	7–8	Cross-country skiing: 4 mph	8–9
Light downhill skiing	6–7	Vigorous downhill skiing	7–8	Handball: social	8–9
Tennis: singles	6–7	Horseback riding: galloping	7–8	Vigorous basketball	8–9
Badminton: competitive	6–7	Mountain climbing	7–8	Squash: social	8.5
Spading	7	Ice hockey	7–8	Squash: competitive	>10
		Touch football	7–8	Handball: competitive	>10
		Basketball	7–8	Running	
		Paddleball	7–8	6 mph	10
		Canoeing: 5 mph	7–8	7 mph	11.5
				8 mph	13.5
				9 mph	15
				10 mph	17

Table 3.2.
Part of Activity Chart with Steps for Inpatient Rehabilitation After Myocardial Infarction

	Exercise	Ward Activity	Educational & Craft Activity
Step 1	Passive ROM to all extremities (5X ea), teach pt *active* plantar and dorsiflexion of ankles to do several times per day.	Feeding self sitting with bed rolled up to 45°, trunk and arms supported by over-bed table.	Initial interview and brief orientation to program.
Step 2	Repeat exercises of Step #1.	1. Feeding self. 2. Partial AM care (washing hands & face, brushing teeth) in bed. 3. Dangle legs on side of bed (1X).	Light recreational activity, such as reading.
Step 3	Active assistive exercise in shoulder flexion and elbow flexion and extension, hip flexion, extension and rotation, knee flexion and extension, rotate feet. (4X ea).	1. Begin sitting in chair for short periods as tolerated, 2X/day. 2. Bathing whole body. 3. Use of bedside commode.	More detailed explanation of program. Continue light recreation.
Step 4	Minimal resistance, lying in bed do above ROM 5X ea. Stiffen all muscles to the count of 2 (3X).	1. Increase sitting 3X/day. 2. Change gown.	Begin explanation of what is an MI. Give pt pamphlets to read, begin craft activity: 1. Leather lacing, 2. Link belt. 3. Hand sewing, embroidery. 4. Copper tooling.
Step 5	Moderate resistance in bed at 45° above ROM exercises, hands on shoulders elbow circling (5X each arm).	1. Sitting ad lib. 2. Sitting in chair at bedside for meals. 3. Dressing, shaving, combing hair—*sitting down*. 4. Walking in room 2X/day.	Continue education about healing of heart, reasons for early restrictions in activity.
Step 6	1. Further resistive exercises sitting on side of bed, manual resistance of knee extension & flexion, (7X ea movement). 2. Walk distance to nearest bathroom and back (note if patient needs assistance).	1. Walk to bathroom, ad lib if pt can tolerate. 2. Stand at sink to shave.	Continue craft activity or supply pt with another one. Pt may attend group meetings in a wheelchair for no more than 1 hour.
Step 7	1. Standing warm-up exercises: a. Arms in extension and shoulder abduction, rotate arms together in circles (circumduction) 5X each arm. b. Stand on toes, 10X. c. May substitute abduction 5X ea leg. 2. Walk length of ward hall (50 ft) and back to room at average pace.	1. Bathe in tub. 2. Walk to telephone or sit in waiting room (1X/ day).	1. May walk to group meetings on the same floor.

less range, and augmenting range with unwanted movements. These subtle signs, along with the vital signs taken at the end of the activity, will tell the therapist if the endurance training was too difficult. The warning signs to grade down include:

1. Any of the subtle signs listed previously;
2. A heart rate that exceeds the physician's target heart rate;
3. A heart rate that goes up more than 20 bpm from the resting pulse;
4. Failure to return to the resting heart rate after 5 minutes of rest;
5. Systolic blood pressure that does not go up at all; and
6. Systolic pressure that goes up more than 20 mm Hg from the baseline pressure.

The simplest method for obtaining baseline information on endurance is to record the number of repetitions that are performed or the amount of time (duration) that the patient can sustain effort during an activity. Selecting one over the other should be based on which is more practical. Some activities are easier to time, like minutes needed to eat a full meal. On the other hand, counting the number of spoonfuls taken to the mouth may be more useful when only a few repetitions are possible.

Unlike range of motion and muscle testing, which require a decision tree process, the therapist usually chooses only one of the previously mentioned methods for evaluating endurance. The physician may specify which method is to be used, or the doctor may leave it up to the discretion of the therapist.

BIOMECHANICAL POSTULATES REGARDING CHANGE

An example of a biomechanical postulate would be: A *loss of wrist strength* due to *disuse atrophy, pain, and stiffness* secondary to subacute rheumatoid arthritis will be resolved by achieving *Good minus wrist extensor strength*, which will result in the *ability to do flower arrangements on the job*.

Once your evaluation has identified a biomechanical deficit, like a loss of wrist strength, the next step is to select a measurable biomechanical short-term goal. It is very easy to write measurable biomechanical goals because the biomechanical frame of reference uses quantitative evaluation methods, such as muscle grades. However, biomechanical goals are sometimes written incorrectly in the form of service goals that state what the therapist will do (23). Service goals, such as stretching and making a splint, are called therapeutic methods in this text. Biomechanical goals must be written in the form of outcome goals that state what the patient will be able to do, such as exhibit increased strength.

Once you have identified a measurable biomechanical goal, it is time to select an appropriate functional outcome. If the therapist and patient cannot agree on a functional outcome, it doesn't matter how accurately the therapist states the biomechanical goal. The functional outcome is what the patient gets for his/her effort. Patients want to know if they can drive their car again, not how many degrees of finger flexion they will achieve. As discussed in Chapter 2, functional outcomes are ultimately the patient's area of expertise. The therapist's contribution is recognizing how specific biomechanical gains make specific functional outcomes possible.

The relationship between biomechanical goals and functional outcomes requires clinical experience. A therapist has to look at a Manual Muscle Test and decide if the patient has sufficient strength to do a car transfer before actually trying one. Can a patient do a car transfer with Good muscle strength or is Normal strength required? Does a patient need full supination to feed him/herself? There are no published norms to guide the student. The best way to learn is to keep track of both from the beginning of treatment. When the patient can achieve a functional outcome, he/she has the necessary biomechanical skills. It is crucial that you establish a link between biomechanical skills and functional outcomes as soon as possible. This link often influences the choice of activity and is essential for reimbursement (4–6).

SUMMARY

The assumptions and deficits that are addressed by the biomechanical frame of reference define the scope of what you can treat with this approach. The number of deficits have been expanded since the early theorists' work after World War I. For example, structural instability and low-level endurance have been added because of changes in the health care system. In the current medical climate, many patients are so sick when treatment begins that these domains must be treated before more aggressive biomechanical treatment can be implemented. Other deficits have been further refined by subdividing them, like dividing range of motion into controlling edema, maintaining ROM, and increasing ROM.

Biomechanical evaluation protocols are well documented but not always thoroughly critiqued. Biomechanical tests passed into common use before measurement theory became a standard in occupational therapy. Goniometry and Manual Muscle Testing have good reliability, but validity still requires clinical judgment. Therapists must decide how current range and strength impact on function. They must also use intuition to predict future performance, like return to work. The decision tree process can streamline assessment procedures, including biomechanical evaluations. Complete evaluation of every possible deficit is not done unless there is a reason for it.

Probably the biggest change in the biomechanical frame of reference has been the change in focus for reimbursement from biomechanical goals to functional outcomes. Because biomechanical goals are so concrete, they set the early standards for documentation in physical disabilities. Today, however, documentation of functional change must be included in biomechanical progress notes for reimbursement from many third-party payers.

STUDY QUESTIONS

1. What are the four assumptions of the biomechanical frame of reference?
2. What five deficits are addressed by this frame of reference?
3. Why is edema such a devastating deficit?
4. Why does maintenance come before regaining ROM and strength?
5. How reliable is goniometry? When is it the most reliable?
6. What two conditions suggest the need for AROM goniometry?
7. How valid are the norms for ROM?
8. What is the OT's special responsibility for lower extremity ROM?
9. How well do two different therapists agree on the MMT?
10. How valid is the MMT?
11. Why do you need the decision tree process?
12. What are the steps in the decision tree process for ROM/MMT?

13. Name five methods for evaluating endurance.
14. True or False: A therapist will be reimbursed by third-party payers for increasing ROM and muscle strength?

References

1. Reed KL. Models of practice in occupational therapy. Baltimore: Williams & Wilkins, 1984.
2. Glynn JW, Morgan VR. You can do research in the clinic. Advance for Occupational Therapy 1990;6:1.
3. Safaeed-Rad R, et al. Normal functional ROM of upper limb joints during performance of three feeding activities. Arch Phys Med Rehab 1990;71:505.
4. Dahl M. Money and reimbursement versus OT practice. Pennsylvania Occupational Therapy Association workshop. Philadelphia, 1990.
5. Pinson CC. Work programs reimbursement: what is happening across the nation? Physical Disabilities Special Interest Section Newsletter, 1991;14:2.
6. Marmer LA. How to set up a group. Advance for Occupational Therapy 1992;8:11.
7. Pedretti LW, Pasquinelli S. A frame of reference for occupational therapy in physical dysfunction. In: Pedretti LW, Zoltan B, eds. Occupational therapy practice skills for physical dysfunction. 3rd ed. St. Louis: CV Mosby, 1990:7.
8. Affleck AT, et al. Providing occupational therapy in an intensive care unit. Am J Occup Ther 1986;40:323.
9. Trombly CA, Scott AD. Evaluation. In: Trombly CA, ed. Occupational therapy for physical dysfunction. 3rd ed. Baltimore: Williams & Wilkins, 1989: 184.
10. Rothstein JM, Miller P, Roettger RF. Goniometric reliability in a clinical setting: elbow and knee measurements. Phys Ther 1983;63:1611.
11. Horger MM. The reliability of goniometric measurements of active and passive wrist motions. Am J Occup Ther 1990;44:342.
12. Miller PJ. Assessment of joint motion. In: Rothstein JM, ed. Measurement in physical therapy. New York: Churchill Livingstone, 1985.
13. Clarkson HM, Gilewich GB. Musculoskeletal assessment. Baltimore: Williams & Wilkins, 1989.
14. Norkin C, LeVangi P. Joint structure and function. Philadelphia: FA Davis, 1992.
15. Hollis LI. Functional restoration—hand rehabilitation. In: Hopkins HL, Smith HD, eds. Willard and Spackman's occupational therapy 6th ed. Philadelphia: JB Lippincott, 1983:461.
16. Nicholson B. Evaluation of the hand. In: Stanley BG, Tribazi SM, eds. Concepts in hand rehabilitation. Philadelphia: FA Davis, 1992: 58.
17. Lamb RL. Manual Muscle Testing. In: Rothstein JM, ed. Measurement in physical therapy. New York: Churchill Livingstone, 1985:47.
18. Trombly CA. Cardiopulmonary rehabilitation. In: Trombly CA, ed. Occupational therapy for physical dysfunction. 3rd ed. Baltimore: Williams & Wilkins, 1989:595.
19. Kirkendall DT. Mobility: conditioning programs. In: Gould JA, Davies GJ, eds. Orthopedic and sports physical therapy. St. Louis: CV Mosby, 1985:242.
20. Foderaro D, O'Leary S. Cardiac dysfunction. In: Pedretti LW, Zoltan B, eds. Occupational therapy practice skills for physical dysfunction. 3rd ed. St. Louis: CV Mosby, 1990:595.
21. Geiger C. Cardiac rehabilitation. Lecture presented at Temple University School of Occupational Therapy, Philadelphia, 1988.
22. Temple Hospital Exercise Physiology Staff. Lecture presented at Temple University School of Occupational Therapy. Philadelphia, 1988.
23. Denton PL. Psychiatric occupational therapy: a workbook of practical skills. Boston: Little, Brown & Company, 1987.

Biomechanical Postulates Regarding Intervention

The function-dysfunction continua that are addressed by the biomechanical frame of reference are:

1. Structural stability;
2. Low-level endurance;
3. Edema;
4. Passive range of motion;
5. Strength; and
6. High-level endurance.

This chapter is intended to supplement entry-level textbooks by focusing on sequencing treatment and situational thinking.

Biomechanical deficits are treated fairly sequentially. If a broken clavicle lacks structural stability, you can't strengthen shoulder muscles. Working simultaneously on all biomechanical deficits for a *single body segment* is highly unlikely. Instead, therapists focus on deficits that are adjacent to each other in the sequence, such as reducing edema and increasing ROM (Memory Aid 4.1). This "adjacent deficits" approach is less common in other frames of reference. For example, it is hard to predict the exact sequence of treatment for each individual in the model of human occupation. Which would you address first, the patient's values or the attitudes of his family? It isn't possible to rigidly sequence homeostatic treatment. For some patients, cardiovascular dysfunction is the most life-threatening; in others, it may be the immune system. By comparison, the biomechanical frame of reference has a much more predictable treatment sequence.

However, you cannot apply every step of the general treatment sequence listed in Memory Aid 4.1 to a specific individual. Application of general concepts requires situational thinking. When you study the biomechanical case simulation, think about the situational thinking that is modeled in this chapter.

PREVENTING STRUCTURAL DAMAGE

Chapter 3 explains why the assumption that structural stability will be present is outdated and why this concern has become a part of early biomechanical treatment. Prevention of further structural damage is listed first in the treatment sequence because we have an obligation to "do no harm." Yet, hospital staff impose stress forces on unstable or vulnerable body parts during necessary hospital procedures. This can result in additional structural damage. For example, a patient with an unstable cervical spine must be turned without causing additional lacerations of the spinal cord. Further structural damage is prevented by using orthoses and positioning devices that protect a specific vulnerable body part during hospital procedures. Since prevention is paramount, therapists implement orthoses and positioning devices simultaneously rather than sequentially. A few specific examples are listed in Table 4.1.

The physician does the situational thinking about structural stability. The doctor determines if structural stability is present or absent. Therapists in acute care need to consult daily with the physician about the patient's status. Therapists are expected to understand and implement all procedures that enforce rest or provide stress per the doctor's orders.

REGAINING STRUCTURAL STABILITY

The therapist's second priority is to regain structural stability. The four methods listed in Table 4.1 are numbered to indicate a treatment sequence. Initially, structural stability is regained by enforcing rest. Orthoses and positioning devices are introduced together while the patient is still on bed rest. They may continue to be used for an extended portion of the recovery period.

Memory Aid 4.1.
Biomechanical Goals/Methods/Rationales

Old Biomechanical Assumptions	Range of Motion	Strength and Endurance
I. *FURTHER STRUCTURAL DAMAGE* will be prevented by using: *Orthoses* and *Positioning devices* that protect specific vulnerable body parts during hospital procedures.	IV. *PERIPHERAL EDEMA* will be reduced by: 1. *Elevation* which allows gravity to remove excess peripheral fluids, 2. *Pressure* which prevents filtration of fluids out of capillaries, 3. *Temperature control* which stimulates localized vascular responses 4. *AROM* which pumps fluid from periphery.	VII. *STRENGTH* will be maintained by using: 1. *AROM* which prevents disuse atrophy during enforced rest 2. *ADLs* which maintain strength of physically active patient.
II. *STRUCTURAL STABILITY* will be regained by using: 1a. *Orthoses* 1b. *Positioning devices* and 2. *Procedures* that enforce rest temporarily until damaged structures heal 3. *Procedures* that stress healed structures.	V. *ROM* will be maintained by using: 1. *Passive/Active assistive/active ROM* in currently available range which prevents adhesions/elongate collagen 2. *Scar prevention* devices which use compression to slow collagen growth 3. *Orthoses* and *positioning devices* which maintain joints/soft tissue in one or two functional positions.	VIII. *STRENGTH* will be increased by using: 1. *Isometric exercise* 2. *Active assistive exercise* 3. *Resistive exercise* which recruits more motor units and causes hypertrophy of fast twitch muscles.
III. *ENDURANCE TRAINING* will be initiated by using: *Increased duration* *Higher cardiac steps* *Increased intensity and* *Increased repetitions* during daily activities which gradually stress the cardiopulmonary system while ensuring proper rest.	VI. *ROM* will be increased by using: 1. *Heat* to increase elasticity of tissue 2. *Scar remodeling* via stretch pressure which separates structures and via compression to slow collagen growth 3a. *Passive stretch* or 3b. *Active stretch* beyond current the range which elongates collagen fibers 4. *Orthoses/positioning devices* which maintain gains during cool-down and between treatment sessions 5. *Orthotics* which provide prolonged static stretch in graded increments 6. *Role-related activities* which ensure that gains will be generalized.	IX. *ENDURANCE TRAINING* will be completed by using: *Increased duration,* *Increased MET levels* *Increased intensity* and *Increased repetitions* which gradually stress the cardiopulmonary system and local muscle metabolism.

However, the debilitating effects of prolonged bed rest are well documented (1). Therefore, at the doctor's discretion, bed rest is quickly replaced by procedures that enforce rest of *only* a specific body part, like not weight-bearing on a fractured leg. Eventually, procedures that gradually stress healed structures are implemented.

The therapist's role in regaining structural stability is vital. Therapists make many of the orthoses and order some of the positioning devices. The therapist is obligated to end every treatment session with the proper placement of these devices. If therapists don't use these devices consistently and properly, how can we expect other health care professionals to use them?

INITIATING ENDURANCE TRAINING

Chapter 3 explains why the assumption that endurance will be present is outdated and why this concern has become a part of early biomechanical treatment. First, you should anticipate endurance deficits whenever the following systems are impaired: (*a*) local muscle metabolism (e.g., diabetes), (*b*) cardiovascular system (e.g., congestive heart failure), and (*c*) respiratory system (e.g., emphysema). Second, the need for early endurance training is also likely in any patient who has been on total bed rest for 6 or more days (1). Third, patients who have paralysis will also have early endurance problems. These patients have fewer muscles to do the same job as

Table 4.1.
Postulates Regarding Intervention: Biomechanical Frame of Reference

Goals	Method/Rationale	Application: Examples
I. *Further structural damage* will be *prevented* by using	Orthoses, which protect a specific vulnerable body past during hospital procedures	1. Cock-up splint for hemiplegia 2. Sling for UE injury
	Positioning, which protects a specific vulnerable body part during hospital procedures	1. Spinal board 2. W/C arm trough with cone
II. *Structural Stability* will be *regained* in damaged structures by using	1a. Orthoses, which are worn temporarily to enforce rest until the damaged structures are healed	1. Dorsal rubber band splint for flexor tendon repair 2. Body jacket/body cast
	1b. Positioning, which temporarily enforces rest until damaged structures are healed	1. Stryker frame 2. Wedge for hip replacement
	2. Procedures, which temporarily enforce rest of a specific body part until the damaged structures are healed	1. Nonweightbearing for hip replacement patient 2. No resistive exercise during arthritic flare-up
	3. Procedures, which gradually stress structures that are healed	1. Stump toughening and shaping 2. LE weightbearing for fracture
III. *Endurance training* will be *initiated* by using	Increased duration, which gradually stresses cardiopulmonary system while ensuring rest	1. Sitting tolerance in minutes 2. Tolerance for evaluation
	Increased level in cardiac step program, which gradually stresses cardiopulmonary system while ensuring rest	1. Graduate to eating while sitting up in a chair 2. Stand instead of sit to shave
	Increased intensity, which gradually stress cardiopulmonary system while ensuring rest	1. Cardiac target heart rate 2. Dress in 10 fewer minutes
	Increased repetitions, which gradually stresses cardiopulmonary system while ensuring rest	1. Feed self 10 addition bites of food 2. Walk 10 additional steps

a healthy person. Their remaining overworked muscles will fatigue quickly at first.

Cardiac charts are very helpful when you are initiating low-level endurance training with an acutely ill patient. Cardiac charts break activities down into very small steps. For example, it would be unwise to have a patient comb his/her hair if he/she is exhausted just from feeding him/herself with arms supported on an over-the-bed table (2). The sensitive basement (see Appendix) of a cardiac chart helps you grade down for very low endurance. On the other hand, if a patient does most of his/her ADLs sitting down, *skip* this step in the biomechanical treatment sequence! The aerobic demands of ADLs will be sufficient to maintain low-level endurance without a therapist's intervention.

The four methods that initiate endurance training are listed in Table 4.1. These methods are not numbered because they can be used in any order. All four methods gradually stress the cardiopulmonary system while ensuring proper rest (3).

While a loss of endurance may not be life-threatening, it is still very upsetting to the patient and staff. A therapist may have only 5 minutes to mobilize a patient before the patient tires. An acutely ill patient may not even have sitting tolerance for sedentary activities. If the patient has to repeatedly lie down and rest, therapy is constantly interrupted.

REDUCING PERIPHERAL EDEMA

Sequencing

The four methods for reducing edema are not numbered because they are often used simultaneously. Therapists are very aggressive about treating edema because it is so dangerous. Table 4.2 lists a few examples of methods to treat edema.

While edema control is the fourth step in the biomechanical treatment sequence, it is not a discrete step that is pursued in isolation. Therapists often strive simultaneously to regain structural stability and reduce edema. Similarly, edema control may extend into the early stages of treatment to increase range of motion. This step can be skipped for those fortunate patients who have minimal or no edema.

Situational Thinking About Edema

Situational thinking needs to be used when choosing the various methods to reduce edema. For example, elevation is a commonly used method, but it is most practical when the patient is at rest. Devices such as arm slings can be detrimental once the patient can use the involved extremity because the sling prevents active motion. The sling not only turns the physically active patient into a "functional hemiplegic," but it prevents

Table 4.2.
Biomechanical Postulates Regarding Intervention

Goals	Method/Rationale	Application: Examples
IV. *Peripheral edema* will be *reduced* by using	Elevation, which allows gravity to remove excess accumulation of peripheral fluids	1. Arm sling 2. W/C arm trough
	Pressure, which prevents filtration of fluids from capillaries into interstitial tissues	1. Coban wrap 2. Retrograde massage
	Temperature control, which stimulates localized vascular responses	1. Icing 2. Contrast baths
	Active ROM, which pumps fluids out of interstitial and joint structures	1. Gentle active ROM 2. Active assistive ROM
V. *Passive range of motion* will be *maintained* by using	Passive ROM through the CURRENTLY AVAILABLE range, which prevents adhesions and molds collagen into orderly chains	1. PROM to ONLY 90° of shoulder flexion for patient with SCI who is still in Pope halo 2. Continuous passive motion (CPM) Machine
	Assisted active ROM through the CURRENTLY AVAILABLE range, which prevents adhesions and molds collagen into orderly chains	1. Assisted AROM of burned hand within the limits of the IV needles
	Active ROM through CURRENTLY AVAILABLE range, which prevents adhesions and molds collagen into orderly chains	1. Gentle AROM of hand for a patient in acute flare-up of arthritis
	Scar prevention devices, which use compression, which may slow collagen synthesis	1. Pressure dressings 2. Elastomer molds 3. Transparent face mask 4. Pressure garments
	Orthoses, which maintain joints and soft tissue in a single functional position	1. Foot-drop splint 2. Neck conformer splint
	Positioning, which maintains joints and soft tissue in two or three comfortable positions	1. Arthritic patient will sleep supine with as little flexion as possible

active motion, which helps pump out excess fluids. Less cumbersome elevation devices, such as wheelchair troughs and pillows, should be considered for the active patient.

Pressure is another method requiring situational thinking. For example, Coban wrap is contraindicated for patients with open skin wounds. Its ribbed contour would leave an uncosmetic imprint on grafted skin. Pressure garments are smooth but expensive and may take time to receive from the manufacturer. This makes pressure garments more practical for maintaining a reduction in edema than for reducing edema with a series of garments.

Active ROM to reduce edema also requires situational thinking. AROM can aggravate edema if the therapist or patient is too aggressive during the early stages of recovery. This method can cause an already overstressed vascular system to collapse (4).

MAINTAINING JOINT RANGE OF MOTION

Sequencing

Maintaining joint ROM is the fifth step in the biomechanical treatment sequence. Every patient doesn't need this step, so give yourself permission to skip it when it is appropriate. This step is crucial *only* for patients who experience extended periods of bed rest, like a patient in a coma, *or* for patients who have the potential for scarring due to wound healing.

If extended bed rest is required, ranging is sufficient to maintain joint ROM. There are several methods for maintaining ROM. While I have listed passive ROM first on Table 4.2, followed by active assistive ROM and active ROM, this is not a treatment progression. The method you choose depends on what your patient can do. If the patient cannot move him/herself at all, the therapist obviously has to use passive ranging. If the patient can actively move without assistance, you may choose active ranging. Or, you may need to use the intermediate technique of assisted ranging if the patient is weak.

When wound healing is present, there is a great potential for massive hypertrophic scarring. Scar growth can be rampant; almost like a cancer. Hypertrophic scarring can produce a severe loss of range of motion. Physicians used to believe that wounds were moldable only during the first 3 weeks, when the wound rapidly fills up with collagen fibers. Today, we know that collagen continues to be replaced at a high metabolic rate for up to 18 months, like water that is constantly changing behind a dam (5). Unfortunately, the collagen fibers tend to chemically bind together in bulbous tangles and adhere adjacent structures together. Stretch is needed to force new collagen fibers into orderly chains. Collagen fibers that have been stretched into orderly chains have considerably more strength than immobilized fibers, which makes them less fragile and prone to tear (5).

When even wound healing is present, scar prevention must be implemented to maintain ROM. Scar prevention is difficult to implement because it requires patient compliance for as many as 18 months. Patients may be especially noncompliant in the early stages when ROM is still normal and visible scars are not yet present. Yet, the physician may order scar prevention even before wound closure and scar formation begin because scar management is less effective once the scar tissue matures (6).

Scar prevention devices that use compression may be ordered. These devices, such as pressure garments and Elastomer molds, may decrease blood flow enough to slow collagen synthesis (6). However, they also increase the risk of ischemia and produce friction and shearing forces. The therapist must monitor the vascularity of the wound and look for breakdown of surrounding tissues and discontinue these devices when necessary (6).

Scar prevention also includes orthoses, such as a neck conformer splint, and positioning, like sleeping supine to prevent flexion contractures. These methods prolong the effects of ROM and are most effective when applied soon after ROM is done. Compression devices, orthotics, and positioning are often used simultaneously because scar prevention must be aggressive to keep up with the high metabolic rate of scar formation.

Situational Thinking About Maintaining Range

Ranging is defined as motion that goes through the *currently available range* only. Currently available range is often partial range of motion. Even if partial ROM permits small losses in range to occur, it is still better than the profound contractures that were seen following prolonged periods of enforced rest. Of course, the currently available range may already be normal, so this phrase does not preclude ranging to the end of normal limits. When in doubt, ask the physician to specify how much of the range is "currently available."

Depending on the situation, partial range may be preferred, required, and sufficient. Partial range of motion for the hand of a patient with a quadriplegic spinal cord injury is *preferred*. This promotes tightness of the finger flexor tendons, which then produces a functional light grasp by tenodesis action (7). Partial range of motion may be *required*. Range of motion for recently repaired peripheral nerves must be kept well within the

elastic limits of the nerve. Repeated overstretching of the nerve is known to cause interneural fibrosis (8). In other instances, partial range of motion may be *sufficient*. Partial excursion of recently repaired tendons may be sufficient to prevent adhesions from forming and may assist in nutrition by producing local circulation of synovial fluid (9).

Selection of active, passive, or active assistive ranging is determined by more than what the patient can do. Selection is also influenced by what is safe. Active ROM can be dangerous because some patients can't be trusted to stop soon enough. They may lack the sensation or cognition needed to comply with treatment precautions, or they may just refuse to accept the precautions. Passive range of motion eliminates these problems, but creates its own problem—fear. Using PROM with a patient who already has active motion requires that patient to tolerate a loss of control. Some therapists prefer active assistive ranging because it is a nice combination of control by the therapist and active participation by the patient.

The use of orthoses and positioning devices to maintain passive range also requires caution. First, these devices can produce skin breakdown. Second, therapists need to remember that these devices do not move body segments through the full or even currently available range. They position the patient in a single comfortable position that can be tolerated for several hours. Therefore, a variety of orthoses and positioning devices may be needed. When patients remain in one position and are not ranged daily, they can become contractured in the position dictated by the orthosis or positioning device.

INCREASING JOINT RANGE OF MOTION

Sequencing

The sixth step in the biomechanical sequence is to increase joint range of motion. The methods for increasing range are numbered to denote a treatment sequence (Table 4.3). Heat is the first method used to increase range. Even if just neutral warmth is used (body heat trapped by warm clothing), heat increases the elasticity of collagen fibers in soft tissue and makes them more amenable to stretch (10).

Traditionally, intense heat modalities such as hot packs, paraffin baths, hydrotherapy, and ultrasound have been used by physical therapists who have a physics background. Physics is especially important for understanding ultrasound waves that heat the bones first and can cause burns, which show up on the surface several hours later. Perhaps this is why a survey of 639 therapists found that ultrasound was the heat modality used least often by occupational therapists (11). Where

Table 4.3.
Biomechanical Postulates Regarding Intervention

Goals	Method/Rationale	Application: Examples
VI. *Joint range* of motion will be *increased* by using:	1. *Heat*, which increases the elasticity of collagen fibers in soft tissue	1. Neutral warmth 2. Warm water
	2. *Scar remodeling procedures*, which provide stretch pressure to separate deeper structures, and *compression*, which slows collagen synthesis	1. Deep friction massage 2. Tendon-gliding exercises See Maintain ROM for devices
	3a. *Passive stretch:* beyond current range, which elongates collagen fibers in soft tissue via Manual stretch: when stretching at end of range, when patient can't actively stretch due to pain/weakness, or when patient consistently substitutes -OR- Static stretch: when patient can tolerate prolonged stretching	1. Joint mobilization 2. Joint manipulation 3. Myofascial release 4. Distraction approach 5. Incentive approach 1. Traction weights 2. SCI hamstring stretch
	3b. *Active stretch* beyond current range against MINIMUM RESISTANCE to elongate collagen via Pure exercise when passive stretch is dangerous or frightens the patient -OR- Purposeful activity when you need to motivate/distract patient who has pain	1. Shoulder wheel 2. PNF diagonals 1. Play checkers overhead to stretch shoulder flexors
	4. *Orthoses/positioning*, which maintain gains from stretching during cool-down/between Rx	See Maintain ROM for examples
	5. *Orthotics*, which provide gradually increasing amounts of prolonged static stretch	1. Joint jacks 2. Serial casting
	6. *Role-related activities* through the increased range, which ensure that gains will be generalized to daily routines	1. Reach for videotapes on third shelf of cabinet at work at TV station

occupational therapists work in isolation, such as in home health and private practice, the interdependence between occupational and physical therapy is not available. Occupational therapists working alone may use heat modalities before they stretch their patients. Facility-based training is the most common way for OTs to learn about heat modalities (11) and may be mandatory to enable a therapist to be covered by the facility's liability insurance.

Once scars have formed, the second step to increase ROM is scar remodeling. Scar tissue needs to be made more pliable to increase the effectiveness of the stretching that immediately follows. Scar remodeling procedures that provide stretch pressure include deep friction massage and tendon-gliding exercises. These procedures help to separate deep structures like tendons, nerves, and blood vessels that are stuck together by collagen bundles. These structures need to move separately instead of moving together as one mass. Stretch pressure has to be done repeatedly to be effective. For example, deep friction massage may be done as much

as 10 times a day. Scar remodeling also includes compression devices like pressure garments. These devices must be worn around the clock, except during bathing. Scar prevention must be done relentlessly. Once scar formation becomes significant, it may have to be surgically removed or forcefully stretched by orthotics.

Stretching is the third step to increase range. **Stretching** is defined as motion that goes beyond the currently available range. Stretching beyond the currently available range should not be done without a physician's order, particularly when the patient has just had surgery or lacks structural stability! Stretching has been divided into passive stretch and active stretch (Table 4.3). They are numbered 3*a* and 3*b* to indicate that these are alternate methods rather than a sequence. The one you use depends on a variety of rationales (see discussion in the sections that follow).

Heat, scar remodeling, and stretch are effective only when stretch is maintained as the tissues cool (12). The idea behind these first three methods to increase ROM is to *prepare* the collagen fibers for elongation (6). Only prolonged but mild stretch at the end of range can produce a *permanent* lengthening of collagen fibers (6). When stretch is prolonged, the collagen fibers form new cross-links in newly elongated patterns during the long periods of metabolic turnover (6).

Therefore, the fourth step for increasing joint range is the use of orthoses and positioning devices. These devices maintain the stretch longer than a therapist can sustain manually. They lock in the gains achieved immediately after stretching and retrain the collagen fibers between therapy sessions. Every session aimed at increasing joint range should end with the application of appropriate orthoses and positioning devices.

The fifth step to increase ROM is the use of orthotics that are specifically designed to provide prolonged passive stretch in increasing amounts. Examples include serial casting and joint jacks that can be progressively tightened. Constant reevaluation is needed because these orthotics can cause skin breakdown, especially when a patient is overzealous. These types of stretching orthoses are usually prescribed only after stretching and customary orthotics have failed.

After gains in ROM are achieved, it is time to introduce the sixth and final step for increasing ROM, which is role-related activities. You cannot assume that a patient will automatically use his/her increased range in daily life. A patient may be so used to loading the dishwasher one-handed that he/she may not use the newly achieved gains in shoulder abduction. Even well-educated patients may believe that faithful compliance with home exercises will maintain their increased range despite constant disuse (13). They can truly be unaware that they are guarding the injured body part during every waking moment by keeping it immobilized. Therapists don't have the time to show a patient how increased range will affect every role-related activity, but a few trials will make the cognitively intact patient aware of his/her substitution patterns. This step may take only one treatment session, but it should not be omitted.

The inability to generalize gains in ROM to daily life is a special problem for patients with chronic pain and cognitive impairment. Patients with chronic pain are afraid to move their body during familiar activities (14). Good body mechanics must be taught to chronic pain patients using a wide variety of role-related tasks to help break the cycle of pain and fear. For the cognitively impaired patient, this last step may require family education to teach family members to prompt the patient to use the newly acquired range.

Situations for Passive Stretch

Three situations make passive stretch particularly useful (13). First, the patient may not be able to actively stretch beyond his/her current restrictions because of weakness. Remember, the patient needs considerable strength to fight against resistive soft tissue when stretching. Second, active stretching requires a conscious effort to prevent substitutions. When patients can't learn to prevent substitutions after you point them out, passive stretch is preferred. Third, if your goal is to increase motion at the end of the range, passive stretch is also preferred. Muscles become actively insufficient at the end of range (15). This decreases the strength they have to stretch the restricted tissues. Activities that require considerable dexterity can also be frustrating to the patient who is asked to work at the end of range. It may be too difficult to knot small pieces of yarn at the end of an arm's length. Passive stretch enables the therapist to prevent substitutions, to assist the patient to the end of range (where muscles are always weakest), and to fight against resistive soft tissue when the patient is weak. When these three situations arise, passive stretch is often more effective.

Once you decide to use passive stretch (2*a*), you then have to choose between manual stretch and static stretch. Manual stretch is done by the therapist. There are different types of manual stretch. *Joint mobilization* consists of passive rocking, oscillatory movements aimed at increasing joint play that is not under voluntary control. For example, you might want to rock a stiff PIP joint side to side in a very small range at a rate of 2 oscillations per second while applying traction to this joint. *Myofascial release* is designed to stretch and break up adhesions of the fascia that surround every muscle and internal organ. *Joint manipulation* is used to break up massive adhesions and is usually done under anesthesia. It is a last resort when other methods have failed. Joint mobilization, myofascial release, and joint manipulation require extensive training. Detailed instructions are absent in introductory textbooks for occupational therapists.

Manual stretch can also be done by what I call the "distraction approach" and the "incentive approach." The incentive approach is manual stretch done a few degrees past the point of discomfort with a visual or verbal goal. Some patients need the incentive of seeing their extremity move one more inch up a finger board or knowing that they have tolerated the stretch for 5 additional seconds. These concrete signs of progress can motivate patients. Yet, many patients have a negative reaction to discomfort and prefer to be distracted. Distractors include talking about something else and sneaking the stretching in between pain-free motions. The incentive and distraction approaches are psychological strategies that do not require specialized training.

Static stretch is less labor-intensive than manual stretch. Static stretch is achieved by positioning the patient so that a body part or heavy object provides the stretch, leaving the therapist free to do other things. Patients with neck and back injuries are often put in traction. Spinal cord patients can be taught to do a static hamstring stretch by leaning their trunk well forward in the bed in a long-leg sit position. Some patients prefer static stretch, but others may not be able to tolerate the duration this technique requires. Manual stretching can be graded to last a few seconds, while static stretch usually lasts for a minute or more. This really focuses the patient's attention on pain.

Situations for Active Stretch

Active stretch is particularly useful in two situations. First, it is helpful when the patient is afraid of passive stretch, which requires a patient to tolerate a loss of control. Second, active stretch is helpful when passive stretch is dangerous. For example, newly grafted skin, sutured tendons, and other vulnerable soft tissue can tear during passive stretch before the patient can warn the therapist to stop.

Once you select active stretch, you must remember that it is done against *minimal* resistance. You don't want to confuse the patient by adding outside resistance, which encourages maximal muscle contractions. You want the patient to relax—not fight you—to achieve maximal soft-tissue excursion.

Active stretch can be done using pure exercise. Examples of pure exercise include the shoulder wheel, the finger board, and proprioceptive neuromuscular facilitation (PNF) diagonals. The PNF approach has proven to be significantly superior to passive stretching in linear planes in two out of three studies (16). If this trend continues, we need to reconsider the traditional approach to stretching in anatomical planes. The disadvantage of PNF is that the patient must be able to follow three- to four-step verbal commands and perform complex multi-joint movements that may be too difficult for some patients.

Active stretch can also be done using purposeful activities. There are advantages to using a purposeful activity instead of exercise to provide active stretch. The activity may (*a*) distract the patient who has pain; (*b*) motivate the patient who values purposeful activity; and (*c*) provide diagonal movements, which are more natural than the linear movements inherent in exercise (13). Purposeful activity may also reduce psychological dependence on the therapist, which manual stretching promotes. Active stretch makes the patient responsible for change.

However, modifying purposeful activities to provide active stretch requires skill. Remember, to increase range you must keep resistance to a minimum to keep the muscles relaxed! For example, positioning an activity

overhead may increase shoulder range, but it also requires gravity-resisted strength. It might be better to place the patient in a side-lying position so that reaching above shoulder height is done in a gravity-eliminated plane. Adding springs and rubber bands that help the patient stretch during purposeful activity also requires skill. Repeated adjustments are needed to provide just the right amount of assistance as stretching increases ROM.

Situational Thinking About Stretching

Before you begin to focus on increasing joint range, you need to consider the patient's potential for return of strength. If there is no hope of motor return, you must carefully consider whether the patient can maintain the gains produced by aggressive stretching. For example, a patient with severely spastic elbow flexors may not be able to maintain full passive elbow extension. Is it worth it to painfully stretch this patient's elbow to *full* range every day? This kind of dilemma requires considerable situational thinking. There are no easy answers.

Heat modalities also require situational thinking. Heat always produces some localized edema, so it may be contraindicated for patients with edema (10). If stiffness is due to edema, you should consider using ice instead. Intense heat can also cause rebound pain in some patients (17). Too much heat can also make the patient feel limp and tired. If I want to follow the heat with a resistive activity, I might use warm tap water instead of an intense heat modality.

Stretching also requires situational thinking. Students often have a negative emotional response to stretching because it must be done in the range where the patient feels discomfort. This means stopping just short of intolerable pain, which is difficult to identify until it is too late. If a patient grimaces or says "Ow, that hurts," the student may stop short. Understretching can eventually lead to more pain and stiffness. To stretch safely when you are in the "discomfort zone," you need to move so slowly that motion is almost imperceptible.

When you use a *slow* speed for stretching, it gives you more time between the moment danger signs appear and when you stop stretching. Several nonverbal danger signs you should watch for include a sudden increase in sweat, visual signs of stretching on the skin, a gradual loss of slack, the patient suddenly looking away, and a sudden constriction of the pupils. As these signs emerge, the student should *not* ask "does it hurt?" Many patients have discomfort even before you touch them. Instead, the student should tell the patient, "Tell me when to stop." Your part of the verbal contract is to stop whenever the patient says "stop." Once the patient trusts you enough to able to relax, you can usually feel when the soft tissue runs out of slack even before he/

she says "stop." If the patient says "stop," but you don't feel any restrictions or see nonverbal signs of discomfort, you can always ask, "Can I go a little farther?" Once you establish rapport, the patient will usually let you stretch farther and farther into the range. This combination of nonverbal danger signs and verbal contracting makes it possible for the student to have confidence in his or her stretching techniques on the very first attempt.

The number of repetitions achieved also requires situational thinking. Initially, maximum stretch may be achieved only once because you are stretching so slowly. You need to remember that maximum safe excursion is more important than many repetitions if the goal is to increase ROM. When scar tissue is placed under low amounts of stretch that are administered slowly, the tissue responds by relaxing and elongating; when scar tissue is stretched quickly, the scar tissue resists the stretch and then tears (6). Slow stretching that produces small gains is more effective than aggressive overstretching (16).

Overstretching is a real possibility (16). Shortened soft tissues are at risk for injury because of a loss of tensile strength, inflammation, weakened blood vessels, and osteoporosis. Clinical signs of overstretching include pain that persists after the release of the stretch and redness and swelling that persists for several hours.

MAINTAINING MUSCLE STRENGTH

Maintenance of muscle strength is the seventh step in the biomechanical sequence, but every patient doesn't need it. Loss of strength is a problem only when a patient has his/her activity completely restricted from 6 to 10 days of bed rest (1) or a specific body part is restricted for extended periods of time.

Fortunately, maintenance is easy to implement. While still on bed rest, the patient can perform active range of motion (AROM) exercises of intact muscles to maintain at least Fair strength (Table 4.4). Even if the patient doesn't have showering or tub privileges, he/she can maintain Fair plus to Good minus strength by doing all a.m. care at bedside. For the patient who is already physically active, I recommend skipping this box.

An additional benefit of maintaining muscle strength is that it also maintains joint ROM. By definition, Fair or greater strength means active motion through the full range. Ranging to maintain full range would be redundant for joints that have Fair strength and above.

INCREASING MUSCLE STRENGTH

Sequencing

Increasing strength is the eighth step. The four methods on Table 4.4 are numbered to indicate a treatment sequence. The sequence begins with isometric exercise and ends with Progressive Resistive Exercise (PREs). The specific method you use for a particular patient depends on the patient's initial muscle grades. A detailed discussion of how to use these methods can be found in Chapter 8 of Trombly (16).

Situational Thinking About Strengthening

Precautions must be observed when implementing strengthening programs. Fatigue is believed to be a potential source for additional structural damage in the acute stages of rheumatoid arthritis, multiple sclerosis, and Guillain-Barré syndrome (18).

Strengthening programs can be designed by varying (a) the amount of resistance, (b) the type of contraction used, (c) the speed of the movement, and (d) the use of purposeful activity vs. pure exercise. Situational thinking is required to use these design factors to develop a prescriptive, individualized strengthening program.

First, strengthening programs can be graded by the amount of resistance (load) from none to "repetition maximum" (RM). **Repetition maximum** is the maximum load a muscle group can lift a given number of times before fatigue sets in (19). For example, if a person can lift a given weight eight times, that weight is an eight-RM load.

Research does not provide clear guidelines for how to choose the correct repetition maximum. Significant gains in strength have been made with repetition maximums of two to 10, done in sets of two to six (19). By convention, three sets of 10 repetitions with 2- to 4-minute rest periods between each set have been used. Longer sets and rest periods may take up too much therapy time.

Whether you use two-RM sets or 10-RM sets, the ultimate goal of a strengthening program is to approach failure-to-lift. Approaching failure-to-lift ensures that all the motor units in a muscle are strengthened. As fatigue sets in, motor units that initially rested are recruited and have the opportunity to hypertrophy (16). Patients need to understand that approaching failure-to-lift is a sign of success, not "failure."

Clinical signs that the patient is approaching failure-to-lift include *mild* shaking of the extremity, difficulty completing the full movement, grimacing, grunting, and sweating. If these signs become pronounced, the patient may be recruiting adjacent muscles groups because the load is too great for the weak muscles that have been targeted. Substituting with muscles that are already strong defeat the purpose of a strengthening program. Of course, as a particular amount of resistance becomes too easy, the therapist increases the load to make the clinical signs reappear.

Table 4.4.
Biomechanical Postulates Regarding Intervention

Goals	Method/Rationale	Application: Examples
VII. *STRENGTH* will be *MAINTAINED* by using	*Active range of motion* by currently intact muscles and joints, which prevents disuse atrophy and stiffness during periods of enforced rest	1. AROM in anatomical planes
	ADLs, which maintain the strength of the patient who is already physically active	1. a.m. care activities 2. Wheelchair propulsion
VIII. *STRENGTH* will be *INCREASED* in a trace muscle using	1. *Isometric exercise* against no resistance, which recruits more motor units and increases proprioceptive awareness of individual muscles as they contract	1. Electric stimulation 2. Biofeedback machine 3. Vibrators 4. Manual contacts
in a Poor minus or Fair minus muscle by using	2. *Active assistive exercise* with assistance to complete the motion, which recruits more motor units and causes hypertrophy of glycolytic fast-twitch muscle fibers	1. Therapeutic skate 2. Deltoid aide 3. Mobile arm support 4. Manual assistance
in a Poor or Fair muscle by using	3. Active exercise through full ROM but against minimal resistance, which recruits more motor units and causes hypertrophy of glycolytic fast-twitch muscle fibers	1. Shoulder wheel 2. Combining short hair 3. Electric typewriter 4. Clothespin races
in a Poor plus, Fair plus, or Good minus and above muscle by using	4. *Progressive or regressive resistive exercise* against the maximum resistance needed to produce failure-to-lift, which recruits more motor units and causes hypertrophy of glycolytic fast-twitch muscle fibers	1. Weight well 2. Theraplast/dental dam 3. Theraputty 4. Weighted weaving 5. Overhead rug knotting

Second, strengthening programs require situational thinking to choose the appropriate type of muscle contraction. Muscle contractions are divided into isometric, concentric (shortening), and eccentric (lengthening) types. Strengthening programs tend to be either isometric or concentric/eccentric. This dichotomy creates a problem with carryover. Concentric exercises increase concentric and eccentric strength (19–21), but do not increase isometric strength (19, 22–25). Eccentric exercises increase only eccentric strength (21, 26). No one type of muscle contraction has a general strengthening effect.

If the exercise program does not match the patient's occupational demands, the program may not produce functional gains. If a secretary needs to perform isometric contractions to stabilize the shoulder girdle and concentric contractions to move the fingers to type, then the strengthening program should reflect these needs. Exercise protocols can't anticipate every patient's needs. Ultimately, the therapist must use situational thinking to ensure a good match between the type of muscle contraction used in treatment and the patient's occupational demands.

Three sources of movement determine what type of contraction is demanded in a therapeutic activity. **Gravitational moment** is the movement that gravity will produce if acting alone by pulling on the body (15). Gravity will produce this movement suddenly and completely,

whether or not a full or sudden motion is desired. The **desired motion** is the movement that the person needs to successfully perform the activity, like partially flexing the knees to walk down stairs. **Objects**, like a hammer in the hand, can increase the gravitational pull on the body. An object can also block the desired movement when it interacts with the environment. For example, a nail can provide resistance by means of friction when the hammer pulls the nail out of the wood.

Three rules will help you determine what type of contraction these three sources of movement acting together will produce in a therapeutic activity (15):

Rule #1. When the gravitational moment and what the object wants are the same as the desired motion, the contraction is eccentric;

Rule #2. When either the gravitational moment or what the object wants is different from the desired motion, the contraction is concentric; and

Rule #3. When no visible movement occurs, but the muscle shortens, the contraction is isometric.

Once you have identified the type of contraction being used, you must identify the muscle group that is producing the motion. Remember, anatomists named the muscles for the movements they produce during a concentric contraction. However, many normal movements are the result of eccentric contractions. You must be able to visualize which muscle group is getting long or short to correctly identify the muscle group being used. Two examples of activity analysis for type of contraction are presented in Figure 4.1.

If the therapist incorrectly identifies the type of contraction or the muscle group used, he/she may design activities to further strengthen the strong muscles that are already overpowering the weak muscles. An inappropriate strengthening program can actually make the muscle imbalance worse.

Speed is the third design factor that requires situational thinking for a strengthening program. Fast *eccentric* contractions produce more torque than slow *eccentric* contractions (15). However, fast eccentric contractions produce ballistic motions, like rapidly slamming a glass down on a table-top. Fast eccentric contractions may be appropriate for athletes, but not for burn patients with newly grafted skin, or for arthritic patients with weak collateral ligaments, and so on. Slow eccentric contractions are safer.

We also know that slow *concentric* contractions produce more torque than fast *concentric* contractions (15). Kinesiologists believe that shortening the muscle at low speed provides enough time for all of the available cross-bridges to form. Ironically, patients frequently prefer fast concentric contractions because speed recruits assistive muscles. If we want a patient to develop maximum tension in the weak muscles and cut down on substitution by adjacent muscle groups, we need to ask for *slow* concentric contractions.

ELBOW MOVEMENT WHILE SETTING A GLASS DOWN ON THE TABLE:

| | = What glass wants is <u>extension</u> |
| Desired motion is <u>extension</u> | = Gravitational moment <u>extension</u> |

Therefore, the contraction must be <u>eccentric</u> of <u>elbow flexors</u> (muscle group that is getting long as the elbow extends). Gravity will break the glass on the table-top with sudden and complete motion, unless the elbow flexors slow down the motion.

ANKLE MOTION WHILE DEPRESSING ACCELERATOR PEDAL OF A CAR:

| | ≠ What pedal wants is <u>no movement</u> |
| Desired motion <u>plantar flexion</u> | = Gravita. moment <u>plantar flex.</u> |

Therefore, contraction must be <u>concentric</u> of <u>plantar flexors</u>. Here the object resists rather than helping the movement.

Figure 4.1.

The use of purposeful activity vs. pure exercise is the fourth factor that requires situational thinking for a strengthening program. Pure exercise provides no cognitive or emotional challenge (13). This enables patients to watch their body parts and to think about the movements they are performing without distractions. Pure exercise is most practical at the two extremes of the strength continuum (13). If a patient has a Trace muscle, you have no choice. A Trace muscle cannot produce a visible joint motion or take any resistance from objects. You must use isometric exercises. Pure exercise is also more practical when above-average strength is needed. A spinal cord patient can perform more functional tasks if he/she has above-average upper extremity strength to compensate for lower extremity paralysis. Above-average strength is achieved by using excessive weight. Yet, excessive weight can significantly interfere with smooth, coordinated movements. Knitting with a 30-lb weight on each forearm would be a chore.

Purposeful activities to strengthen muscles become practical once the patient has Poor to Fair range strength (13). To offset the resistance offered by objects, therapists can:

1. Use gravity-eliminated motions for Poor range muscles;
2. Provide manual assistance; and
3. Use orthoses.

First, gravity-eliminated motions can be incorporated into purposeful activity by using activities that require movements that are parallel to the floor. For example, a patient with Poor shoulder strength might be able to move small tiles horizontally to place them on a tile trivet. Second, it is easy for the therapist to provide manual assistance. The therapist's proprioceptive system enables the therapist to constantly monitor how much assistance is needed to complete a motion. Third, assistance can be provided by a variety of orthoses such as Deltoid aids and skateboards (27).

Purposeful activities are especially practical to strengthen muscles in the Good range. Strength is ultimately needed for natural movements that require coordinated use of several muscle groups to produce arrhythmical, asymmetrical, diagonal movements (13). Pure exercise tends to isolate specific movements and is usually performed in rhythmical, symmetrical, linear patterns (13). Picture how you would repeatedly lift a free weight while flexing your elbow. While it is possible to have a patient use a free weight to perform complex, arrhythmical motions in nonsense sequences, why not use a purposeful activity that shows the patient how to move? Since research has shown that cross-training between different types of exercise programs may be poor, why not strengthen with activities that are identical to the ones that will be used at home or at work? Purposeful activity also tells the therapist how much resistance is enough—whatever it takes to successfully complete the activity.

COMPLETING ENDURANCE TRAINING

Sequencing

You need to know that the complete separation of strength and endurance training is not valid. Some gains in endurance from strengthening programs have been proven (19). Yet, highly resistive strengthening programs don't seem to completely remediate the skill we call "endurance." Endurance requires the efficient use of energy that strengthening ignores. Without good endurance, gains in strength are not functional!

There are four methods for increasing the ability to sustain effort (Table 4.5). All four methods gradually stress the cardiopulmonary system and local muscle metabolism of oxidative slow-twitch muscle fibers (28). These methods are not a treatment sequence. Choose the method that is most practical for the type of activity you are using.

Situational Thinking About Endurance

While endurance training requires low resistance with high repetitions, there is little agreement about what low resistance means. Kottke (29) suggested that 15 to 40% of repetition maximum is appropriate for endurance training. Trombly (16) suggested that less than 50% of maximum intensity be used. However, some jobs may require more than 50% of maximum strength. The therapist should not ask what the work-hardening equipment can provide, but what the patient's roles and interests require! Situational thinking must be used to identify the amount of resistance that is appropriate for endurance training for a particular patient.

The use of pure exercise vs. purposeful activity to increase endurance also requires situational thinking. Steinbeck (30) reported that a significantly greater number of repetitions were done during a purposeful activity than during an exercise. Some patients find that doing the same exercise over and over is boring. Endurance cannot be improved without patient commitment to sustain effort. The patient should choose a meaningful activity that inherently requires repetition or duration. Playing wheelchair basketball to increase endurance may facilitate more compliance than doing wheelchair laps up and down the hospital corridors. Conversely, a patient may be more motivated to persevere if he/she keeps track of the number of "reps" or minutes of exercise. The therapist needs to assess which type of activity creates the most incentive for each particular case.

Occupational therapists are in a unique position to assess and remediate endurance because of their activity orientation. Many purposeful activities have inherent endurance requirements. For example, a patient can have normal strength to walk 20 feet, but still have to sit down in the middle of cooking a meal. The absence of cooked food at the end of the cooking session is a concrete reminder that walking endurance is still inade-

---

Table 4.5.
Biomechanical Postulates Regarding Intervention

Goals	Method/Rationale	Application: Examples
IX. *ENDURANCE TRAINING* will be *COMPLETED* by using	*Increasing the MET levels* of daily activities, which gradually stress the cardiopulmonary system and local muscle metabolism of oxidative slow-twitch muscle fibers	1. Use MET charts as an initial guide for grading and sequencing activities
	Increasing intensity during monitored activities against less than maximal resistance, which gradually stress the cardiopulmonary system and local muscle metabolism of oxidative slow-twitch muscle fibers	1. Perform activity at 70% of maximum heart rate 2. Eat breakfast 10 minutes faster than baseline
	Increasing the number of repetitions during monitored activities against less than maximal resistance, which gradually stress the cardiopulmonary system and local muscle metabolism of oxidative slow-twitch muscle fibers	1. Gradually increase number of spoonfuls of food per meal 2. Increase number of wheelchair push-ups
	Increasing duration during monitored activities against less than maximal resistance, which gradually stress the cardiopulmonary system and local muscle metabolism of oxidative slow-twitch fibers	1. Increase time doing an activity in standing table 2. Increase time during day that patient walks

Deficit/Cause/Goal/FO	Method/Rationale	Specific Modality: Name, Description, Precautions
Deficit: loss of strength in wrist is due to *Stage specific cause:* disuse atrophy, pain, and stiffness secondary to sub-acute rheumatoid *Short-term Goal:* increase wrist extensors from F+ to G− *Functional outcome:* ability to prepare flower arrangements at florist's shop	*Heat* which will decrease pain and stiffness	*Warm water bath:* submerge hands and wrists in bowl of warm water for 5 minutes. Gently move hands around in the water.
	Resistive exercise which will recruit more motor units and cause hypertrophy of glycolytic fast twitch muscle fibers	*Velcro checkers:* Place arm in trough of mobile arm support in full pronation. Have patient pick up velcro checker from board using wrist extension and three jaw chuck. Patient is allowed to remove arm from trough to place checker on board. The board is placed medially to hand to inhibit ulnar drift. Patient will switch hands after moving each piece.

Figure 4.2. Biomechanical Postulate Regarding Intervention

quate. However, not all purposeful activities lend themselves to endurance training. For example, self-care activities often require few or no repetitions. How many times can you ask patients to tie their shoes without making them wonder if they are being punished for doing it badly? That is why occupational therapists frequently switch to hobbies, games, and crafts to get the repetitions that are needed to increase endurance.

Endurance is defined as the ability to sustain effort (19) and to recover quickly (31). Nevertheless, all four methods for increasing endurance focus only on sustaining effort. Scientific guidelines for how much rest should be provided are not available. There are vague references to "fatigue being the enemy" (19). By tradition, rest periods of 2 to 4 minutes between sets of exercise are used. Cardiac surgeons may recommend a return to the resting heart rate 5 minutes after the activity ceases. Yet, controlled studies of "quick recovery" in medically ill patients with a wide variety of diagnoses have not been done. Recovery is a complicated problem because fatigue is not a single entity. Fatigue can be the result of synaptic fatigue, depletion of glycogen, build-up of lactic acid, shunting of blood to the skin to control body temperature, electrolyte imbalance, increased blood viscosity due to dehydration, and blood flow constricted by prolonged muscle action (28). Situational considerations about the speed of recovery need to be investigated.

EXAMPLE OF A BIOMECHANICAL POSTULATE REGARDING INTERVENTION

See Figure 4.2 for a specific example of a biomechanical postulate regarding intervention. The deficit can be general because the short-term goal will be specific and measurable. Deciding on the general method before selecting a specific treatment modality is not an academic nicety. The general method enables you to narrow down the wide range of activities. For example, the goal in Figure 4.2 is to increase strength from Fair plus to Good minus. Active assistive exercise would not provide enough resistance to achieve this goal. Yet, maximal resistance would overwhelm the Fair plus muscle group. This eliminates two categories of exercise before you begin. Knowing that light resistive exercise is needed helps us picture what type of specific activities would strengthen this particular patient.

SUMMARY

Even this lengthy discussion of the biomechanical postulates regarding intervention leaves many questions unanswered. For example, more research is needed to validate accepted biomechanical methods such as the use of three sets of ten to strengthen. In addition, many situations that require situational thinking were not discussed. Use Memory Aid 4.1 to stimulate your thinking with the biomechanical case simulation.

STUDY QUESTIONS
1. Who does the situational thinking about structural stability?
2. Why are cardiac step charts more appropriate than MET charts when endurance training is initiated?
3. What is the difference between ranging and stretching?
4. Passive stretch can be applied by what three agents?
5. When would you use passive vs. active assistive ranging?
6. What strategies enable you to perform stretching safely?
7. What conditions make the use of active stretch difficult?
8. Which speed of movement would you use for strengthening?
9. When is pure exercise most helpful for increasing strength?
10. Why can't you let work-hardening equipment determine endurance goals?

References

1. Affleck AT, et al. Providing occupational therapy in an intensive care unit. Am J Occup Ther 1986;40:323.
2. Trombly CA. Cardiopulmonary rehabilitation. In: Trombly CA, ed. Occupational therapy for physical dysfunction. 3rd ed. Baltimore: Williams & Wilkins, 1989:595.
3. Foderaro D, O'Leary S. Cardiac dysfunction. In: Pedretti LW, Zoltan B, eds. Occupational therapy practice skills for physical dysfunction. 3rd ed. St. Louis: CV Mosby, 1990:595.
4. Bruening L. Reflex sympathetic dystrophy. Paper presented at the Surgery and Rehabilitation of the Hand Annual Symposium, Philadelphia, 1987.
5. Madden JW. Wounds and Wound Healing. Paper presented at the Surgery and Rehabilitation of the Hand Annual Symposium, Philadelphia, 1987.
6. Stanley BG, Tribuzi SM. Concepts in hand rehabilitation. Philadelphia: FA Davis, 1992.
7. Wilson DJ, et al. Spinal cord injuries: a treatment guide for occupational therapists. rev ed. Thorofare, NJ: Slack, Inc, 1984.
8. Schultz RJ. Management of nerve gaps. In: Omer GE, Spinner M, eds. Management of peripheral nerve problems. Philadelphia: WB Saunders, 1980.
9. Salter R. Textbook of disorders and injuries of the musculoskeletal system. 2nd ed. Baltimore: Williams & Wilkins, 1983: 5.
10. Santiestaban AJ. Physical agents and musculoskeletal pain. In: Gould JA, Davies GJ, eds. Orthopedic and sports physical therapy. St. Louis: CV Mosby, 1985:199.
11. Taylor E, Humphrey R. Survey of physical agent modality use. Am J Occup Ther 1991;45:924.
12. Sapega A, et al. Biophysical factors in range of motion exercise. Physicians and Sports Medicine 1982;9:57.
13. Dutton RE. Guidelines for using both activity and exercise. Am J Occup Ther 1989;43:576.
14. Mayer TG, Gatchel RJ. Functional restoration for spinal disorders: the sports medicine approach. Philadelphia: Lea & Febiger, 1988.
15. Norkin CC, Levangie PK. Joint structure and function. Philadelphia: FA Davis, 1989.
16. Trombly CA. Treatment. In: Trombly CA, ed. Occupational therapy for physical dysfunction. 3rd ed. Baltimore: Williams & Wilkins, 1989:287.
17. Trombly CA. Arthritis. In: Trombly CA, ed. Occupational therapy for physical dysfunction. 3rd ed. Baltimore: Williams & Wilkins, 1989:543.
18. Spencer EA. Functional restoration: neurologic, orthopedic, and arthritic conditions. In: Hopkins HL, Smith HD, eds. Willard and Spackman's occupational therapy. 7th ed. Philadelphia: JB Lippincott, 1988:503.
19. Fox EL. Sports physiology. 2nd ed. New York: Saunders College Publishing, 1984.
20. Komi PV, Buskirk ER. Effect of eccentric and concentric muscle conditioning on tension and electrical activity in human muscle. Ergonomics 1972;15:417.
21. Petersen S, et al. Influence of concentric resistance training on concentric and eccentric strength. Arch Phys Med Rehabil 1990;71:101.
22. Duncan W, et al. Mode and speed specificity of eccentric and concentric exercise training. JOSPT 1989;11:70.
23. Kraemer WJ, Fleck SJ, Deschenes M. A review: factors in exercise prescription of resistance training. NSCA J 1988;10:36.
24. Lindl H. Increase of muscle strength of isometric quadriceps exercises at different knee angles. Scand J Rehabil Med 1979;11:33.
25. Kanehisa H, Miyashita M. Effect of isometric and isokinetic muscle training on static strength and dynamic power. Eur J Appl Physiol 1983;50:365.
26. Friden J, et al. Adaptive response in human skeletal muscle subjected to prolonged eccentric training. Int J Sports Med 1983;4:177.
27. Trombly CA. Orthoses: purposes and types. In: Trombly CA, ed. Occupational therapy for physical dysfunction. 3rd ed. Baltimore: Williams & Wilkins, 1989:329.
28. Kirkendall DT. Mobility: conditioning programs. In: Gould JA, Davies GJ, eds. Orthopedic and sports physical therapy. St. Louis: CV Mosby, 1985:242.
29. Kottke FJ. Therapeutic exercise. In: Krusen FH, Kottke FJ, Ellwood PM. Handbook of physical medicine and rehabilitation. 2nd ed. Philadelphia: WB Saunders, 1971.
30. Steinbeck TM. Purposeful activity and performance. Am J Occup Ther 1986;40:529.
31. Perinchief J. Work hardening. Lecture presented at Temple University School of Occupational Therapy, Philadelphia, 1988.

CHAPTER / 5

Biomechanical Case Simulation

CREATING NARRATIVE HYPOTHESES AND AN EVALUATION PLAN

Harley is a 29-year-old white male automechanic who has a L3 complete spinal cord injury due to an automobile accident 10 days ago. He had a laminectomy with posterior fusion. He is wearing a left hip spica cast that extends from just below his armpits to just above his right hip and left knee. He also suffered a left clavicular fracture and a fracture of the fourth digit of his right hand. He did not lose consciousness. He still has a nasogastric (NG) tube, but food supplements have been started. He has a Foley catheter and is on a bowel training program. The staff have begun to explain skin inspection and are turning him every 2 hours in bed and letting him sit in a wheelchair for only 1 hour. He is divorced and lives alone in a third-floor apartment with no elevator.

Student's Narrative Hypotheses

Use this space to write your narrative hypotheses. Restrict yourself to ±7 hypotheses by chunking related concerns. Read an entry-level chapter on spinal cord injury before you start. Use Memory Aid 2.2 to guide you.

Suggested Narrative Hypotheses

Based on the diagnosis and date of onset, I would expect:

1. Structural instability and pain of newly fused lumbar spine and fractured left clavicle and right finger
2. Disuse atrophy of his fractured left arm and right hand, but Normal strength of his right arm and left hand
3. At L3, weakness of "key" muscles, which are partially enervated
4. Below L3, complete loss of sensation and "key" muscles, which are totally de-enervated
5. Loss of endurance
6. Dependence in lower extremity ADLs, bed mobility, and transfers
7. Potential homeostatic deficits such as bladder infections, bowel incontinence, decubiti, and insufficient protein ingestion
8. Psychosocial issues such as stress reactions
9. Concern about his social and financial resources to overcome living alone in a third floor apartment

Student's Evaluation Plan

Use this space to design an evaluation package. Identifying the domains of concern you would test. Name the test you would use, and justify why you would choose these tests. Remember, in-depth testing is not indicated all the time.

Concern	Name of Tests	How the Data Will Be Used

Suggested Evaluation Plan

Based on the narrative hypotheses, I recommend initial evaluation of:

Concern	Name of Tests	What/How the Data Will be Used For
Structural instability and pain	Physician evaluates structural instability; patient report of pain	Must implement precautions for UE fractures and excessive trunk motions
Weak LUE & R hand	Eyeball AROM of shoulder *with no* resistance; clinical observation of R grasp during ADLs	Precautions for clavicular and fourth finger fracture preclude resistance but you need a baseline to guide ADL training
Normal RUE & L hand	Screen strength for RUE; Grip strength L hand	Quickly rule out disuse atrophy of intact RUE and left hand
Weak "key" muscles at L3 level	Eyeball AROM of hip flexion/abduction of RLE and extension of both knees	P.T. will do complete LE MMT when body cast no longer blocks left LLE; need baseline to plan compensation for LE movements during ADLs
Sensory-motor loss below L3	Complete sensory eval; watch for hip abduction knee flexion/ ankles motions during ADLs	Any sensation spared below the level of the lesion increases probability for additional motor return
Endurance	ADL's on cardiac step chart; check vital signs	Will homeostatic concerns, disuse, and fractures impede endurance during early treatment sessions?

Homeostatic issues addressed by looking at chart & talking to nurses

ADLs	Transfers NOT TESTED!	Clearance for UE weightbearing needed from physician; Fracture of clavicle and UE weakness will impair ability to push up
	Screen UE and LE ADLs in bed; evaluate bed mobility	Rule out unnecessary dependence; need to maintain UE conditioning without overstressing patient
Psychosocial Issues	C.O.T.E. and clinical observation	I don't want to upset the patient with an in-depth interview until I get to know him better
Environment	Talk to social worker	Same as psychosocial issues

EVALUATION RESULTS

Active ROM for BUEs is "within functional limits" except for his left shoulder, which is limited to 140° of flexion, 150° of abduction, and 20° of horizontal adduction. LUE strength: shoulder is Fair; distal segments are Normal. RUE strength: shoulder is Good; elbow and wrist are Normal. His dominant right hand is black and blue, especially the fourth digit. See the MMT form for LE test results (Fig. 5.1). Sitting balance was not tested.

Sensation was not tested between T2 and L2 on the left and between T2 and T12 on the right because of the body cast. Light touch and sharp/dull are intact at L3, impaired at L4–L5, and absent at S1–S2 (S1–S2 include soles and lateral sides

CLINICAL RECORD—MANUAL MUSCLE EVALUATION

Name _____ *Hanley* _____

Age _____

Diagnosis _____ L3 complete SCI _____

LEFT							RIGHT
		Examiner's Initials					
		Date					
		ACTION	PRIME MOVERS	INNERVATION	SP. C. LEVEL		
	N E C K					N E C K	
		Flexion	STERNOCLEIDOMASTOID	Spinal Accessory.	C 2-3		
		Extension	EXTENSOR GROUP	Spinal Accessory.	C 1-8		
NOT Tested	T R U N K	Flexion	RECTUS ABDOMINIS		T 5-12	T R U N K	Not tested
		Rotation	EXTERNAL OBLIQUE		T 5-12		
			INTERNAL OBLIQUE		T 5-12		
		Extension	Thoracic	Post. Rami Spinal Nerves			
			Lumbar				
		Pelvic Elevation	QUADRATUS LUMBORUM		T 12 L 1-3		
Not Tested	H I P	Flexion	ILIOPSOAS	Femoral	L 2-4	H I P	Fair –
			SARTORIUS	Femoral	L 2-4		
		Extension	GLUTEUS MAXIMUS	Inf. Gluteal	L 5 S 1-2		
		Abduction	GLUTEUS MEDIUS	Superior Gluteal	L 4-5 S 1		
			TENSOR FASCIA LATAE	Superior Gluteal	L 4-5 S 1		Not Tested
		Adduction		Obturator	L 2-4		
		External Rotation			L 3 S 3		
		Internal Rotation			L 4 S 1		
	K N E E	Flexion	BICEPS FEMORIS	Sciatic	L 5 S 1-2	K N E E	
			SEMITENDINOSUS SEMIMEMBRANOSUS	Tibial	L 5 S 1-3		
		Extension	QUADRICEPS	Femoral	L 2-4		Fair –
	A N K L E	Inversion	ANTERIOR TIBIALIS	Deep Peroneal	L 5 S 1-2	A N K L E	
			POSTERIOR TIBIALIS	Tibial	L 4-5 S 1-2		
		Eversion	PERONEUS LONGUS	Sup. Peroneal	L 4-5 S 1		
			PERONEUS BREVIS	Sup. Peroneal	L 4-5 S 1		
		Plantar Flexion	GASTROCNEMIUS	Tibial	S 1-2		
			SOLEUS	Tibial	S 1-2		
	T O E S	Flexion	DIGITORUM LONGUS	Tibial	L 5 S 1-2	T O E S	
			DIGITORUM BREVIS	Tibial	L 5 S 1-2		
		Extension	DIGITORUM LONGUS & BREVIS	Deep Peroneal	L 4-5 S 1		
	H A L L U X	Flexion	HALLUCIS LONGUS	Tibial	L 5 S 1-2	H A L L U X	
			HALLUCIS BREVIS	Tibial	L 5 S 1-2		
		Extension	HALLUCIS LONGUS	Deep Peroneal	L 4-5 S 1-2		

KEY:
5	N	NORMAL	Complete range of motion against gravity with full resistance
4	G	GOOD	Complete range of motion against gravity with some resistance
3	F	FAIR	Complete range of motion against gravity
2	P	POOR	Complete range of motion with gravity eliminated
1	T	TRACE	Evidence of slight contractility. No joint motion
0	0	ZERO	No evidence of contractility

Figure 5.1.

A. ENGAGEMENT
  0 -Needs no encouragement to begin task
  ①-Encourage once to begin activity
  2 -Encourage two or three times to engage in activity
  3 -Engages in activity only after much encouragement
  4 -Does not engage in activity

B. CONCENTRATION
  ⓪-No difficulty concentrating during full session
  1 -Off task less than one-fourth time
  2 -Off task half the time
  3 -Off task three-fourths time
  4 -Loses concentration in less than 1 minute

C. RESPONSIBILITY
  ⓪-Takes responsibility for own actions
  1 -Denies responsibility for 1 or 2 actions
  2 -Denies responsibility for several actions
  3 -Denies responsibility for most actions
  4 -Denial of responsibility; messes up project and
     blames therapist or others

D. FOLLOW DIRECTIONS
  ⓪-Carries out directions without problems
  1 -Occasional trouble with more than three-step
     directions
  2 -Carries out simple directions; has trouble with two-
     step directions
  3--Can carry out only very simple one-step directions
     (demonstrated, written, or oral)
  4 -Unable to carry out any directions

E. ACTIVITY NEATNESS
  ⓪-Activity done neatly
  1 -Occasionally ignores fine detail
  2 -Often ignores fine detail; materials are scattered
  3 -Ignores fine detail; work habits disturbing to those
     around
  4 -Unaware of fine detail; so sloppy that therapist has
     to intervene

F. PROBLEM SOLVING
  0 -Solves problems without assistance
  ①-Solves problems after assistance given once
  2 -Can solve only after repeated instructions
  3 -Recognizes a problem but cannot solve it
  4 -Unable to recognize or solve a problem

G. SOCIABILITY
  0 -Socializes with staff and patients
  ①-Socializes with staff and occasionally with other
     patients or vice-versa
  2 -Socializes only with staff or with patients
  3 -Socializes only if approached
  4 -Does not join others in activities

H. COMPLEXITY AND ORGANIZATION OF TASK
  ⓪-Organizes and performs all tasks given
  1 -Occasional trouble organizing complex tasks he
     should be able to do
  2 -Organizes simple but not complex tasks
  3 -Can do only very simple activities with
     organization imposed by therapist
  4 -Unable to organize or carry out task when
     materials/directions available

I. INITIAL LEARNING
  ⓪-Learns new activity quickly and easily
  1 -Occasionally has difficulty learning a complex
     activity
  2 -Frequent difficulty learning complex activity but can
     learn simple one
  3 -Unable to learn complex activities; occasional
     difficulty learning
  4 -Unable to learn an new activity

K. INTEREST IN ACCOMPLISHMENT
  ⓪-Interested in finishing activities
  1 -Occasional lack of interest or pleasure in finishing a
     long-term activity
  2 -Interest or pleasure in accomplishment of short-term
     activity; lack of interest in a long-term activity
  3 -Only occasional interest in finishing
  4 -No interest or pleasure in finishing

L. DECISION MAKING
  0 -Makes own decisions
  1 -Makes decisions but occasionally seeks therapist
     approval
  ②-Makes decisions but often seeks therapist approval
  3 -Makes decision when given two choices
  4 -Refuses to or cannot make any decisions

M. FRUSTRATION TOLERANCE
  0 -Handles all tasks without becoming overly
     frustrated
  ①-Occasionally becomes frustrated with complex
     tasks; can handle simple ones
  2 -Often becomes frustrated with complex tasks; can
     handle simple ones
  3 -Often becomes frustrated with any task but
     attempts to continue
  4 -Becomes so frustrated with simple tasks that
     refuses or is unable to function

N. EXPRESSION
  ⓪-Expression consistent with situation and setting
  1 -Occasionally inappropriate
  2 -Inapropriate several times during session
  3 -Expression inconsistent with situation
  4 -Extremes of expression: bizarre, uncontrolled or no
     expression

Figure 5.2. Excerpts from (Comprehensive Occupational Therapy Evaluation): HARLEY

of the feet, buttock, and back of thighs and calves). Proprioception is intact at the knees (L3), impaired at the ankles (L4–L5), and absent at the toes (L5–S1).

Resting heart rate is 84 and resting blood pressure is 130/90. During Triflow exercises he can raise two out of three balls 10 times. He has a functional cough.

He is independent in eating and needs only set up assistance for grooming and minimal assistance for upper extremity (UE) bathing. UE dressing was not evaluated because he can't wear a shirt over the body cast. He needs maximum physical assistance and a long-handled bath sponge and reacher to bathe and dress both legs. He is dependent with shoes and socks and transfers. Transfers were not evaluated; he still experiences clavicular pain during bed push-ups. He sits in a wheelchair with his left leg supported in an elevated position and his buttocks forward in the chair so his trunk can lean back to accommodate the body cast.

He is alert and oriented times three. He follows multiple step verbal instructions. Verbal and written communication skills are intact. Safety awareness "appears good." He is pleasant, cooperative, and hopeful about his future functional ability. He enjoys traveling and drove a car before his accident. See excerpts from the C.O.T.E. for additional information (Fig. 5.2).

INTERPRETING THE TEST RESULTS

Use two pages to list each hypothesis, *but* leave a generous space under each hypothesis to list the evaluation results that you believe are relevant to each hypothesis. In front of each cue, write one of the following symbols. A plus means a cue confirms and a minus means a cue disconfirms a hypothesis. A ± means a cue partially confirms and partially disconfirms a hypothesis. A question mark means the cue's relevance is unclear. Remember, these symbols are feedback to you about the accuracy of your hypotheses! They do not indicate the patient's assets and deficits! At the bottom of each list, conclude that each hypothesis was confirmed as written, *OR* write a revised hypothesis. Cues that are completely unrelated to your hypotheses should be preceded by a capital N for New and added to the end of the list.

Student's Cue Interpretation List

1.

The Student Writes a Problem List

The cue interpretation list and hypothesis evaluation represents an inner dialogue that is too lengthy to put in a medical chart. A facility will want you to write a Problem List that consists of general deficits and dysfunction. On the next page, convert your confirmed hypotheses in to a Problem List. By definition, a Problem List does not include assets and function, so delete them. Feel free to change the numbers and descriptions from the ones used in your hypotheses. Remember, working memory is limited to ± 7 pieces of information, so eliminate unconfirmed hypotheses and chunk related problems. Don't forget to add new problems not anticipated by your hypotheses!

1.

2.

3.

4.

5.

6.

7.

8.

Suggested Cue Interpretation List

1. *Structural instability and pain of spine, clavicle, and finger*
   - \+   Spinal cord injury and laminectomy 10 days ago
   - \+   Wearing left hip spica cast from armpits to right hip and left knee
   - \+   Experiences clavicular pain during bed push-ups
   - \+   Dominant right hand is black and blue, especially the fourth finger

   Confirmed as written

2. *Disuse atrophy of Fx'ed L arm/R hand, but Normal strength of R arm/L hand*
   - \+   L shoulder has Fair strength
   - ±   R shoulder has Good strength
   - \+   Limited AROM of L shoulder
   - \+   R elbow/wrist have Normal strength
   - ?   R pinch strength during self-care not recorded
   - \+   LUE hand has Normal strength
   - ±   No to minimum assistance for UE bathing, grooming, eating, and writing

   Confirmed as written

3. *At L3, weak "key" muscles for hip flexion/adduct/& knee extension*
   - \+   R hip flexors are Fair minus
   - ?   R hip adductors not tested
   - \+   R knee extensors are Fair minus

   Confirmed as written

4. *Below L3, total loss of sensation/AROM*

    −   Light touch & sharp/dull are impaired at L4–L5

    +   Light touch & sharp/dull absent at S1

    −   Proprioception impaired at ankles, which is L4–L5

    +   Proprioception absent at toes, which is L5–S1

    ?   Hip extension/abduction/knee flexion/ankle motions not reported

Revision: Impaired sensation to L4–L5, but AROM below L3 not known

5. *Loss of endurance*

    +   Elevated HR and BP at rest

    +   Triflow: only 2 out of 3 balls lifted

    +   Level of self-care rated at Level 2 of 14 on cardiac step chart

Confirmed as written

6. *Dependence in LE ADLs, bed mobility, & transfers*

    ±   Max assist plus long-handled devices for LE ADLs

    +   Dependent with socks/shoes

    +   Clavicular pain impeded bed push-ups; Transfers too dangerous to test

Revision: dependent to max assist in LE ADL's, bed mobility, & transfers

7. *Homeostatic concerns*

    +   NG tube & food supplements

    +   Foley catheter/bowel training

    +   Skin inspection/turning by staff

    −   Functional cough

Confirmed as written

8. *Expected stress reactions*

    −   Pleasant and cooperative

    −   Only occasionally becomes frustrated with complex tasks

    +   Needs encouragement to begin task

    +   Solves problems with assistance

    +   Often seeks therapist's approval when making decisions

    ±   Socializes with staff but only occasionally with other patients

Revision: Discrepancies in stress reactions need to be investigated

9. *Unknown environmental resources*

    ?   Since he is divorced, is there anyone close to help him

    ?   Does he have financial resources to move from apartment on third floor

Hypothesis needs to be investigated

N. Good safety awareness; Able to learn/organize complex tasks; Interested in finishing tasks; work is done neatly

Suggested Problem List

1. Structural instability and pain of spine, clavicle, and finger
2. Disuse of fractured R hand/L arm and casted trunk
3. At L3, weakness of partially enervated "key" LE muscles
4. LE Sensation impaired at L4–L5 and absent at S1
5. LE AROM below L3 needs to be evaluated during ADL's
6. Low endurance
7. Dependent to max assist for LE ADL's, bed mobility and transfers

8. Homeostatic concerns need to be tracked
9. Stress reactions and environmental resources need to be investigated

Reflection on the Problem List

Note that some numbers have changed from the hypothesis list to the Problem List. This is customary since test results often redefine the therapist's focus. Feel free to chunk the problems differently. Chunking is a personal strategy that helps an individual remember the main treatment issues. Clinicians omit "structural instability" from a Problem List because it seems so obvious to them. Students initially need to list this "red flag" to remind them to identify and then implement precautions.

1. *Structural instability and pain of lumber spine, clavicle, and finger.* The physician often expects the therapist to infer medical precautions from medical procedures, such as a laminectomy and cast applied 10 days ago. The physician also expects the therapist to ask for permission to use potentially dangerous movements before implementing a treatment program, such as transfers.

2. *Disuse atrophy of fractured L arm/R hand.* The fracture of his left clavicle makes him protect his left shoulder, so it has only Fair strength and limited AROM. The strength of the fractured fourth finger is unknown. Right grasp during ADLs was not recorded. He is independent in eating and grooming and needs minimal assistance for UE bathing, so he may be using his right hand during ADLs some of the time. "Intact written communication" is unclear since his dominant right hand has a fracture. Is he able to sign his name left-handed? More information about right hand use is needed. Note that the asset of normal strength of his RUE and left hand are deleted from the Problem List.

3. *At L3, weakness of partially enervated "key" LE muscles.* The student should be prepared to provide assistance if his partial range is not sufficient to achieve LE self-care.

4. *LE Sensation impaired at L4–L5 and absent at S1.* He is classified as an L3 complete lesion, but he has impaired sensation at L4–L5. Recovery of function up to 3 levels below the level is possible because of overlapping dorsal roots, which duplicate muscle enervation. A "zone of partial preservation" below the level of the lesion is consistent with a diagnosis of complete SC lesion.

5. *LE AROM below L3 needs to be evaluated during ADLs.* LE AROM below L3 should be eyeballed to confirm spared L4–L5 function. The word "eyeball" was not used on the Problem List because it is less professional sounding than "evaluate," but in fact, it is what therapists do.

6. *Loss of endurance.* His heart rate and blood pressure are elevated at rest and he still can lift only two out of three Triflow balls. His ADL activity level is only at cardiac Stage 2 out of 14. For a young man with a history of good health, these data show that his remaining muscles are currently overtaxed. The student should be conservative when estimating activity tolerance.

7. *Dependent to max assist in LE ADLs, bed mobility, and transfers.* The student should plan to provide maximum physical assistance and long-handled devices to make early independence possible. This has a positive effect on self-confidence when the patient is emotionally fragile. It will also help to maintain AROM so that strengthening to reverse disuse atrophy is less likely.

8. *Homeostatic concerns need to be tracked.* Homeostatic concerns will interrupt or curtail therapy time, increase his hospital bills, and will produce additional anguish for Harley if they are not prevented. He still has an NG tube so nutritional needs may not be met. He has a functional cough; thus, respiratory infections are less likely to interrupt therapy. He still has a Foley catheter so bladder infections are a realistic concern. The bowel training program doesn't always prevent accidents. The turning schedule will not prevent skin breakdown from shearing forces as he

becomes more physically active, especially during transfers, so daily skin inspection by the therapist is paramount.

9. *Stress reactions and environmental resources need to be investigated.*   Cues show a discrepancy. His need for encouragement, assistance, and approval probably indicate stress. He may be in a stage of denial, as indicated by the fact that he is pleasant and cooperative, rarely shows frustration, and only occasionally socializes with other patients. His behavior at 10 days postinjury may not fully indicate the level of stress he is experiencing. Support from environmental resources is still unclear this early in his recovery. Environmental resources will make the differences between a successful and unsuccessful transition to the community.

NOTE.   Cognitive assets are not included on the Problem List. These assets are logical since the car accident producing the caudal spinal cord injury was not close to his head and he didn't lose consciousness.

IDENTIFYING DEFICITS NOT ADDRESSED BY THE BIOMECHANICAL FRAME OF REFERENCE

Before you design biomechanical treatment activities, it is important to identify the blind spots that will be present in your treatment plan because the biomechanical frame of reference doesn't address homeostatic, "sensory-motor," MOHO, psychosocial, or perceptual-cognitive concerns. You don't need to scatter your energy by solving all these problems now, but you do need to identify these unaddressed concerns before you get too involved in the minutiae of biomechanical treatment. Make sure you list BOTH the name of the concern and the specific evaluation results to prove that each specific concern exists. For example, a respiratory infection (specific homeostatic concern) might be supported by the presence of a fever, fatigue, and lost therapy time (specific results).

Student's List of Deficits Not Addressed

One narrative hypothesis raised concerns about his human and nonhuman environmental resources. Use this space to identify two additional MOHO assets or deficits. Name each MOHO concern. Then give an example of a question that needs to be explored in future dialogue with this patient for each MOHO concern. Memory Aid 14.1 should be used as a guide.

1.

2.

One narrative hypothesis raised the issue of stress reactions. Use this space to identify two additional psychosocial assets or deficits that are ignored by the MOHO frame of reference. Name each psychosocial concern. Then write a reasonable question regarding each concern that needs to answered in the future. Memory Aid 14.1 should be used as a guide.

1.

2.

Use this space to identify one neurodevelopmental deficit that was ignored when the narrative hypotheses were formulated. Name the NDT concern. Use a chapter on spinal cord injury as a guide.

One narrative hypothesis identified a loss of somatosensation below the level of the lesion. Use this space to identify one additional "sensory-motor" asset or deficit. Name the sensory-motor concern that needs to be explored. Use Memory Aid 16.1 as a guide.

The narrative hypotheses about homeostasis introduced concern about his nutritional needs, bladder infections, bowel incontinence, and potential for skin breakdown. Use this space to identify two additional homeostatic deficits that are REALISTIC concerns for the future. Name the specific concerns, not just the homeostatic systems. Use Memory Aid 17.1 as a guide.

1.

2.

Use this space to chunk current rehabilitation assets and deficits into two major groups. Substantiate it with specifics from the evaluation results. Use Memory Aid 2.2 as a guide.

Suggested List of Deficits Not Addressed

MOHO assets and deficits.   Note the use of question marks to indicate reasonable question about issues not specifically mentioned in the report.

Locus of control: How much internal control does Harley feel in the midst of the technology and medical procedures he has experienced?

Expectations of success: What does Harley really mean when he says he is "hopeful about his future functional ability"?

Occupational goals: What life-long values will motivate Harley to meet the challenge of spinal cord injury?

Meaning of activities: What does his job as an automechanic mean to Harley? Does he like it? Is it fulfilling?

Interests: What other interests does Harley have besides traveling?

Psychosocial assets and deficits ignored by MOHO.   Note the use of question marks to indicate reasonable questions about issues not specifically mentioned in the report.

Acute care stressors
>   Is he experiencing stress due to mutilation?
>   Is he experiencing stress due to the medical jargon and procedures which create a sense of helplessness?
>   Is he experiencing stress due to the inability to relieve stress with food and recreation?
>   Is he experiencing stress due to sleep deprivation?

Sexuality
>   Has Harley or his physician brought up the issue of sexual dysfunction yet?
>   Are significant others visiting him to preserve his sense of physical and social intimacy?
>   How closely tied is his concept of masculinity to his job as an automechanic?

Neurodevelopmental deficit.   Spasticity of BLE.

Sensory-motor assets and deficits.   Bone pain at fracture sites.

Homeostatic deficits.   Notice the use of questions because substantiating data were not present in the initial evaluation. Notice the omission of autonomic dysreflexia, which is not likely with an L3 lesion.

Possible complications include:
- Deep vein thromboses and pulmonary emboli;
- Osteoporosis and heterotopic ossification; and
- Stress ulcers.

Rehabilitation chunks.
1. Independence to minimal assistance needed for UE ADLs.
2. Dependence to maximal assistance needed for LE ADLs, transfers, and bed mobility.

GENERATING TREATMENT GOALS

Use the next page to generate a biomechanical goal spreadsheet. Focus on the biomechanical deficits from the Problem List. Use Memory Aid 4.1 to help you chunk and sequence short-term goals (possible in 1 week) and long-term goals. Divide your concerns into short- and long-term goals by thinking about what is safe, functional significance, goals that are possible in 1 week, and goals that must be treated directly. Prioritize within short-term and long-term by asking if one goal is a prerequisite for another goal. Make biomechanical goals measurable. Finish each S-T goal with a suggested functional outcome. Be sure to include compensatory devices and procedures in the functional outcomes if your long-term goals indicate that full recovery is not possible.

Student's Goal Spreadsheet

Dysfunction.

To help you write functional outcomes for every S-T biomechanical goal, BRIEFLY list Harley's current dysfunction.

Short-term Biomechanical Goals   (in 1 week seen twice a day)

Long-term Biomechanical Goals   (after as much therapy as patient needs)

Suggested Biomechanical Goal Spreadsheet

Dysfunction

1. No to minimum assistance for eating, grooming, writing, and UE bathing
2. Maximum assistance for LE ADLs; dependent in bed mobility and transfers

Short-term Biomechanical Goals (in 1 week seen twice a day):

1. Structural stability of his spine, left clavicle, and fourth finger of his right hand will improve as evaluated by the physician
   FO: bed mobility and transfers with maximum physical assistance
2. Endurance will improve as seen by a resting blood pressure of 125/85 and a resting heart rate of 75, 5 minutes after an activity
   FO: to permit Level 3 self-care activities on a cardiac step chart
3. AROM will increase for left shoulder abduction from 140° to 160° and horizontal adduction from 20° to 45°
   FO: independence in UE bathing
4. Increase AROM of right hip flexion and knee extension bilaterally
   FO: to the full range needed for bathing in bed with a long-handled bath
       sponge and moderate physical assistance
5. Evaluate AROM for right hip abduction, knee flexion, and ankle motions during self-care
   FO: moderate assistance in LE dressing

Long-term Biomechanical Goals (after as much therapy as patient needs)

1. Structural stability of his spine, clavicle, and fourth finger will be completely regained
2. Strength of BUEs and spared trunk muscles will be above Normal
3. Leg muscles enervated at L3 will increase to Fair
4. Impaired sensation and Poor strength at L4–L5
5. Endurance will be functional for ADLs while seated and for repeated walking for short distances

Reflection on the Goal Spreadsheet

Except for structural stability, which is evaluated by the physician, biomechanical goals are made measurable by upgrading from the baseline scores. The fact that additional testing is needed to establish measurable LE baseline scores is not unusual. Treatment must begin even if the therapist doesn't have every possible piece of information on a patient.

Structural stability must always be the first goal before you can consider stressing peripheral structures. While structural stability is traditionally thought of as a homeostatic concern, nothing can get a student in trouble faster than ignoring structural stability precautions. Experienced therapists don't list structural stability as a goal in their treatment plans because it is such an obvious concern to them. Students need to list it in their initial treatment plans until this concern also becomes automatic.

Sequencing biomechanical goals is straightforward except for endurance. The endurance goal (#2) might be achieved indirectly while working on the strengthening goals (#3 and 4), so endurance could be listed as either #5 or #2.

Regaining high-level endurance is questionable. Walking tolerance may never be normal. He may use a wheelchair for energy conservation even though he can walk short distances to overcome architectural barriers.

Notice that AROM for shoulder abduction and horizontal adduction were chunked together since they will all be strengthened by the method of light anti-gravity movements. It is wrong to make each one of these joint movements a separate goal! This would create an unwieldy list of short-term goals and raise your anxiety level. Try to think of one activity that can be modified to require both shoulder motions at the same time. Notice that shoulder flexion was omitted from the short-term goals. His shoulder will pass through flexion while moving from horizontal adduction to abduction, so it makes sense to wait to see if some improvement in flexion can be gained indirectly.

AROM for hip flexion and knee extension are also chunked together. These motions naturally go together to produce straight leg raises which are useful in many daily activities. Try to think of an activity that requires both of these motions that is not too difficult for his Fair minus strength.

Many LE muscles will be totally deenervated. This means he will need ankle orthoses and crutches or canes. His car will need hand controls to compensate for loss of ankle motions. He may have to return to a modified job like an automechanic service manager. Reaching down to work inside the engine and lifting heavy objects would be difficult to resume.

We can only speculate about what functional outcomes are most important to Harley at this particular time. Waiting for two people to get him in the wheelchair before he can leave his room may be frustrating. Since he likes to travel, car transfers may be important. He may have walking on his mind, so putting on socks and shoes may be important. He may be motivated to start LE bathing training if male aides are not available. Returning to work may be a priority since he is single and doesn't have an income to support himself.

DESIGNING TREATMENT ACTIVITIES

Use the next two pages (Figs. 5.3 and 5.4) to design two biomechanical treatment activities. Choose any two short-term biomechanical goals from your spreadsheet to generate postulates regarding change and postulates regarding intervention. List all of the mini-goals under each short-term goal to remind you to include the entire treatment sequence in your biomechanical modalities.

I encourage you to draw stick figures in the Rationale column. Descriptions of activities can be difficult to understand without visual aids.

Try to use the same purposeful activity for both biomechanical short-term goals. If serendipity strikes and you are able to use the same activity again, you don't need to describe the entire activity a second time. You only need to describe the modifications that make the second biomechanical goal possible. Remember, there are many advantages to using the same activity more than once, such as cutting down on set-up and clean-up time.

See Figures 5.5 through 5.8 for suggested activities after you have written two of your own.

SECTION III

NEURODEVELOPMENTAL FRAME OF REFERENCE

Deficit/Cause/Goal/FO	Method/Rationale	Specific Modality: Name, Description, Precautions

Figure 5.4.   Student's Activity #2

Deficit/Cause/Goal/FO	Method/Rationale	Specific Modality: Name, Description, Precautions
Deficit #1: structural instability of spine, left clavicle, and fourth finger of right hand *Stage-specific cause:* partially healed fractures *S–T biomechanical goal:* Structural stability will be regained as evaluated by the doctor *Functional outcome:* Independent wheelchair transfers to a car	*Orthoses* that temporarily enforce rest of the spine	Wear body cast
	Procedures that prevent excessive pressure on spine, clavicle, and finger	Delay transfer training: dependent transfer to wheelchair with two people so he doesn't bear body weight on left clavicle and right hand Moderate assistance for left shoulder flexion and right grasp during LE ADLs and bed mobility using long-handled devices
	Procedures that safely stress clavicle and finger	Continue with independent feeding and UE bathing using both hands

Figure 5.5. Biomechanical Postulates for Harley

Deficit/Cause/Goal/FO	Method/Rationale	Specific Modality: Name, Description, Precautions
Deficit #2: loss of endurance *Stage-specific cause:* deconditioning and extra demands made on muscles above L3 *S–T biomechanical goal:* Endurance will improve as seen by a resting BP of 125/85 and resting HR of 75 5 minutes after an activity *Functional outcome:* he can visit with friends at the end of day without falling asleep	*Increased duration,* which gradually stresses the cardiovascular system while ensuring proper rest	Sit up in wheelchair in semi-reclining position one more time than the current schedule requires (baseline information is needed to give an exact number). Take vital signs 5 minutes after returning to bed.
	Increased intensity, which gradually stresses the cardiovascular system while ensuring proper rest	Reduce assistance from maximal to moderate during LE bathing using assistive devices except when washing toes and heels (max assist to prevent decubiti). Take vital signs after resting 5 minutes.

Figure 5.6. Biomechanical Postulates for Harley

Deficit/Cause/Goal/FO	Method/Rationale	Specific Modality: Name, Description, Precautions
Deficit #3: loss of AROM in left shoulder *Stage-specific cause:* disuse atrophy and pain due to clavicular fracture *S–T biomechanical goal:* AROM will increase for shoulder abduction from 140° to 160° and horizontal adduction from 20° to 45° *Functional outcome:* able to lift hood on car in standing while leaning against the car and cane in one hand	*Active assistive exercise,* which recruits more motor units and causes muscle hypertrophy of glycolytic fast-twitch muscle fibers	*Basketball practice:* Position hoop directly overhead but within arm's reach so that 150° of shoulder abduction is required when Harley sits under it in a wheelchair in a semi-reclining position. Place him close enough so he can drop the balls in the hoop. Precaution: avoid throwing which will increase bone pain and produce trunk rotation when the throwing, arm follows through. Place nerf balls on table to his far left so he has to reach across his chest with 30° of horizontal adduction. Gradually move hoop higher and farther to his right side and the balls farther to his left on the table as his range increases. Provide physical assistance to increase active range of these Fair minus muscles.

Figure 5.7.   Biomechanical Postulates for Harley

Deficit/Cause/Goal/FO	Method/Rationale	Specific Modality: Name, Description, Precautions
Deficit #4: loss of AROM of RLE muscles enervated at L3 *Stage-specific cause:* disuse atrophy and partial enervation *S–T biomechanical goal:* Right hip flexion and knee extension will increase from Fair − to within functional limits for LE bathing with moderate assistance and a long-handled bath sponge *Functional outcome:* Independence in LE bathing	*Active assistive exercise,* which recruits more motor units and causes hypertrophy of glycolytic fast-twitch muscle fibers	*Kick balloon:* While in bed in a semi-reclining position, have Harley practice right straight leg raises using hip flexion and knee extension. Provide physical assistance for these Fair minus muscles. Then give him a long-handled bath sponge to see how far he has to lift his right leg if assistance is reduced from maximal to moderate. Replicate this same leg position for balloon kicking. Place a balloon directly over his right foot at a height similar to that required for LE bathing. Ask him to kick the balloon with his right foot while you physically assist him as needed. Have him keep track of how many hits and misses he has.

Figure 5.8.   Biomechanical Postulates for Harley

SECTION III

NEURODEVELOPMENTAL FRAME OF REFERENCE

CHAPTER 6

Neurodevelopmental Treatment

INTRODUCTION

Dr. and Mrs. Bobath designed the Neurodevelopmental Treatment approach to address the motor problems of patients with neurological deficits. The title Neurodevelopmental Treatment (NDT) tells you that the Bobaths used neurophysiological and developmental theories as the basis for their frame of reference. The Bobaths developed NDT during a storm of clinical thinking that took place from approximately 1940 to 1960. This was a frustrating but exciting time because so many options were created for therapists.

Several sensorimotor frames of reference were developed to remediate children and adults with brain damage (1). Some of these frames of reference are not used today. These include patterning (Doman-Delacato), neurobehavioral treatment (Banus), synergy-based treatment (Brunnstrom), and perceptual-motor treatment (Frostig and Kephart). Others, such as sensory integration (Ayres) and sensorimotor treatment (Rood), have been accepted primarily in pediatric settings. The work of two clinicians has endured in the form of reflex evaluation (Fiorentino) and synergy evaluation (Brunnstrom). Two frames of reference are still used today in a wide variety of settings. They are proprioceptive neuromuscular facilitation (PNF), which was developed by Knott and Voss, and neurodevelopmental treatment. NDT is well known because of its wide network of certified instructors in America, Europe, and other countries.

ASSUMPTIONS OF NEURODEVELOPMENTAL TREATMENT

Models of Motor Control

The Bobaths based their clinical work on a model of motor control developed by an English neurologist, J.H. Jackson (2). This model states that the nervous system is organized hierarchically, with the spinal cord being the lowest level, the brainstem being intermediate, and the cortex being the highest level of motor control.

Brain lesions were believed to damage higher centers, which normally inhibited the primitive movements of lower centers. These primitive mass movements include hyperactive tonic reflexes and pathological limb synergies. This loss of inhibition was referred to as the release phenomenon (3). Since primitive movements were associated with spasticity, the first goal of treatment was to inhibit both spasticity and pathological limb movements. Unlike Brunnstrom, who recommended using pathological synergies to facilitate early limb movements (4), the Bobaths believed that these synergies are too hard to get rid of once patients learn how to use them. After the inhibition of spasticity and pathological movements, treatment progresses to stimulation of automatic reactions, such as righting reactions. Once automatic reactions were present, the Bobath's assumed that normal voluntary movements would naturally emerge (3).

Today, new research supports a distributed model of motor control (5, 6). Rather than a strict hierarchy, the nervous system communicates simultaneously along ascending and lateral pathways in addition to the descending pathways (5, 7). Neural communication is believed to be organized around the accomplishment of specific tasks (2). Therefore, motor control is distributed over the entire nervous system. Which site controls a particular movement depends on what task is to be executed (8). This makes it very difficult to picture how a specific lesion would then affect a specific movement (2). However, the distributed model of motor control does suggest modification of NDT assumptions.

Skill Acquisition

While the Bobaths let developmental theory influence their thinking, NDT is *not* a pure developmental frame of reference. The Bobaths believed that teaching normal motor milestones is *NOT* the proper focus for the treatment of brain-damaged individuals (3). Some normal motor milestones are dangerous for brain-damaged patients. These patients often get stuck in primitive behaviors that are safe only for normal infants (3). For example, normal infants first attempt head control while prone on elbows. However, this posture strengthens the flexion synergy of the arms, which can dominate the brain-damaged individual. Similarly, the Asymmetrical Tonic Neck Reflex is a normal stage of motor development that normal infants pass through quickly. Yet, this reflex can quickly dominate brain-damaged children and produce severe deformities. Practicing motor milestones in brain-damaged individuals can reinforce abnormal patterns of movement that become more stereotyped with repetition.

Therefore, the first assumption of the NDT frame of reference is the belief that it is important to remediate foundations skills that make normal skill acquisition possible (3). These foundation skills include midline symmetry, righting reactions, trunk rotation, plus many more. The Bobaths believed that if brain-damaged patients acquired these foundation skills, a minimum of practice would be needed to achieve normal motor milestones. For example, if midline symmetry is achieved, little practice would be required to acquire the skill of sitting.

The Bobaths also believed that skill acquisition begins with automatic reactions, such as vertical head righting, and later progresses to voluntary control (5). NDT treatment has traditionally facilitated automatic reactions in isolation from any purposeful activity. Keshner objects to teaching balance on tilt boards because she thinks they are unrelated to the normal environment (7). The normal environment often provides little advance warning and usually challenges us when our attention is divided. This is a different task from the expected tilt of therapeutic equipment that moves in only one or two planes while patients are concentrating solely on their balance.

Focusing only on foundation skills and teaching automatic reactions in isolation have recently been challenged. Carr and Shephard researched a motor learning theory which divides tasks into open or closed tasks (9). During **open tasks,** the patient, objects, and other people are in motion, and the conditions change with each performance. Motor examples of open tasks include catching a ball and walking down a crowded hallway. During **closed tasks,** the objects are stationary, and performance does not change from one attempt to the next. Motor examples include walking alone down the stairs at home or brushing your teeth.

Since our therapeutic goals include skill acquisition for both open and closed tasks, it is not enough to retrain foundations skills in isolation. Repetitive practice of

foundation skills is effective only with closed tasks (10). While weight shifts in standing are necessary for normal gait, they are not sufficient for walking around unpredictable obstacles in a shopping mall. Open tasks can be learned only by performing functional movements in a variety of environmental contexts (11, 12). Patients are not memorizing repetitive weight shifts or other foundation skills during open tasks. They are learning to solve motor problems (13).

These new theorists are not saying that teaching foundation skills are improper. Carr and Shephard call this initial step "practicing missing components" (9). They believe that this foundations approach is a good starting place that does not go far enough. Carr and Shephard recommend practicing foundation skills followed immediately by open tasks in a changing environment to achieve carryover.

For instance, teaching balance as an isolated foundation skill is an appropriate first step. Initially, teaching balance during purposeful activity may be too dangerous for very low functioning patients. No one wants to fill out an accident form. Remember, a purposeful activity divides the therapist's attention as well as the patient's. However, teaching isolated foundation skills is not sufficient. It is essential to progress as quickly as possible to using automatic reactions for problem solving in the natural environment if our goal is to make our patients functional (14). If neural communication is organized around specific tasks, then foundation skills must be learned during specific purposeful tasks.

A lack of carryover has been one of the main criticisms of NDT. As you will see in Chapter 8, NDT preparation and functional application can be used together for skill acquisition.

Role of Sensation

The second assumption is the belief that normal movement is learned by experiencing what a normal movement feels like (3). A child learns how to ride a bicycle by learning how it feels to ride the bike correctly, not by having a parent describe or demonstrate how to do it. According to Mrs. Bobath, "the therapist controls and guides the child's motor output to her sensory input, but she withdraws her help gradually and systematically so that the child finally learns to control his movements unaided" (3). Various sensory modalities, such as brushing and vibration, are not the answer to teaching normal movement (15). It is the sensory feedback of normal movement itself that teaches a patient how to move normally again.

Clearly, Mrs. Bobath did not see motor learning as a passive process imposed by the therapist. The ability to respond to sensory input from handling techniques requires different skills from the ability to initiate voluntary movement (10). The patient must experience the sensation of self-initiated movement and eventually take total responsibility for active movement. This active approach is supported by research on motor learning. Roy and Diewert found that it is easier to relearn movements if the patient actively plans, initiates, executes, and terminates the motor sequence (16).

One aspect of sensory input that was not addressed by the Bobaths is the belief that vision guides movement (9). The Bobaths placed a strong emphasis on proprioceptive feedback for learning. Proprioception is important when learning is taking place, but the visual system is more important once a movement is learned and can be executed by motor memory (18). Visual input allows the patient to anticipate the need for change and to reprogram motor output before errors occur. You don't wait to bump into people on the stairwell. You see where they are and how quickly they are moving and modify your own movements accordingly. Vision is very important for the feedforward mode.

Feedforward mode is used for habitual movements, such as walking, or fast ballistic motions, such as throwing a ball (18). The cerebellum runs a "stored tape" and does not monitor any proprioceptive feedback. During feedforward movements, the muscle spindle is electrically silent! The motor cortex presets the muscle spindle to whatever the task will require based on previous experience. Presetting the muscle spindle independently of extrafusal length or load is called gamma bias (19).

Feedforward enables people to predict the consequences of an action to *avoid* errors rather than waiting to detect and react to them (10). Feedforward mode is very important for everyday life. If we had to consciously think about every movement, we would not be able to attend to important abstract ideas. Since many skilled movements are dependent upon preplanned motor programs (9), our patients must learn to work in feedforward mode. Once they can use feedforward, they can carry over their gains in therapy to daily life (14).

If an error is made while in feedforward mode, the cerebellum switches to feedback mode. The **feedback mode** is important for correcting errors, learning unfamiliar movements, and relearning skilled movements (18). When we are trying to analyze a movement in feedback mode, we tend to move slowly and activate the muscle spindle afferents (18).

The old concept of using sensory feedback from normal movement is now combined with the new concept that sensory patterns can initiate centrally programmed movements in feedforward mode (6). The old concept of sensory feedback being primarily proprioceptive has been revised to include other sensory modalities such as vision (5).

Postural Control

The third assumption states that postural control is essential for limb movements (3). As Mrs. Bobath noted, "the automatic movements of postural adjustment accompany voluntary movements like a shadow" (15, p. 20). The Bobaths originally believed that these adjustments were based on reflexes, so they called them a "postural reflex mechanism." When the distributed model of motor control replaced the hierarchical model, the belief that reflexes control these axial movements was abandoned (5). However, research still supports the fact that postural control produces an axial adjustment that precedes limb movement and occurs simultaneously with the impulse to act (10). For example, if you plan to move the arm forward while reaching for an object, axial contractions occur prior to forward sway and while reaching for the object (9, p. 1).

During early attempts to learn a new movement, postural control is inadequate to support limb movements. Bly says that initially, limb movements are "yoked" or linked to axial movements (14). For example, when a normal infant first tries to sit up unsupported, trunk extension is accompanied by an obligatory retraction of the upper extremities. This retraction impedes hand function since the hands are drawn back away from objects in the midline. If the arms are brought back to the midline, the trunk slumps forward. Extension with retraction is a transition phase of normal development that normal infants quickly outgrow. Unfortunately, brain-damaged patients often get stuck in this transition stage. The chapter on NDT evaluation ensures that you will be able to recognize this dangerous transition strategy.

Infants with intact brains quickly develop proximal stability of the neck and trunk, which make skilled limb movements possible. For example, normal infants learn how to maintain back extension while "unyoking" the arms to reach for objects. The hand can reach for an object, and the foot can take a step because they have a stable neck and trunk. When this stable but independent foundation is missing, hand and foot function suffer noticeably.

While the Bobaths abandoned the idea that postural control is reflex-based, the importance of postural control has stood the test of time. The main modification of the third assumption about postural control is the new emphasis on teaching postural movements during functional activities. The distributed model of motor control suggests that practicing postural adjustments in isolation on therapy balls and mat tables is not sufficient. Postural reactions are task-specific. For instance, arm control in supine may not carry over to control in sitting because the postural movements needed to support limb movement are totally different in these two positions (14).

It is easier to use purposeful activity to help patients learn how to make repeated postural adjustments. Purposeful activity tells the patient why he/she has to make all those funny little movements of the head and trunk. This is especially helpful with cognitively impaired patients who cannot generalize abstract concepts. It even helps family members understand the need for these new axial movements. Purposeful activity also tells the patient what postural adjustments to make and when to make them: whatever it takes to complete the activity successfully.

Role of Muscle Tone

A fourth assumption of NDT states that you cannot impose normal movement on abnormal muscle tone (3). Brain damage often results in a loss of the normal balance between inhibition and facilitation of flexor and extensor tone. Therefore, a top priority in NDT is to normalize muscle tone before and during the patient's attempts to move.

Normalizing tone includes inhibiting spasticity. Spasticity is a major problem in patient management (3, 15). **Spasticity** is defined as abnormal resistance to passive stretch due to an exaggerated stretch reflex. Initially, it manifests as a classic clasp-knife phenomenon. Passive movement elicits a sudden "catch," followed by a full release. However, the Bobaths did not perceive spasticity as a localized muscular phenomenon: "When observing a spastic patient, one is struck by the fact that spasticity shows itself in definite patterns of abnormal coordination" (15, p. 2). In NDT, abnormal coordination includes the lack of reciprocal enervation.

Lack of reciprocal control causes unwanted cocontraction in spastic conditions (15). **Cocontraction** is the simultaneous contraction of all muscles around a joint that blocks movement. Unwanted cocontraction has been confirmed by EMG studies. Sahrmann and Norton found that 16 patients with CVAs, TBIs, and MS demonstrated unusually slow eccentric extension of the elbow when lowering their arms to their sides (20). Slowness was caused by a prolonged recruitment of biceps and brachioradialis that began during elbow flexion and continued even when the patient wanted to extend his/her elbow. Prolonged recruitment of flexors was gradually overcome by the triceps as the arm was lowered. This resulted in cocontraction of opposing muscle groups. When normal subjects eccentrically extended the elbow, the triceps were electrically silent while minimal flexor tone was used to lower the forearm. McLellan found similar results regarding cocontraction during voluntary knee flexion and extension of 11 spastic patients (21).

Their quadriceps and hamstrings were not silent at any stage of knee movement.

However, abnormal cocontraction is not present in all brain-damaged patients. Milner-Brown and Penn studied muscle activity in children with cerebral palsy (22). Mildly involved children exhibited normal alternating electrical activity and reciprocal elbow flexion and extension. Moderately involved children had normal performance at slow speeds, but at fast speeds, a "complete breakdown in reciprocal enervation occurred, and cocontraction appeared" (22, p. 616). Severely involved children exhibited electrical activity in flexors and extensors at the initiation of elbow movement, which severely impaired movement due to cocontraction.

Knutsson and Richards reported similar results in 26 adults with spastic hemiparesis (23). Mildly involved adults demonstrated normal muscle activity except for premature activation of the calf muscles, which produced minimal gait disturbance. However, severely involved adults had abnormal cocontraction of several limb muscles with a complete disruption of reciprocal enervation and disorganization of the gait sequence. Abnormal cocontraction appears to be a characteristic of more severely involved patients.

The concept of spasticity is complicated by fixing (5, 14). **Fixing** is a voluntary holding of body parts in rigid postures once voluntary movement emerges (3). Unlike spasticity, fixing comes and goes, depending on how threatened the patient feels. Fixing is often seen when the patient experiences a fear of falling. The patient doesn't actually have to fall; the mere thought of falling can trigger this phenomenon.

Fixing may be an attempt to reduce the degrees of freedom of complex motions (5, 14). Degrees of freedom are the number of planes each joint moves through (24). For example, the upper extremity has nine degrees of freedom: three planes in the shoulder, one in the elbow, two in the wrist, two in the metacarpophalangeal (MCP) joints, and one in the IP joints. Nine degrees of freedom creates a control problem. Engineers solved a similar control problem by making the steering wheel of a car turn both front wheels together (10). Fixing also reduces the variety of motor responses required by a changing environment. Yet this lack of variety is unacceptable for people who locomote through unpredictable environments. Therefore, prevention of fixing is a top treatment priority. Physical support from handling and environmental surfaces reduces degrees of freedom, which in turn decreases the need for fixing (5).

Abnormal muscle tone can eventually lead to shortening of soft tissue. Clinicians have reported that the classic clasp-knife phenomenon becomes masked by stiffness, so that eventually the clasp-knife release is no longer felt in spastic patients. Lee et al. found significantly increased resistance to passive elbow extension in three spastic hemiparetic patients, even though EMG activity in the biceps was decreased (25). These authors concluded that this increased stiffness was due to subclinical muscle contractures that had not yet produced a visible loss of range of motion. Tardieu et al. (26) found that muscles that were immobilized in a shortened position rapidly lost the normal number of sarcomeres and that the remaining sarcomeres became resistant to stretch. If left untreated, shortening can result in permanent contractures that are not amenable to NDT (3).

Keshner suggests that normalization of tone has a doubtful impact on recovery (7). However, after the flaccid stage, brain-injured patients often develop tight, painful muscles. Whatever the cause of the tightness, it is not helpful to quickly elongate painful muscles. Cooperation is difficult to achieve when a patient is severely distressed. While the tightness that clinicians feel is probably some combination of spasticity, abnormal cocontraction, compensatory fixing, and viscoelastic shortening, common sense dictates that we gently elongate what is tight and painful before asking the patient to move.

However, the overemphasis on inhibition of spasticity has been replaced with a more balanced approach. Today, NDT instructors emphasize the immediate use of complex, purposeful movements as soon as any normalization of muscle tone can be achieved (5, 14). "As soon as possible" means within seconds, not hours or days. That is why the Memory Aid for NDT goals in Chapter 9 repeatedly pairs passive elongation and initiation of active movement in a single treatment sequence. This pairing creates a better balance of inhibition and facilitation than lumping all inhibition goals in one column and all facilitation goals in a second column. Chapter 8 introduces you to the idea that handling techniques must be followed immediately by purposeful activity within the same treatment session.

Facilitation is needed because spastic muscles can also be weak. The cause of this weakness is still debated. EMG studies have shown that spastic muscles, such as the biceps, exhibit muscle atrophy and decreased firing rates of the remaining motor units (20, 27). It is still not known if the decreased firing rate of a spastic muscle is the cause of its weakness. Tang and Rymer found no significant correlation between weakness and decreased firing rates in the biceps of hemiparetic patients (27). This means the weakest muscles did not necessarily demonstrate the slowest firing rates. Perhaps the weakness of spastic muscles is due to their shortened length, which results in a contraction at the end of range where all the muscles have a short moment arm. Muscles are strongest when the moment arm is longest, which is usually in mid-range (24).

Facilitation is also needed to strengthen hypotonic muscles that have abnormally low muscle tone. **Hypotonia** is characterized by joint hypermobility, muscles that feel very soft to the touch, the inability to hold a limb up after it is placed by the therapist, poor endurance, and weakness (28). During the early stage of recovery from stroke, muscle tone is often hypotonic. Bohannon et al. found that cerebral vascular accident (CVA) patients with a median onset time of 19 days demonstrated little or no spasticity in 75% of the muscles tested (29). During the early stage of recovery, the Bobaths recommend facilitation of weak hypotonic muscles.

Therefore, the Bobaths developed facilitation techniques for weak muscles. However, facilitation must be carefully graded down whenever muscle tone becomes too high (3). Overstimulation, such as moderate to maximal resistance, can overstrengthen spastic muscles and perpetuate the imbalance of muscle power around a joint. Fetters reported that while the quadriceps responded monosynaptically to normal levels of stimulation, excessive stimulation recruited elbow, knee, and ankle flexors, in addition to the targeted quadriceps (30). Excessive stimulation can produce a pattern of irradiation that is undesirable (30). Unlike the biomechanical frame of reference, which uses maximum resistance to strengthen weak limb muscles, NDT judiciously facilitates hypotonic and weak spastic muscles to reestablish a balance of flexor and extensor muscle tone.

In summary, there are two modifications in the assumption that you cannot produce normal movement when abnormal muscle tone is present. First, it is probably more accurate to say that you cannot produce normal movement when muscles are tight and painful. Tightness can take the form of spasticity, abnormal cocontraction, fixing, or viscoelastic shortening. NDT techniques can inhibit the spasticity, cocontraction, and fixing. Second, a more balanced approach to inhibition and facilitation is now emphasized.

Plasticity of the Brain

The Bobaths' optimism about the plasticity of the human brain is the final assumption of this frame of reference. While it was a controversial idea when the Bobaths first began, there are now substantial amounts of data to support this final assumption. A number of mechanisms make recovery possible beyond the early recovery associated with a reduction of brain swelling and shock.

Collateral sprouting is one mechanism that supports brain plasticity. Within 3 to 5 days of the injury, collateral axons from nearby neurons begin to bypass the damaged area to reconnect broken synapses (31). Unlike regenerative sprouting of damaged neurons, these collateral sprouts appear to produce functional gains.

Regenerative sprouting is unsuccessful because of glial scarring, which misguides new growth to inappropriate targets.

Plasticity is also supported by silent synapses. The brain appears to have silent synapses that do not function until damage occurs. These silent synapses are part of bilateral systems (32). In the past, systems were labeled ipsilateral or contralateral, but today many systems are known to have bilateral enervation. As Moore notes, "For example, many of the secondary sensorimotor centers of the neocortex are now known to send (or receive) bilateral pathways" (32, p. 461).

Plasticity is also related to sex differences. Males have significantly greater hemispheric specialization than females (9). For example, language is a specialized function of the left hemisphere in males. Females have language centers on both sides of their brains and a larger corpus callosum to carry information back and forth between these two language centers. If the primary language center is damaged in women, the other language center appears to be able to perform some language functions. This permits more recovery in female brains following brain damage.

Finally, plasticity is made possible by uncommitted areas in the brain. At birth, many areas of the cortex are not fully myelinated. Poor conductivity delays the commitment of brain areas to their special functions. If brain damage occurs in one area while other areas are not yet committed, these uncommitted areas may take over the functions of the damaged area. For example, children with left hemisphere damage to the primary language center exhibited spared language function when given the Wechsler Test of Intelligence (33). However, maintenance of a function by an uncommitted area may be at a cost. These same children had depressed visual-spatial skills, which suggests that the right hemisphere sacrificed some of its normal visual function when it took over language function.

Young children are not the only patients with uncommitted areas. Incomplete myelination delays commitment in some areas for several years after birth (34). The corticospinal tracts associated with motor control are not fully myelinated until 2 years of age. The reticular formation, which controls muscle tone, and the cerebellum, which coordinates movements, are not fully myelinated until early adulthood.

Collateral sprouting, silent synapses, sex differences, and uncommitted areas of the brain are only four mechanisms that explain brain plasticity. As more is learned with new cellular technology, additional mechanisms may be discovered. While the anatomy of the brain has been mapped for some time, we are still learning about the true functions that these structures perform.

DEFICITS ADDRESSED BY NEURODEVELOPMENTAL TREATMENT

The deficits addressed by the NDT frame of reference include axial control, automatic reactions, and limb control. These function-dysfunction continua identify the unique domains of concern that are recognized by NDT. Each continuum has a specific sequence of development that enables you to identify the patient's current level of skill. The assumptions of NDT apply to all three continua. You are relying on facilitation of skill acquisition during closed and open tasks, the sensation of what normal movement feels like, postural control to support limb movements and automatic reactions, normal muscle tone before and during patient-initiated movement, and brain plasticity.

Axial Control

Axial control is defined as the control of neck and trunk. Axial control is one of NDT's major contributions to our understanding of motor control. Other frames of reference mention axial control in passing or ignore it completely. The biomechanical frame of reference, for instance, primarily evaluates the limbs. Consensus for assessing range of motion of neck and trunk does not exist. Neck and trunk muscles are often deleted from manual muscle testing forms. It's as though the limbs are suspended in the air, able to function without a trunk.

Conditions that produce brain damage often affect axial control. Since the trunk provides the foundation for all limb movements, deficits that affect the neck and trunk can profoundly affect limb function. Treating limb dysfunction in patients with brain damage without addressing axial control issues constitutes a major blind spot. While we can see that our patient spills his/her food when using utensils, the solution may require treating the neck and trunk as well as the limb.

Automatic Reactions

Automatic reactions have been a part of evaluation tools for some time (35), but the Bobaths determined their importance for normal movement. **Automatic reactions** include righting reactions, equilibrium reactions, and protective extension of the limbs. They are called automatic because they occur without having to consciously think about them. They enable us to safely return to midline where we have a large, stable base of support. Without this safety, we would not be free to risk the movement needed to explore our environment (3).

Automatic reactions require both postural and limb control. To reach out with protective extension, an individual needs limb extension and trunk lateral flexion with anterior pelvic tilt (3). Automatic reactions require a person to coordinate these separate movement components into one swift response. Even if the individual components are present, the patient still may not be capable of the speedy melding of movements from widely dispersed body segments. This is like rubbing the top of your head and patting your stomach while hopping on one foot. It takes practice to put these complex automatic reactions together.

Limb Control

The Bobaths encouraged the therapeutic community to look at the scapula and pelvis as essential contributors to limb control (3). Mobility of the scapula and pelvis add significantly to the degrees of range of motion in both the shoulder and hip. For example, the scapula contributes 60° of the 180° for shoulder abduction (24). If scapular muscles are paralyzed, patients can no longer fully abduct the shoulder to 180°, even if shoulder abductors like the middle deltoid are still intact (36). This proximal contribution to full shoulder and hip range is called scapulo-humeral rhythm and lumbar-pelvic rhythm (24).

In addition to contributing to full range of motion, the scapula and pelvis also provide proximal stability, which is needed for skilled distal movements. For example, scapular muscles contract to stabilize the scapula during the first 60° of shoulder flexion while the hand reaches forward for an object (24). Not until mid-range does the scapula contribute 60° of the 170° for full shoulder flexion (24). Voss called this sequence of events "distal timing" (17). Distal timing is made possible by proximal stability of the shoulder and pelvic girdles early in the range.

Stability of the scapula is problematic because it has little bony contact with the axial skeleton and weak ligaments holding it to the clavicle (24). Stability of the scapula comes primarily from the same muscles that mobilize the scapula (24). Therefore, paralysis of scapular muscles has a profound effect on scapular stability as well as humeral mobility.

Unfortunately, brain-damaged individuals tend to initiate movement from the scapula and pelvis instead of stabilizing these proximal structures during the early phases of limb movement (3). This is a reversal of normal distal timing. Proximal key points of control like the shoulder and pelvis are used to inhibit this early proximal movement while leaving the distal end of the extremity to free to move. These proximal key points also enable the therapist to facilitate scapular and pelvic movements to supplement shoulder and hip motion.

NEUROPHYSIOLOGY OF MOTOR CONTROL

Motor control requires far more than the sensory-motor strip in the cortex. While conflicting theories of motor control are still being debated, there are three major centers of motor control that are well recognized. Skeletal muscles are under voluntary, subcortical, and local spinal cord control. The student must be able to identify all the sites for motor control that exist within these three levels. The sensory-motor strip is just the tip of the iceberg when it comes to motor control.

Voluntary Control

Voluntary control of skeletal muscles can be divided into three functions: (*a*) the impulse to move, (*b*) direct control, and (*c*) indirect control. The **impulse to move** is the result of complex decisions made in the association areas of the cortex.

Direct cortical control is the function of the well-known **pyramidal system** (18). This is the direct pathway from the sensory-motor strip in the cortex to the gamma-motor neurons. Note that this system controls the limb and axial muscles in separate tracts. Limb control is mediated by the lateral corticospinal tract, which crosses in the pyramidal decussation. Seventy-five percent of these fibers synapse with upper extremity motor neurons, so damage here primarily produces loss of contralateral fine finger movements, while the proximal muscles are less severely affected. Neck and trunk control, however, are mediated by the anterior corticospinal tract, which does not cross, so loss of axial function is ipsilateral.

However, poor bilateral trunk control is possible in hemiplegia because of (*1*) ipsilateral paralysis of trunk muscles and (*2*) contralateral paralysis of the arm and leg. First, trunk control is poor on the same side as the brain lesion due to damage of the anterior corticospinal tract, which does not cross. This brain damage initially produces hypotonia, followed by spasticity of the ipsilateral trunk muscles. Second, trunk control can also be poor on the contralateral side from the brain lesion because the hemiplegic arm and leg cannot efficiently push against the support surface to steady the trunk. Immediately after a stroke, the hemiplegic limbs are hypotonic, which may cause the patient to fall towards the hemiplegic side. Later, the leg may develop extensor spasticity and push the trunk away from the hemiplegic side.

Indirect cortical control is a function of the **extrapyramidal system**. This motor system smoothes movement and suppresses unwanted movements (18). In addition to sending motor commands directly to the anterior horn cells, the cortex also sends an efferent copy of the motor commands down indirect, multineuronal extrapyramidal tracts (6). These tracts, like the corticopontocerebellar tract, terminate in the basal ganglia and neocerebellum. While damage rarely hits these subcortical centers directly, their multineuronal connections with the cortex are often damaged.

The first function of the extrapyramidal system is to smoothe out movements. Smoothness is controlled by the neocerebellum, which monitors peripheral feedback, such as muscle spindle input (37). The cerebellum is able to interpret muscle spindle data while in feedback mode because of **alpha-gamma coactivation** (37). Since the muscle spindles are parallel to the skeletomotor fibers, the muscle spindles would no longer be on stretch if the skeletomotor fibers contracted alone (gamma activation). Once the muscle spindle goes slack, its stretch receptors stop firing. To prevent this loss of input, the intrafusal muscle fibers contract (gamma activation) at the same time as the skeletomotor fibers contract. Gamma activation maintains tension on the muscle spindle's stretch receptors located in the central region of the spindle, which keeps it firing. Ideally, alpha-gamma coactivation makes the extrafusal and intrafusal muscle fibers shorten at the same rate.

If there is a difference between the intended length that the muscle spindle was told to expect and the actual length the muscle contracts to, the discrepancy is noted by the cerebellum. Such a discrepancy occurs when you expect to lift a heavy suitcase, but the suitcase turns out to be light (38). The intrafusal muscle fibers of the spindles would contract slowly because they were preset for a heavy suitcase. The extrafusal muscle fibers, however, would shorten faster than programmed because the suitcase was light. This would put the muscle spindles on slack and decrease their firing rate. This discrepancy in firing rates between intrafusal and extrafusal fibers tells the neocerebellum that an error was made. Once the discrepancy is noted, the neocerebellum smoothes out subsequent motor attempts. Our patients need to work in feedback mode when we are trying to teach them what high-quality, normal movements feel like.

The second function of the extrapyramidal system is to suppress unwanted movement (18). This function is mediated by the basal ganglia. If there is too much suppression, it is difficult to initiate movement, especially preprogrammed ballistic movements (38). Parkinson's disease is a classic example of too much suppression. On the other hand, if there is too little suppression, irregular gross movements such as athetoid movements appear. While the Bobaths designed a treatment approach for the athetoid type of cerebral palsy (3), no one has tested the value of NDT for progressive conditions that exhibit too much suppression, such as Parkinson's disease.

Subcortical Facilitation

The skeletal muscles are also under the subcortical control of brainstem nucleii. These nucleii have *no* corti-

cal projections. They facilitate muscles; they never inhibit muscles. Facilitation can be phasic or tonic.

Phasic extension and flexion are the result of changing head positions that stimulate the vestibular end-organs (47). Linear acceleration stimulates the otoliths, which activate the lateral vestibular nucleus. This lateral nucleus activates the lateral vestibulospinal tract, which facilitates ipsilateral phasic extension of the limbs, neck, and trunk (39). Rotary acceleration stimulates the semicircular canals, which activate the medial vestibular nucleus. This medial nucleus activates the medial vestibulospinal tract, which facilitates bilateral phasic neck flexion when the whole body is rotated (34).

Tonic extension is the result of constant gravitational pull on the haircells of the otoliths (34). Tonic extension is needed to maintain an upright posture against the constant pull of gravity. This constant input is sent indirectly to the extensors by way of the reticular formation, which controls sleep and arousal. When we are awake, the reticular formation permits the extensors to be stimulated to maintain an upright position. When we are asleep, the reticular formation shuts down outside stimuli so the muscles can relax. Since we cannot turn gravity off, the only way to let the extensors rest is to have the reticular formation turn off the input. Tonic extension is divided into axial and limb pathways. Tonic limb extension is mediated by the lateral reticulospinal tract (34) while tonic axial extension is mediated by the medial reticulospinal tract (39).

Tonic flexion affects only the limbs. Tonic flexion is created by constant firing of the red nucleus. This center tonically facilitates the contralateral limb flexors via the rubrospinal tract (39).

Local Spinal Cord Control

Motor efferents from higher centers eventually synapse on spinal cord interneurons. These descending commands are subject to local influence by the spinal cord interneurons before the descending input can arrive at the anterior horn cell (37). The spinal cord is now seen as a control site, not just as a passive part of the final common pathway (40). Local influence is mediated by the monosynaptic stretch reflex, the spinal cord control of reciprocal enervation, and convergence of afferent and efferent tracts on spinal cord interneurons.

The muscle spindle monitors muscle *length* and acts on the anterior horn cell via the stretch reflex. When a muscle is stretched quickly, such as by tapping just below the kneecap, the muscle spindle is also stretched. This produces the **stretch reflex** that fires monosynaptically to make the tapped muscle contract.

Local spinal cord control also occurs in the form of reciprocal enervation. **Reciprocal enervation** produces reciprocal movement by making the muscles on one side of a joint contract, while the muscles on the other side of the joint relax. Reciprocal enervation is controlled locally by spinal cord "half-centers" (41). These centers are networks of interneurons between flexor and extensor motoneurons that have a mutually inhibitory function (Fig. 6.1).

Finally, instructions coming down from higher centers via the efferent tracts, and input coming up from the periphery via the afferent tracts converge on spinal cord interneurons (37). Descending commands from the pyramidal tracts, extrapyramidal tracts, and excitatory brainstem nucleii have to be weighed against ascending feedback from the muscle spindles, Golgi tendon organs (GTO), joint receptors, cutaneous receptors, vestibular receptors, visual receptors, and auditory receptors. Local input via the stretch reflex and "half-centers" have to be weighed. Whether the final message given to the alpha-motor neuron is facilitory or inhibitory depends on the summation of all the messages converging on the spinal cord interneurons.

SUMMARY

You must understand the assumptions of the NDT frame of reference to understand the contributions of this frame of reference. The assumptions include the concepts of distributed motor control, skill acquisition, sensory input during feedforward and feedback, postural control, normalizing muscle tone, and brain plasticity. You also need to understand the three deficits that are addressed by NDT. This will make you aware that this frame of reference is limited to axial control, automatic reactions, and limb control.

Finally, you need to understand the neurophysiology of motor control to understand why NDT works. NDT inhibition techniques are used to modify the excitatory effects of the stretch reflex, spinal half-centers, and tonically active subcortical facilitory tracts on resting muscle tone. Our handling will inhibit these abnormal excitatory influences until plasticity permits recovery. Our handling also helps the patient initiate normal movements. As the patient pays attention to normal proprio-

ceptive, tactile, vestibular, visual, and auditory input, the extrapyramidal system regains the ability to smoothe out and suppress unwanted movements. This will eventually enable the patient to run normal preprogrammed movements in feedforward mode, using the cerebellum. Plasticity of the sensory-motor strip is the tip of the iceberg when it comes to recovery through NDT.

STUDY QUESTIONS

1. What is the value of studying normal motor development?
2. What is the difference between an open and closed task?
3. What is the difference between feedforward and feedback?
4. NDT says what type of sensory input is crucial for motor learning? What type of sensory input does NDT ignore?
5. Why is postural control important?
6. How does muscle tone differ in mildly vs. severely involved brain-injured patients?
7. What is "fixing," and when is it seen?
8. What is dangerous about facilitating weak muscles in brain-injured patients?
9. Name four mechanisms that make brain recovery possible.
10. What contribution does axial control, automatic reactions, and proximal limb control make to motor control?
11. Name the three major levels for motor control.
12. How is bilateral trunk involvement possible in hemiplegia?
13. What are the two functions of the extrapyramidal system?
14. Subcortical control of muscle tone is influenced by what type of input?
15. What is alpha-gamma coactivation?
16. How is reciprocal enervation controlled locally?

References

1. Reed KL. Models of practice in occupational therapy. Baltimore: Williams & Wilkins, 1984.
2. Horak FB. Assumptions underlying motor control for neurologic rehabilitation. In: Contemporary management of motor control problems: Proceedings of the II Step Conference. American Physical Therapy Association, 1991:11.
3. Adams M. Bobath certification (8-week) course. Memphis, TN, 1982.
4. Brunnstrom S. Movement therapy in hemiplegia. Philadelphia: Harper & Row, 1970.
5. Bly L. A historical and current view of the basis of NDT. Pediatric Physical Therapy, 1991;3:131.
6. Stockmeyer SA. Overview of current motor control theories. NDT Northeast Regional Conference. Providence, RI, 1993.
7. Keshner EA. How theoretical framework biases evaluation and treatment. In: Contemporary management of motor control problems: Proceedings of the II Step Conference. American Physical Therapy Association, 1991:37.
8. Craik RL. Recovery process: maximizing function. In: Contemporary management of motor control problems: Proceedings of the

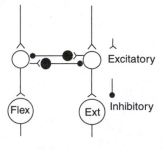

Figure 6.1.

II Step Conference. American Physical Therapy Association, 1991:175.

9. Carr JK, Shephard RB, eds. Movement science: foundations for physical therapy in rehabilitation. Rockville, MD: Aspen Publications, 1987.

10. Sabari JS. Motor learning concepts applied to activity based intervention with adults with hemiplegia. Am J Occup Ther 1991; 45:523.

11. Higgins JR, Spaeth RK. Relationship between consistency of movement and environmental conditions. Quest 1972;17:61.

12. Smyth, MM: Memory for Movements. In: Symth MM, Wing AM, eds. The psychology of movement. San Diego: Academic Press, 1984:83–117.

13. Bernstein NA. The coordination and regulation of movements. New York: Pergamon, 1967:127–134.

14. Bly L. Motor control and more. NDT Northeast Regional Conference. Providence, RI, 1993.

15. Bobath B. Adult hemiplegia: evaluation and treatment. 2nd ed. London: William Heinemann Medical Books Limited, 1978.

16. Roy EA, Diewert GL. Encoding of kinesthetic extent information. Perception & Psychophysics 1975;17:559.

17. Voss DE, Ionta MK, Myers BJ. Proprioceptive neuromuscular facilitation. 3rd ed. Philadelphia: Harper & Row, 1985.

18. Carpenter MB. Human neuroanatomy. 7th ed. Baltimore: Williams & Wilkins, 1976:287.

19. Gowitzke BA, Milner M. Scientific basis of human movement, 3rd ed. Baltimore: Williams & Wilkins, 1988:255.

20. Sahrmann SA, Norton BJ. The relationship of voluntary movement to spasticity in the upper motor neruone syndrome. Ann Neurol 1977;2:460.

21. McLellan DL. Cocontraction and stretch reflexes in spasticity during treatment with baclofen. J Neurol Neurosurg Psychiatry 1977;40:30.

22. Milner-Brown HS, Penn RD. Pathophysiological mechanisms in cerebral palsy. J Neurol Neurosurg Psychiatry 1979;42:606, 616.

23. Knutsson E, Richards C. Different types of disturbed motor control in gait of hemiparetic patients. Brain 1979;102:405.

24. Norkin CC, Levangie PK. Joint structure and function. Philadelphia: FA Davis, 1989.

25. Lee WA. Broughton A, Rymer WZ. Absence of stretch reflex gain enhancement in voluntarily activated spastic muscle. Exper Neurol 1987;98:317.

26. Tardieu C, Lespargot A, Tarbary C, et al.: For how long must the soleus muscle be stretched each day to prevent contractures? Dev Med Child Neurol 1988;30:3.

27. Tang A, Rymer WZ. Abnormal force-EMG relations in paretic limbs of hemiparetic human subjects. J Neurol Neurosurg Psychiatry 1981;44:690.

28. Zoltan B, Pedretti LW. Evaluation of muscle tone and coordination. In: Pedretti LW, Zoltan B, eds. Occupational therapy practice skills for physical dysfunction. 3rd ed. St. Louis: CV Mosby, 1990:132.

29. Bohannon RW, Larkin PA, Smith MB, Horton MG. Relationship between static muscle strength deficits and spasticity in stroke patients with hemiparesis. Phys Ther 1987;67:1068.

30. Fetters L. Cerebral palsy: contemporary treatment concepts. In: Contemporary management of motor control problems: Proceedings of the II Step Conference. APTA, 1991:219.

31. Neito-Sampedro M, Cotman CW. Growth factor induction and temporal order in CNS repair. In: Cotman CW, ed. Synaptic plasticity. New York: Guilford Press, 1985:407–455.

32. Moore JC. Recovery potentials following CNS lesions: a brief historical perspective in relation to modern research data on neuroplasticity. Am J Occup Ther 1986;40:459, 461.

33. Milner B. Sparing of language function after early unilateral brain damage. Neurosci Res Prog Bull 1974;12:213.

34. Powers W. Functional neuroanatomy. Graduate course at Boston University, Boston, 1978.

35. Barnes MR, Crutchfield AC, Heriza CB. The neurological basis of patient treatment. Vol. II: Reflexes in motor activity. Morgantown, WV: Strokesville Publishing, 1978.

36. Lehmkuhl LD, Smith LK. Brunstrom's clinical kinesiology. 4th ed. Philadelphia: FA Davis, 1983.

37. Vander AJ, Sherman JH, Luciano DS. Human physiology—the mechanisms of body function. 4th ed. New York: McGraw-Hill, 1985:685.

38. Trombly CA. Motor control therapy. In: Trombly CA, ed. Occupational therapy for physical dysfunction. 3rd ed. Baltimore: Williams & Wilkins, 1989:72.

39. Gilman S, Newman SW. Manter and Gatz's essentials of clinical neuroanatomy and neurophysiology. 7th ed. Philadelphia: FA Davis, 1987.

40. Craik RL. Abnormalities of motor behavior. In: Contemporary management of motor control problems: Proceedings of the II Step Conference. APTA, 1991:155.

41. Jankowska E, Lundberg A. Interneurones in the spinal cord. Trends Neurosci 1981;4:320.

CHAPTER 7

Neurodevelopmental Treatment Evaluation Critiqued

If you can't see it and you can't feel it, you can't treat it with NDT! Unlike other approaches, the Bobath approach does not tell you specifically what to do with your hands. You must know what the result should look like and feel like to tell you if your handling is correct. The extensive discussion that follows should help you understand what NDT-certified therapists look at and what they feel when they assess movement.

Evaluation is a good place to teach new terminology. NDT jargon is often misunderstood because it makes us look at our patients in a way that is very different from the biomechanical frame of reference. Classic NDT terms will be defined throughout this chapter.

Procedures that assess axial control, automatic reactions, and limb control come from three different sources: (a) formal evaluation tools, (b) clinical observation, and (c) normal developmental trends. These evaluation procedures are still evolving, and each one solves only part of the puzzle. References are given when procedures are already described in the literature. Detailed descriptions are provided when no other resource is available.

REFLEX DEVELOPMENT

Abnormal reflex development is commonly seen in children with brain damage, such as cerebral palsy. It is rarely seen in adult patients. If adult patients have abnormal tonic and phasic reflexes, they quickly disappear. Therefore, reflex development is primarily discussed in the pediatric literature.

Reflexes have three essential characteristics (1). First, they can produce realignment of the head and limbs but do not move the body through space. For example, the ATNR can move the arms and legs into a fencer position. Second, they are triggered by outside stimuli, like a noise making an infant turn his/her head to look for the sound. Third, these reflex movements are stereotyped but never obligatory in normal infants. The stimu-

lus always produces the same predictable movement or posture, but with repetition, the reflex loses its ability to provoke a response. Tonic reflexes are considered to be normal as long as they disappear at the appropriate time and are not obligatory.

Procedures for reflex evaluation have been published in numerous texts. However, many of these sources cite Fiorentino's *Reflex Testing Methods for Evaluating CNS Development* (2). Her text is well organized and beautifully illustrated. It provides pictures of test positions, test stimuli, and positive and negative responses.

Remember that reflexes become inhibited gradually. If you feel or see an inconsistent or weak response, it probably means that higher centers are gradually inhibiting the spinal cord and brainstem reflexes. However, just because you observe a weak or inconsistent reflex doesn't make it clinically significant. Clinical observation of voluntary movements is necessary to assess the influence of reflexes at this final stage of recovery.

The decision tree process needs to be applied to defuse your anxiety when you see the long list of reflexes. This list can be broken down into small groups that have varying significance. *Oral reflexes*, such as the rooting, gag, and suck reflexes, are vital only if you are heavily involved in feeding and speech issues. *Neonatal reflexes* such as Stepping Reactions and the Galant Reflex are fascinating, but their clinical significance is unknown. *Phasic reflexes*, like the Moro, Flexor Withdrawal, and Crossed Extension, need to be formally assessed only when they produce strong motor responses that consistently interfere with evaluation and early treatment.

However, *tonic reflexes*, like the Asymmetrical Tonic Neck, the Symmetrical Tonic Neck, the Tonic Labyrinthine, the Positive Supporting, the Palmar Grasp, and the Plantar Grasp, need to be routinely evaluated in children. These tonic reflexes can linger for long periods of time in brain-damaged children and have devastating effects. They can impede motor development and produce severe deformities that eventually interfere with autonomic functions like breathing. In brain-damaged adults, they are rarely seen or are present in a mild version once the coma lifts.

AUTOMATIC REACTIONS

Essential Characteristics

Righting reactions have three essential characteristics (1). First, righting reactions are initiated by the person for a purpose instead of by outside stimuli. Second, movement produced by the reaction facilitates movement through space like rolling. Third, the movement is a "chain reaction" that cannot be stopped in mid-sequence. For example, once you start rolling you may roll off the bed because you can't stop. Righting reactions persist for life and become incorporated into equilibrium reactions rather than becoming inhibited, like tonic reflexes.

Righting reactions are confusing because there are so many kinds. Some of them have more than one name. I have divided them into vertical and rotary types. Vertical righting reactions enable us to move away from a vertical orientation to the ground and then safely return. They are our first line of defense when we want to safely move within a posture without falling. Vertical righting reactions include optical and labyrinthine righting. **Optical righting** is tested with the eyes open and it returns the head to a vertical upright position. Optical righting is often called **vertical head righting**. Labyrinthine righting produces the same head adjustment, but is tested with vision occluded. Labyrinthine righting is rarely tested because tilting patients with their eyes closed is very threatening.

Rotary righting reactions enable us to twist body parts out of alignment from the longitudinal axis of the body and then return to a symmetrical alignment. The ability to untwist is very helpful when we use rotation to make a transition from one posture to another, like sitting up on the edge of the bed. Rotary righting includes **neck righting** which enables us to **log-roll,** and **body righting,** which enables us to **roll segmentally**.

Equilibrium reactions and protective extension have three essential characteristics (1). First, these reactions enable a person to quickly prevent or minimize falls without having to think about it. Second, the person can stop the movement anywhere in the sequence. For example, a person can stop in mid-roll as soon as the hand touches the alarm clock. Third, the movement can be modified for each new situation. For example, coaches teach football players to suppress protective extension so they can concentrate on catching the ball instead of putting out their hand to break their fall.

Test Modification

The Fiorentino book is the best resource for learning the administrative and scoring protocols for automatic reactions (2). However, procedures for testing equilibrium reactions may have to be modified. It is especially difficult to keep brain-damaged children from falling off the tilt board. To prevent accidents, therapists have modified tilt-board procedures. One modification involves getting on the tilt board to hold the child and determining if his/her response matches your normal response. This type of physical assistance limits the therapist's ability to interpret the results. Only the potential for a normal response can be reported since you don't know if the patient would have actually fallen. At least it gives you a baseline estimate so you don't have to report that the patient was untestable. Be sure to report any modifications you make.

It is dangerous to evaluate rotary righting in adults by twisting their heads to make them roll. Therefore, I have added the Derotative Procedure (3) to righting reactions during rolling on the clinical observation sheet (see Table 7.1). This procedure involves turning the patient from supine to prone by holding onto the legs. If the patient does not log-roll (i.e., he/she leaves the shoulder girdle behind on the mat), axial tone is usually very low. This is an early warning sign that neck and body righting will be delayed. Rolling onto the sound side is the most important way to evaluate rolling in a stroke patient. This elicits retraction of the hemiplegic arm and leg while the sound side is pinned underneath the body.

Evaluation of equilibrium reactions in adult patients is especially difficult. Adult-size balls and bolsters are available, but they are even more unstable and difficult to control than tilt boards if you have a severely impaired adult patient. Adult patients are usually tested sitting on a matt table or standing. Initially, the patient is gently moved away from vertical while the therapist holds the shoulders. If the patient can tolerate this, distal segments, like the lower leg, can be used. Using the distal body parts produces a more valid response because they stress the patient more and therefore have the most potential for eliciting a visible automatic reaction. While the use of distal body parts blocks abduction of the uphill leg, it also gives the therapist something to hang onto if the patient starts to fall.

Scoring Patient Performance

Automatic reactions have traditionally been scored as present or absent. Clinical observations provide a more sensitive scoring system for automatic reactions (4). It is essential to evaluate *all* of the movement strategies that make up a quality response (see Table 7.1).

Table 7.1.
Neurodevelopmental Clinical Observations

Yes = patient is able to perform	No = patient is not able to perform
PA = physical assistance (max/mod/min)	I = independent
± = partial performance	NT = Not Tested

Sits Symmetrically:
_____ Head in midline & erect
_____ Shoulder height is even: R > ? < L (circle 1)
_____ Neutral pelvic tilt
_____ Equal weight on both hips: R > ? < L
_____ Symmetrical hip abduction: R > ? < L
_____ Both feet flat on floor

SUBLUXATION: _____ fingers wide on _____ side
_____ Scapula downwardly rotated
_____ Lateral trunk flexion _____ side
_____ Arm internally rotated/pronated

AUTOMATIC REACTIONS WHILE ROLLING: Choose only one!
_____ No log-roll during LE Derotative procedure (trunk is flaccid)
_____ Log-rolls upper body during LE Derotative procedure
_____ Log-rolls using unsafe arching and limb retraction (Neck Righting)
_____ Log-rolls safely with neck, shoulder, and hip flexion (Neck Righting)
_____ Segmentally rolls but can't stop roll, even at edge (Body Righting)
_____ Can stop segmental roll at any point in space (Equilibrium Reactions)

LE EXTENSION SYNERGY DURING ADLs IN SITTING: P = Present   A = Absent
_____ Resists external rotation when legs cross or foot rests on opposite knee
_____ Resists knee flexion when crossing hemiplegic leg over sound leg
_____ Knee extends so hemiplegic foot rests in front of sound foot on floor
_____ Resists hip flexion when patient tries to touch hemiplegic foot on floor
_____ Resists ankle dorsiflexion when trying to put shoes on

PLACING REACTION of _____ arm:
_____ Arm in RIP at side
_____ Arm in RIP diagonally
_____ Arm in front of body

EQUILIBRIUM IN SITTING: tilt to

Left	Right
_____ Vertical head righting	_____
_____ Trunk elongation of weightbearing side	_____
_____ Rotation w/posterior tilt	_____
_____ Abduct uphill arm/leg	_____

ACTIVE WEIGHT SHIFT IN SITTING:
_____ Lean forwards with (circle 1) anterior/neutral/posterior tilt
_____ Lean 1/3 way back towards supine with (circle 1) posterior/neutral/anterior tilt
Higher functioning patients:
_____ Sideways to R/trunk elong
_____ Sideways to L/trunk elong
_____ Active trunk rotation to R
_____ Active trunk rotation to L

ECCENTRIC CONTROL of _____ arm:
_____ Lower arm at side of body
_____ Lower arm diagonally
_____ Lower arm in front of body

PROTECTIVE EXTENSION IN SITTING:

Left	Right
_____ Vertical head righting	_____
_____ Lateral trunk flexion of weightbearing side	_____
_____ Rotation w/anterior tilt	_____
_____ Extend downhill arm/leg	_____

Patients often have some quality movements while lacking others. Each movement component should be individually scored as present, impaired, or absent (+, ±, −). This profile of assets and deficits enables you to treat each patient's specific need for automatic reactions.

Trunk elongation is an important characteristic that distinguishes an equilibrium response from protective extension (see Table 7.1). **Trunk elongation of the weightbearing side** is the NDT solution to the confusion about the two sides of the trunk. Right and left change, depending on whether you are facing or sitting next to the patient. Auto mechanics solved a similar problem by referring to the driver's and passenger's side of a car.

The Bobaths identified the weightbearing side of the trunk by first identifying the limb that bears the most weight. For example, if you lean to your right side while sitting, you put more weight on your right hip and thigh. If the trunk on the same side as your right weightbearing leg becomes longer, you exhibit trunk elongation of the weightbearing side. However, if the trunk on the same side as the right weightbearing leg becomes shorter, you exhibit **lateral trunk flexion**. Trunk lateral flexion is a part of a protective extension response rather than an equilibrium response, so it is important to know which of the two axial strategies the patient is using in order to score these two automatic reactions correctly.

It is often difficult to see whether the trunk is getting longer or shorter because adult patients wish to remain fully dressed. To make it even harder, patients often use rigid fixing when they are tilted off balance. This restricts their automatic reactions to very small movements instead of the large movements shown in textbooks.

I recommend watching the shoulder on the weight-bearing side. If the SHOULDER on the weightbearing side goes UP, the trunk is elongating. If the SHOULDER on the weightbearing side goes DOWN, the trunk is shortening (see Fig. 7.1). Sometimes you can see fat rolls form on the side that is shortening if the patient has his/her shirt off.

Pelvic tilt is another characteristic that distinguishes equilibrium reactions from protective extension (see Table 7.1). Posterior tilt is associated with an equilibrium reaction, while anterior tilt is associated with protective extension (4). **Anterior pelvic tilt** is defined as a forward movement of the anterior superior iliac spine (ASIS). It is produced by a **force couple,** which is two muscles pulling in opposite directions to create a rotary movement (5). The force couple for anterior tilt involves the low back extensors pulling up and the hip flexors pulling down on the pelvis (see Fig. 7.2). **Posterior pelvic tilt** is defined as a backwards movement of the ASIS. The force couple for posterior tilt involves the hamstrings pulling down and the abdominals pulling up on the pelvis.

Pelvic tilt is even harder to see than trunk elongation because patients who fix exhibit only a small range of motion unless tilted far enough to actually fall. Again, I recommend watching the shoulders. When the pelvis tilts, the center of gravity is disturbed, so the patient pulls his/her SHOULDER(s) in the OPPOSITE direction from the PELVIS to use his/her trunk as a counterweight to keep from falling.

The patient's trunk must be tilted *behind* vertical to observe the following shoulder movements. When you tilt the patient straight backwards until the trunk is *behind* vertical, you know the patient is using posterior

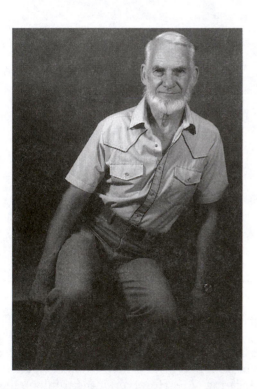

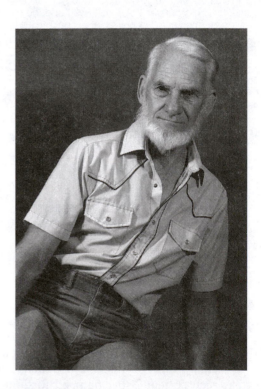

Trunk Elongation

1. The shoulders don't catch your eye because they remain level—*BUT:*
2. The left shoulder has moved up relative to the left hip to produce trunk elongation of the weightbearing side and
3. The right shoulder has moved down toward the right hip to produce trunk shortening of the non-weightbearing side.
4. Note the full hip hiking on the non-weightbearing side. This response is not always this pronounced. You may have to slide one hand under this hip to feel if hip-hiking is present.

Lateral Trunk Flexion

1. Now the shoulder on the weightbearing side catches your attention. The left shoulder has moved down towards the left hip to produce trunk shortening of the weightbearing side.
2. The right shoulder has moved up relative to the right hip, BUT the trunk elongation is not as pronounced as the elongation shown in the left hand picture because the right hip has also hiked upwards.

Figure 7.1.   Trunk elongation (*left*) and lateral trunk flexion (*right*).

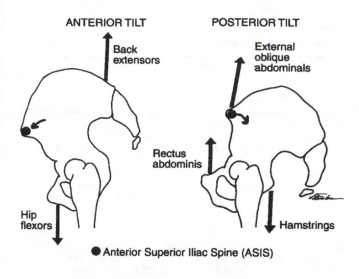

ANTERIOR TILT

Back extensors

Hip flexors

POSTERIOR TILT

External oblique abdominals

Rectus abdominis

Hamstrings

● Anterior Superior Iliac Spine (ASIS)

Figure 7.2 Force couples for pelvic tilt.

pelvic tilt if BOTH SHOULDERS move FORWARD. However, when tilted diagonally backwards, the shoulders respond asymmetrically. When you tilt the patient diagonally backwards until the trunk is *behind* vertically, you know the patient is using posterior tilt if the SHOULDER on the WEIGHTBEARING side moves FORWARD. Conversely, when the SHOULDER on the WEIGHTBEARING side moves BACKWARDS, the patient is using anterior tilt and is prepared to use protective extension in the arm that is thrown backwards (see Fig. 7.3). If you're not sure what the patient is doing, imitate the patient's shoulder motions and weight-shift to feel what your pelvis is doing.

Decision Tree Process

The decision tree process also needs to be applied to the long list of automatic reactions. If you test every patient for every automatic reaction, you may spend too much time evaluating this skill. It helps if you prioritize

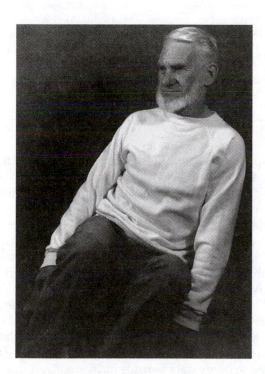

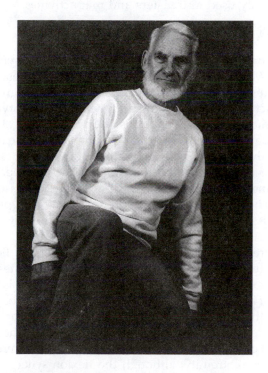

Posterior Pelvic Tilt

1. Because the shoulder on the weightbearing side (*left*) has moved forward relative to the right shoulder, we know that the pelvis has tilted in the opposite direction (i.e., backward).
2. Note the trunk rotation.
3. Imagine both arms coming forward to help pull the body back up to midline.

Anterior Pelvic Tilt

1. Because the shoulder on the weightbearing side (*left*) has moved backward relative to the right shoulder, we know that the pelvis has tilted in the opposite direction (i.e., forward).
2. Note the trunk rotation.
3. Imagine the left arm reaching for the floor to break his fall (i.e., protective extension).

Figure 7.3. Posterior (*left*) and anterior (*right*) pelvic tilt.

the list. *Early righting reactions,* like neonatal body righting, the Amphibian Reaction, and the Landau, are most commonly used in early intervention programs for infants.

Other automatic reactions can be tested only in *high-level patients.* Labyrinthine righting requires blindfolding, which is too dangerous with most patients. Equilibrium on all-fours and kneel-standing are also difficult to do safely with a low-functioning adult unless you have two strong people to support the patient. Protective extension may be too dangerous for patients with even average recovery. The patient must be pushed off balance QUICKLY and FORCEFULLY to assess if the response is FAST enough and POWERFUL enough to actually slow down a real fall. Few patients recover quick, powerful arm extension on the hemiplegic side.

However, vertical righting in the form of optical righting, rotary righting reactions, and equilibrium in sitting and standing should *routinely be evaluated.* These tests are very important because they tell us how safe it is to move a patient within and between postures that are commonly used in transfers and mat activities.

EVALUATION OF SYNERGY

Brunnstrom described how to evaluate limb synergies in *Movement Therapy in Hemiplegia* (6). These are **pathological synergies** in which several muscle groups contract together to produce a primitive, stereotyped, mass movement. There is no isolated movement of one body part, like the wrist moving alone. If even one muscle in the group is activated, all the other muscles are also recruited. The Bobaths call this lack of separate movement of two adjacent body parts a **lack of dissociation.** The Brunnstrom procedure evaluates both proximal dissociation of scapula, shoulder, and elbow and distal dissociation of forearm, wrist, and fingers.

There are two types of pathological synergies: flexor and extensor. The flexor synergy usually dominates the upper extremity, although the extension synergy is also present in the arm. This UE flexor dominance is probably due to the repeated concentric and eccentric contractions of the flexor muscles needed to raise and lower the arm against gravity. The extensor synergy usually dominates the lower extremity, although the flexion synergy can also be seen in the leg. This LE extensor dominance is probably caused by the repeated concentric and eccentric contractions of the extensor muscles needed to straighten and bend the leg while walking. The essential characteristics of these two synergies are listed in Table 7.2. It helps to memorize this table so you know what positions to avoid during early treatment.

Patients rarely exhibit the full range of motion for every movement. For example, one patient with the flexion synergy may be able to fully flex her elbow but

Table 7.2.
Pathological Synergies

Upper Extremity (UE) Synergies	
UE Flexion Synergy	*UE Extension Synergy*
1. Scapular elevation	1. Some scapular protraction
2. Shoulder abduction to 90°	2. Can adduct arm across chest
3. Shoulder external rotation	3. Shoulder internal rotation
4. Elbow flexion to an acute angle	4. Elbow extension
5. Full supination	5. Full pronation
6. Wrist usually flexed	6. Wrist usually extended
7. Fingers flexed	7. Fingers often flexed

UE Flexion Variations

1. Scapular elevation/shoulder abduction replaced with scapular retraction and shoulder hyperextension. All other components are the same as listed above under UE Flexion Synergy.
2. Shoulder external rotation/supination replaced with internal rotation and pronation. All other components are the same as listed above.

Lower Extremity (LE) Synergies	
LE Flexion Synergy	*LE Extension Synergy*
1. Hip ABduction	1. Hip ADDuction
2. Hip flexion	2. Hip extension
3. Hip external rotation	3. Hip internal rotation
4. Knee flexion to 90°	4. Knee extension
5. Ankle dorsiflexion	5. Ankle plantarflexion
6. Toe dorsiflexion	6. Toe plantarflexion although big toe may extend

not supinate at all, while another patient can only flex his elbow 45° but is able to fully supinate. The Brunnstrom scoring protocols are designed to detect these individual differences. In Stage 3, estimates of active range are recorded such as ''½ range'' or ''about 90°.'' These estimates enable the therapist to identify the overactive muscles that need inhibition and their weaker antagonists that need facilitation. It is especially important to identify which version of the UE flexion synergy is present. The shoulder abduction/supination, shoulder abduction/pronation, and shoulder extension variations require slightly different Reflex Inhibiting Patterns (discussed in Chapter 8). Learning how to gather detailed synergy data permits individualized treatment rather than a cookbook approach.

Brunnstrom's protocol sheet (6) is rarely seen in its original form because many clinics have incorporated her procedures into a general evaluation packet. These packets usually omit the instructions for administration and scoring. Since these instructions have been lost over the years, they are listed in Tables 7.3. Be sure to replicate the movements for Stage 4 and 5 exactly as they are written. These movements gradually introduce components of both the flexion and extension synergies. For

Table 7.3A.

Hemiplegia—Classification and Progress Record—Chart 1

Upper Limb—Test Sitting

Name _____ Age _____ Date of onset _____ Side affected _____
Date

_____ Passive motion sense, shoulder _____ elbow _____
_____ pron.-supin. _____ wrist flex.-ext. _____
_____ 1. No movement initiated or elicited _____
_____ 2. Synergies or components first appearing. Spasticity developing _____
_____   Flexor synergy _____
_____   Extensor synergy _____
_____ 3. Synergies or components initiated voluntarily. Spasticity marked _____

	Flexor Synergy	Active Joint Range		Remarks
_____ Shoulder girdle	Elevation			
_____	Retraction			
_____ Shoulder joint	Hyperextension Abduction			
_____	Ext. rotation			
_____ Elbow	Flexion			
_____ Forearm	Supination			
Extensor Synergy				
_____ Shoulder	Pectoralis major			
_____ Elbow	Extension			
_____ Forearm	Pronation			
_____ 4. Movements deviating	Hand to sacral region			
from basic synergies	Raise arm forw.-horiz.			
_____ Spasticity decreasing	Pron.-supin. elbow at 90°			
_____ 5. Relative independence	Raise arm side-horiz.			
of basic synergies	Raise arm over head			
_____ Spasticity waning	Pron.-supin. elbow extended			

6. Movement coordination near
   normal. Spasticity minimal

example, raising the arm above 90° of abduction requires shoulder abduction from the flexor synergy and elbow extension from the extension synergy. Other motions, like placing the hand on the sacral area, include movements that are not a part of either synergy. Patients often exhibit characteristics of two adjacent stages. This is recorded as Stage 2/3, 4/5, etc.

As occupational therapists, we need to assess the effect of lower extremity synergies on ADLs. ADLs involve greater range of motion than gait, particularly hip external rotation and flexion. Rather than using Brunnstrom's leg procedures, I recommend using the procedures listed on the clinical observation sheet (see Table 7.1).

MUSCLE TONE EVALUATION

Four methods have been developed to evaluate muscle tone:

1. Manual assessment of resistance to passive motion;
2. Mechanical devices, such as strain gauges, to measure resistance to passive motion;
3. Visual observation of restrictions in active movement;
4. Electromyography (EMG) to assess the electrical activity of muscles during movement.

Mechanical devices and EMG machines are very reliable, but the time needed to calibrate the equipment and perform a thorough evaluation is unrealistic for the clinic.

Table 7.3B.

Instructions for Administering Brunnstrom's Synergy Evaluation

Stage 1. NO MOVEMENT INITIATED OR ELICITED. Passively move the extremities through the actual synergy patterns. There should be no resistance to passive movement. Then ask the patient to assist you. No active motion should be felt.

Stage 2. SYNERGIES FIRST APPEAR. Passively move the extremities through the actual synergy patterns. Now you will feel resistance. Ask the patient to assist you. Now you should feel some active movement.

Stage 3. SYNERGIES INITIATED VOLUNTARILY. Demonstrate the full synergy pattern. Ask the patient to imitate it. Estimate how much range is exhibited for each motion (e.g., 1/2 range). If any motions are missing, demonstrate that motion specifically and ask the patient to imitate you.

Stage 4. MOVEMENTS DEVIATING FROM BASIC SYNERGIES. Ask the patient to imitate each motion. Raise the arm forward until it is horizontal to the floor with the elbow fully extended. Perform pronation and supination bilaterally. Full ROM, not speed, is emphasized in this alternating motion.

Stage 5. RELATIVE INDEPENDENCE. When patient raises arm over head, arm is forwards in full shoulder flexion with the elbow fully extended. During pronation/supination with elbow extended, the arm may be held in the forward-horizontal or side-horizontal position.

Stage 6. MOVEMENT COORDINATION NEAR NORMAL. Some spasticity may emerge during quick active movements. No synergies are present, but some awkwardness may be noted.

Page 2. SPEED TESTS. The fist must touch both chin and knee. One stroke equals one round trip. The forearm is held in neutral.

Page 2. WRIST STABILIZATION FOR GRASP. Watch for wrist flexion when the elbow flexes which would interfere with retrieval of objects.

Page 2. WRIST FLEXION AND EXTENSION. Performed with fist closed around an object. Watch for finger extension when the wrist flexes (unwanted tenodesis).

Page 2. WRIST CIRCUMDUCTION. Elbow is stabilized against trunk with forearm in pronation to prevent elbow and forearm substitution.

Page 2. GRASP. Release is not required to pass the hook grasp, but it is required to pass for lateral prehension up to spherical grasp.

Page 2. INDIVIDUAL THUMB MOVEMENTS. Hand is in patient's lap with forearm resting in neutral position. Wiggle extended thumb up and down for vertical motions and side-to-side for horizontal motions.

Page 2. OTHER SKILLED ACTIVITIES. Examples: writing, threading a needle.

The muscle tone procedure used in this text assesses spasticity by evaluating resistance to passive motion. This procedure requires the therapist to record separately (a) the amount of resistance felt and (b) where in the range the resistance is first felt. The test items, administrative procedures, and scoring criteria are listed in Table 7.4. Each specific passive motion that elicits resistance is circled. For example, if wrist extension is circled, this would mean that the wrist flexors are tight. This notation system is identical to goniometry forms where a lack of full elbow extension indicates a contracture of elbow flexors.

Unlike passive ROM goniometry, the examiner estimates where in the range the resistance is first felt, not whether the patient has full range of motion. To estimate where in the range resistance is first felt, you must know the norms for full range of motion. These are listed in parentheses in Table 7.4. Only estimates of where resistance is first felt are recorded, such as "at mid-range" or "about 90°". Recording the exact degrees of motion is not reliable because of subject variability. Muscle tone can vary slightly because of room temperature, pain, fear, and fatigue. Of course, if the resistance you feel is due to fixed contractures rather than spasticity, you should indicate that on the muscle tone form.

One study found that muscle tone varied within a single session for the large joints of children with cerebral palsy. The smallest variation in hip motions was 5°, and the readings commonly varied by 10°(7). Another study concluded that a difference of ±10° to 15° in large joints, such as the shoulder and elbow, is not a significant indication of change in children with cerebral palsy (8). Variable spasticity could explain the low inter-rater reliability found in a study of adults with hemiplegia. Worley et al. asked two therapists who immediately followed each other to measure where they first felt resistance by reporting exact degrees measured with a goniometer (9). The inter-rater reliability coefficient was .60 (see Appendix) for degrees of shoulder motion and .52 for degrees of wrist motion.

However, inter-rater reliability was moderate when therapists were asked to *estimate where* in the range resistance was first felt (10). The correlation between different raters estimates was .847. In another study, subjective *estimates of how much* resistance was felt were made during passive ankle motions (11). These subjective estimates were compared to units of torque recorded by a mechanical device during the passive ankle motions. The correlation was .84.

Even though slow passive elongation is generally safe, there are three instances where passive elongation may not provide a reliable indication of muscle tone. Adult patients often resist passive elongation of the neck, trunk, and pelvis. Invasion of these three private body zones and a fear of falling may make the patient try to protect him/herself by fixing.

Adult patients tend to resist passive neck and trunk movements. Instead, ask the patient to look up, down, and to both sides. If active neck range is incomplete,

Table 7.3C.
Hemiplegia—Classification and Progress Record, p. 2

Upper Limb—Test Sitting—Chart 1, continued

Name _____

Date

_____ SPEED TESTS for classes 4, 5, 6   <u>Strokes per 5 sec.</u>

| | Hand from | Normal | _____ _____ |
| _____ | lap to chin | Affected | _____ _____ |

| | Hand from lap | Normal | _____ _____ |
| _____ | to opposite knee | Affected | _____ _____ |

_____ Passive motion sense, digits _____

_____ Fingertip recognition _____

_____ Wrist stabilization for grasp   1. Elbow extended _____
                                             2. Elbow flexed _____

_____ Wrist flexion and extension   1. Elbow extended _____
        fist closed   2. Elbow flexed _____

_____ Wrist circumduction _____

DIGITS

_____ Mass grasp _____   Dynamometer test   Normal _____ lb.
                                                                                   Affected _____ lb.

_____ Mass extension _____

_____ Hook grasp (handbag, 2 lb.) _____

_____ Lateral prehension (card) _____

_____ Palmar prehension (pencil) _____

_____ Cylindrical grasp (small jar) _____

_____ Spherical grasp (ball) _____ catch _____ throw _____

_____ Indiv. thumb movements hands   1. Vertical movements _____
        in lap ulnar side down   2. Horizontal movements _____

_____ Individual finger movements _____

_____ Button and unbutton shirt   Using both hands _____
                                        Using affected hand only _____

_____ Other skilled activities _____

---

gently assist the patient to complete the motion and note any resistance. To evaluate muscle tone of the trunk, you may have to use active assistive weight shifts. Note the amount of resistance and where in the range you felt it.

Adult patients also tend to resist passive pelvic tilt. They find it difficult to understand verbal instructions or even visual demonstration. It is easier to get a patient to permit active, assistive pelvic tilt if you coordinate your manipulation of the pelvis with looking, leaning, and breathing. Start by standing in front of the patient who is sitting with his/her sound hand resting on your shoulder. Have the patient look up at the ceiling, take a deep breath and lean forward while you step backwards and use your flattened hands in the small of his/her back to pull the pelvis forward. Then have the patient look down at his/her navel, blow out, and lean back behind vertical while you step forward and gently push on the ASIS to make the pelvis tilt posteriorly.

If you block the patient's movement by standing still yourself or pump the patient's pelvis out of synchrony with breathing, looking, and leaning, it is much more difficult to get the patient to follow your lead.

Note that movement of the scapula cannot be assessed in degrees. The normal scapula elevates 10 to 15 cm (6). The normal scapula protracts 13 to 15 cm (6), unless the person has developed a resting position that rounds the shoulders forwards. When it isn't practical to expose the patient's back to measure scapular movement directly, you can estimate scapular movement by measuring how far the humerus moves. Find a clothing seam or make an X high on the side of the patient's shoulder. Use a ruler to estimate how many centimeters the seam or X moves. This will give you an estimate of where in the range resistance is first felt during scapular motions.

Finally, a full cephalocaudal evaluation of muscle tone is essential for individualized treatment planning.

Table 7.4.
Muscle Tone Evaluation

Name: _____   Date: _____

SLOWLY move body part passively from zero position. *STOP* as soon as you feel resistance. Estimate where in the range you stopped (e.g., about 90°). Estimate how much resistance you feel by going beyond where resistance started.

Minimal	= therapist easily moved body part beyond point of resistance
Moderate	= therapist moved body part past initial resistance by moving slowly and with effort; patient may experience discomfort
Maximal	= therapist is unwilling to use the full force needed to break through resistance; patient will definitely experience discomfort

CIRCLE RESISTED MOTION	Where Resistance First Felt	Min/Mod/Max
lateral flex R (0°–45°)		
lateral flex L (0°–45°)		
Neck flexion (0°–45°)		
R (0°–60°)		
Neck rotation L (0°–60°)		
posterior		
Pelvic tilt anterior		
R		
Trunk elongation L		
R		
Trunk rotation L		
depression (3 cm)		
Scapular elevation (4″)		
Scapular protraction (4″)		
Shoulder flexion (0°–170°)		
Shoulder abduction (0°–170°)		
Scap upward rota. starts at 30°		
horz. ADduction (0°–40°)		
Sh. horz. ABduction (0°–130°)		
internal (0°–90°)		
Sh. rota. external (0°–90°)		
flexion (0°–135°)		
Elbow extension (0°–135°)		
pronation (0°–90°)		
Forearm supination (0°–90°)		
flexion (0°–80°)		
Wrist extension (0°–70°)		
CMC Abduct (0°–50°)		
Thumb CMC exten. (0°–50°)		
MP flexion (0°–90°)		
Finger IP flexion (0°–110°)		
knees bent		
Hip flexion (0°–120°)		
internal (0°–45°)		
Hip rota. external (0°–45°)		
flexion (0°–135°)		
Knee extension (0°–135°)		
plantarflexion (0°–50°)		
Ankle dorsiflexion (0°–15°)		

Using a few muscle groups to sample muscle tone assumes that patients are generally spastic or flaccid, which is false. Mixed muscle tone in brain-damaged patients is the rule rather than the exception. You need to know specifically which muscles to inhibit, which to facilitate, and which muscles are already close to normal.

DEFICITS IGNORED BY FORMAL EVALUATIONS

The clinical observations listed in Table 7.1 were generated by the NDT approach (4). They include observation of sitting symmetrically, axial weight shifts, placing and eccentric control, and shoulder subluxation that are ignored by formal assessments.

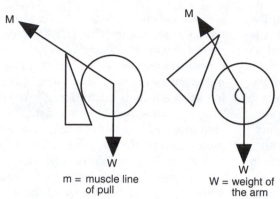

On the left, the scapula is slightly upwardly rotated. The rotator cuff muscles easily hold the head of the humerus on an inclined ramp.

On the right, the scapula is downwardly rotated so the humerus no longer sits on an incline ramp. The angle between lines M and W approach 180° so the two forces cancel each other out by pulling in opposite directions. Now the humerus falls out of the socket.

m = muscle line of pull

W = weight of the arm

Figure 7.4. Subluxation = downward rotation of the scapula.

Assessment of symmetrical sitting can be done visually except for "equal weight on both hips." This characteristic is often difficult to assess by visual inspection alone. It helps to physically lift each buttock to feel if one hip is easier to lift than the other.

Be prepared to offer some physical assistance during active weight shifts in sitting. The patient can have full passive elongation of trunk muscles and still not be able to independently initiate axial weight shifts. Note that axial weight shifts forwards and backwards require observation of pelvic tilt.

Shoulder subluxation is also ignored by formal assessments. **Shoulder subluxation** is a visible separation of the glenohumeral joint. It is reported by how many fingers fit into the gap between the scapula and the head of the humerus. For example, you might be able to get three fingers into this space. Subluxation has several causes. Until you know which cause is operating in a particular patient, treatment of subluxation cannot be individually prescribed.

Subluxation can be caused by downward rotation of the scapula. Downward rotation of the scapula can be caused by paralysis of any of the muscles that make up the force couple for upward rotation. This force couple includes the upper and lower trapezius and serratus anterior. These muscles constantly contract to produce SLIGHT upwards rotation which is the normal resting position of the scapula. This position allows the head of the humerus to rest on an inclined ramp (see Fig. 7.4). However, when the scapula rotates downward, the head of the humerus gets dumped out of its socket (see Fig. 7.4).

Fortunately, you can detect downward rotation very early by measuring the distance between the inferior and superior angles of the scapulae. If the distance between the two superior angles is shorter than the distance between the two inferior angles, the scapulae are upwardly rotated. If the reverse is true, they are

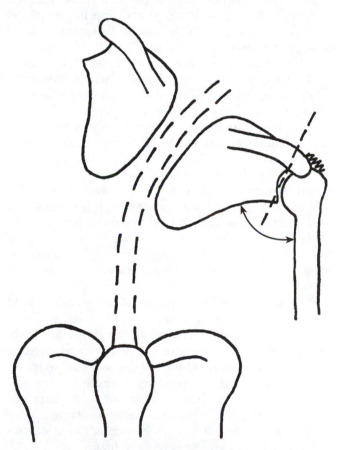

Lateral trunk flexion abducts the humerus (see *arrow* on medial side of humerus). Now the coracohumeral ligament is slack and no longer helps hold the humerus in the glenoid fossa.

Lateral trunk flexion also downwardly rotates the scapula (see *dotted line* through shoulder joint). Now the rotator cuff muscles no longer hold the head of the humerus on an included ramp.

RESULT = SUBLUXATION

Figure 7.5. Subluxation = lateral trunk flexion.

downwardly rotated. Even if the distance between the superior angles is equal to the distance between the inferior angles, the scapula is not upwardly rotated as it should be.

Subluxation can also be caused by paralysis of the rotator cuff muscles. These horizontal muscles are responsible for holding the heavy humerus in the very shallow glenoid fossa (5). They have a better mechanical advantage than the vertical deltoid group when it comes to keeping the head of the humerus on the inclined ramp of the upwardly rotated scapula.

Downward rotation of the scapula can also be caused by consistent shortening of the trunk on the involved side while sitting. This encourages the head of the humerus to fall out of the socket (see Fig. 7.5).

Subluxation is enhanced by shoulder internal rotation. Unfortunately, internal rotation is part of the normal resting position of the dependent arm (hanging) or supported arm (e.g., on a lapboard). The glenohumeral ligament, which is a horizontal ligament in front of the joint, is taut only when the arm is externally rotated (see Fig. 7.6). Slack in this ligament eliminates one of the important sources of structural stability in the shoulder joint. Internal rotation is not easy to see, so use the **shoulder-forearm link**. Shoulder and forearm rotation are always linked except when the elbow is flexed at 90° and tucked against the side of the trunk (5). When the arm is not in this position, internal shoulder rotation is associated with pronation. It is easier to see the hand turn palm down than to see the humerus roll. The peg shown in Figure 7.6 partially supinates the forearm, which in turn partially externally rotates the humerus and puts the glenohumeral ligament on stretch.

Placing is the ability to quickly stop a motion to hold a position and then to quickly move again to a new position (4). **Eccentric control** is the ability to slowly and smoothly lower an extremity. Placing and eccentric control make an extremity feel light and easy to move. Note that the first test position for both placing and eccentric control is with the arm out to the side and above shoulder height (4). This position is farthest from the position preferred by both synergies, so early dissociated movement will be seen here first.

NORMAL GROSS MOTOR TRENDS

Normal gross motor development has been divided into four trends. Each trend shows how normal children mature from primitive to transitional to mature behavior. Each stage has its own essential characteristics, which you should memorize.

The essential characteristics of normal motor trends are important because they identify the movement strategies that your patient is using. These movement strate-

gies are not made clear on even well-accepted developmental assessments. The ability to recognize these movement strategies is what makes a therapist different from other team members who can only report whether motor milestones were passed or failed. Even therapists working with adults need to observe normal motor trends. These trends supplement the data from passively evaluated muscle tone. The essential characteristics of normal motor trends pinpoint the active movement strategies you want your patient to relearn.

The essential characteristics for each stage are listed at the top of every motor trend sheet. Study these motor sheets until you can readily identify the different movement strategies during developmental test items and informal observation of functional movements. Circle the primitive, transitional, or mature box or individual movement strategies observed during each test item.

Developmental ages for motor milestones have been included simply to validate the sequence of maturation. These developmental ages should also remind therapists who are working with adult patients that many of the motor skills that require retraining normally develop in the first three years of life.

Gross Motor Trend I

This trend is entitled ''Hypotonic to Strong Axial Flexion.'' The essential characteristics are listed in Table 7.5. The primitive stage is called ''physiological flexion.'' This refers to the tightly flexed limbs of full-term newborns due to the prolonged flexion of the fetus in the uterus. This limb tightness is accompanied by hypotonic axial flexors.

Neck flexors are hypotonic and elongated during physiological flexion because their antagonist is shortened. Normal infants are born with shortened neck extensors because prenatal myelinization favors early enervation of the upper trapezius (12). We normally think of the upper trapezius as elevating the scapula, but it can also hyperextend the neck by **reverse action**. Reverse action occurs when the distal attachment stays still while the proximal attachment pulls the head back. The lower trapezius, which opposes the upper trapezius by pulling down on the scapula, is not myelinated in normal infants until 6 months of age (12). Brain-damaged adults often exhibit this same sequence of recovery: scapular elevation, which is part of the flexion synergy, leaves the upper trapezius unopposed.

Abdominals are also hypotonic and elongated during physiological flexion because their antagonists are shortened. The hip flexors and low back extensors are tight at birth. These two muscle groups constitute the force couple for anterior tilt. Anterior tilt stretches out the abdominals, which gives them a poor mechanical

Since the arm naturally hangs and rests on armrests in internal rotation/pronation, the therapist must position the arm to make this ligament at least partially taut. This increases structural stability of the shoulder joint and assists the rotator cuff to prevent subluxation.

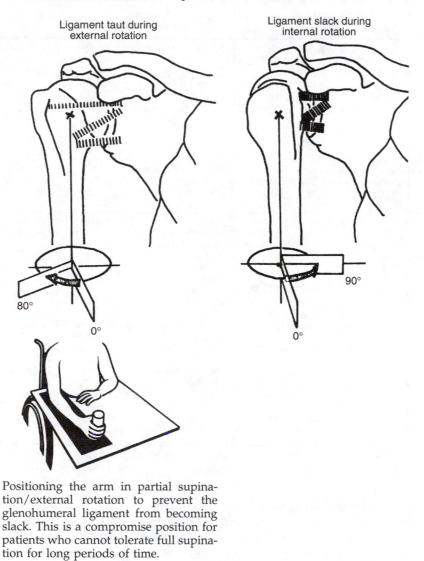

Positioning the arm in partial supination/external rotation to prevent the glenohumeral ligament from becoming slack. This is a compromise position for patients who cannot tolerate full supination for long periods of time.

Figure 7.6. Glenohumeral ligament.

advantage. While brain-damaged adults may or may not have tight hip flexors and low back extensors, they never develop spasticity of the abdominals.

Normal infants strengthen their abdominals by playing with their legs in supine. However, these leg lifts that recruit the abdominals cannot be performed until the hamstrings begin to elongate. Hamstring tightness is present at birth in normal full-term infants. Hamstring tightness can be seen in the Heel-to-Ear Procedure (3). This procedure pulls on the hamstrings by stretching them over both joints that they cross (i.e., extending the knee while flexing the hip). To get relief from this painful

stretch, the infant posterior-tilts the pelvis to give the hamstrings some slack over the hip joint, since the examiner won't permit any slack over the extended knee. Hamstring tightness is brief in normal infants. When it is prolonged, it prevents infants from doing leg lifts in supine with knees straight to play with their legs, which strengthens their abdominals.

Modifications for adults must be used to assess axial flexion (see Table 7.6). Pull-to-sit, which is the time-honored way to assess neck flexors in children, is too stressful for adults. An adult's head weighs too much. Hemiplegic patients may also have shoulder subluxa-

Table 7.5.
Gross Motor Trend I: Hypotonic to Strong Axial Flexion

Pediatrics	Physiological Flexion = NO![a]	Emerging Axial Flexion	Mature Axial Flexion
Essential Characteristics → Test Procedures ↓	1. Arms and legs are tightly flexed 2. Tight neck/low back extensors and hamstrings 3. Neck flexors and abdominals are hypotonic and elongated ↓	1. Arms and legs are partially flexed 2. Emerging elongating of neck/low back extensors and hamstrings 3. Emerging tone in neck flexors and abdominals ↓	1. Arms/legs now fully extended 2. Full elongation of neck and low back extensors and hamstrings 3. Graded control of neck flexors and abdominals ↓
Tight Neck Extensors Block Neck Flexion	Resistance to passive neck elongation felt at beginning of range in supine 0–2 mo	Resistance to passive neck elongation not felt until mid-range in supine 3 mo	No resistance to passive neck elongation anywhere in range 4 + mo
Neck Flexors Activate	Pull-to-sit: full head lag (behind shoulders) 0–3 mo	Pull-to-sit: head held in a line with elevated shoulders 4 mo	Pull-to-sit: head flexed in front of depressed shoulders 5+ mo
Tight Hamstrings Prevent Leg Raises Used to Strengthen Abdominals in Children	Heel-to-Ear: pelvis lifts off bed as soon as heels are in a line with naval during passive leg raising 0–3 mo	Heel-to-Ear: pelvis lifts off bed as soon as heels are in a line with nipples during passive leg raising 3–6 mo	Heel-to-Ear: pelvis lifts off bed as soon as heels are in a line with neck during passive leg raising 6–9 mo
Abdominals Activate to Produce Posterior Pelvic Tilt	Supine: BUE/BLE tightly flexed; low back arched; abdominals elongated 0–3 mo	Supine: actively lifts legs; raises pelvis off bed to touch knees 4 mo	Supine: actively lifts legs; raises pelvis off of bed to touch feet 5 + mo

[a]NO = Not recommended for treatment! Not safe for brain-damaged patients.

tion, which makes pulling on the arms dangerous. Lowering to supine from sitting while holding onto both shoulders is safer and less frightening. Even many normal adults cannot perform a full sit-up independently, so abdominal strength should be assessed with the lowering-to-supine procedure. How far back the patient can lean is only one criterion for evaluating abdominals. Leaning back in sitting with the pelvis in neutral or anterior pelvic tilt also indicates abdominal weakness. Leaning back in sitting with visible axial fixing or reaching for support also constitutes poor abdominal control.

Elongation of tight neck extensors can be evaluated in the adult patient, but the Heel-to-Ear Procedure is omitted for adult patients because even most healthy adults would fail this test. Normal adults don't maintain this level of flexibility because they don't have to long-leg sit as part of their daily routine. However, normal adults should have enough slack in their hamstrings to be able to sit in a chair without having to tilt the pelvis posteriorly! Brain-damaged adults often have spastic

hamstrings, which makes them sit with posterior tilt to relieve the painful stretch on their tight hamstrings. See "sit symmetrically" in Table 7.1 for evaluation of posterior tilt due to hamstring tightness in sitting.

Gross Motor Trend II

This trend is called "Flexor to Extensor Tone." The primitive stage of this trend and Trend I are the same. From the common beginning of "physiological flexion," the normal infant develops mature flexion and extension in equal amounts. However, brain-damaged patients often lack this normal balance, so flexors and extensors have to be evaluated with two separate trends. During the primitive stage extensor tone is present in the neck and low back but absent in the thoracic region. Extension develops later in the thoracic region of the trunk. This is an exception to the cephalocaudal development of extensor tone seen in the limbs.

The transition phase of this trend is called "extension with retraction" because of the retraction of the head,

Table 7.6.
Adult Modifications of Gross Motor Trends

Gross Motor Trend I: Hypotonic to Strong Axial Flexion			
Neck Flexors Activate	Lower-to-Supine: brief or no head control	Lower-to-Supine: head held in a line with elevated shoulders	Lower-to-Supine: head flexed in front of depressed shoulders
Abdominals Activate	Lower-to-Supine: loss of trunk control during 1/3 way back	Lower-to-Supine: controls trunk for 1/3 way back with _____ tilt	Lower-to-Supine: controls trunk for 2/3's way back; posterior tilt
Gross Motor Trend II: Flexor to Extensor Tone			
Lean on One Elbow	Places elbow on mat but arm is easily moved in a circle by the OT; hand is fisted	Puts full weight on elbow with cues but scapula elevates/retracts; hand is loosely fisted	Spontaneously puts full weight on elbow; scapula depressed/ protracted; hand is open
Lean on One Extended Arm	Places hand on mat but arm is easily moved in a circle by the OT; hand fisted	Puts full weight on hand with cues but scapula elevates/retracts; hand is loosely fisted	Spontaneously puts full weight on hand; scapula depressed/protracted; hand is open
Sitting to Test Axial Extension	Sits supported: head completely sags forward; rounded back; hand is fisted	Sits unsupported: head forward but steady; only upper trunk extended; scap. elevated; hand loosely fisted	Sits unsupported: head erect/steady; full trunk extension; scapula depressed; hand is open
Standing to Test LE Extension	Stands supported: hips & knees flexed; takes most of weight; hand is fisted	Stands supported: knees extend BUT hips flex; trunk leans forward; hand loosely fisted	Stands supported: BLE fully extend so feet are directly under trunk; hand open
Gross Motor Trend IV: Mobility Superimposed on Stability			
Reach on One Elbow	Reach on elbow: collapses onto trapped arm	Reach: scap. elevates/retracts; elbow is not directly under shoulder	Reach: scap. is depressed/ protracted; elbow is directly under shoulder
Reach on Extended Arm	Reach on extended arm: collapses onto elbow	Reach: scap. elevates/retracts; hand is not directly under shoulder	Reach: scapula is depressed/ protracted; hand directly under shldr
Sitting	See Clinical Observations for Axial Weight Shifts in Sitting		
Walking	Pulls self up to standing with _____ P.A.; leans heavily on UE's	Sits down smoothly holding onto support Steps sideways during walking pivot transfer Walks with _____ P.A. & _____ aids; leg circumduction; foot drop; wide base	Walks independently with _____ aids; stops; only with advance notice Walks with reciprocal elbow swing Walks safely: makes sudden stops/ turns

scapula, and pelvis. The essential characteristics are listed in Table 7.7. Neck hyperextension and scapular elevation combine to give the characteristic look of "no neck." **Hands loosely fisted** means the MP joints are in neutral position while the PIP and DIP joints are still flexed. This produces weightbearing on the heel of the hand, the thenar eminence, and the knuckles, but not on the center of the palm.

Extension with retraction is a safe transitional stage for normal infants, but it quickly disappears as flexion emerges to balance extensor activity. It is very dangerous for brain-damaged patients because they get stuck in this stage. They refuse to give up this transitional strategy because it gives them the ability to hold a posture stiffly. Extension with retraction quickly leads to neck, shoulder, and pelvic blocks.

The last stage of Gross Motor Trend I is called "mature extension." It includes neck elongation. **Neck elongation** is a classic NDT term that means the back of the neck becomes long. It is different from full neck flexion, where the chin rests on the sternum so the patient looks down at his/her stomach. Neck elongation is important because it produces just enough chin tucking to permit the eyes to gaze down at the hands (see Fig. 7.7). It is different from **jaw-jutting,** where the neck hyperextends but the chin juts forward so the head is in front of the body. Jaw-jutting often goes undetected because it allows the patient's eyes to look straight ahead at the therapist rather than at the ceiling, as in classic neck hyperextension. We all jaw-jut when we put our elbows on the table and rest our chins on our hands. Don't be fooled by the direct eye

Table 7.7.
Gross Motor Trend II: Flexor to Extensor Tone

Pediatrics	Physiological Flexion = NO![a]	Extension with Retraction = NO![a]	Mature Extension
Essential Characteristics → Test Procedures ↓	1. Neck/lumbar extensors are shortened BUT thoracic extensors are floppy! 2. Scap elevators and retractors short 3. Hips flexed and widely ABducted 4. Elbows/knees are fully flexed 5. Hands are tightly fisted ↓	1. Neck hyperextends 2. Scap retracts/elevates during active movement 3. Trunk hyperextends except in sitting 4. Hips retracted; flexed; ABducted to sh width 5. Elbows/knees now partially extend 6. Hand: loose fists ↓	1. Neck elongated; trunk extended except in prone 2. Scap depressed and protracted when shoulder is 0°–60° 3. Hips do not retract; fully extend and ADduct 4. Elbows/knees fully extended 5. Hands open ↓
Prone on Elbows	Prone: Weightbear on FACE: hands are fisted; BUE/BLE are flexed 1 mo	Neck hyperextends; scap elevat/retract; weight on asymmetrically ABducted FOREARMS; hands are loosely fisted; legs flex and ABduct beyond sh width 2–3 mo	Neck elongated; scap depressed and protracted; weight on ADducted ELBOWS so chest is off floor; hands open; legs ABducted less than sh width 4 mo
On All-Fours	Unable to maintain all-fours position	Neck hyperextended; scap elevated; stomach sags; hands loosely fist; knees widely ABducted 6 mo	Neck elongated; scap depressed; back erect; hands open; knees less than sh width 7 mo
Sitting to Test Axial Extension	Sits supported with fully rounded back: —Head sags 0–1 mo —Head bobs 2 mo —Head held forward but steady 3 mo	Sit propped on arms: head erect, steady; scap elevated 4–6 mo Sit supported: only upper back extends; loose fists 4–6 mo	Sits independently: full back extension; neck elong; arms free; hands open 7 mo
Standing to Test LE Extension	Supported: refuses to bear weight or takes some weight 3–4 mo Supported: takes most of weight, but hips and knees flex; positive supporting; UE's flex; hands fisted 5 mo	Stands supported: knees extended BUT hips flexed so trunk leans forward; feet flat on floor; hands loosely fisted 9 mo	Stands supported: BLE fully extended so feet are directly under trunk; feet flat; hands open 10 mo

[a]NO = Not recommended for treatment! Not safe for brain-damaged patients.

contact that jaw-jutting affords the patient in sitting and standing.

Most adults have to be evaluated for mature extension of the arms while weightbearing on one elbow or on one extended arm in side-sitting on a mat table (see Table 7.6). They often won't tolerate the prone on elbow position and are too heavy for one therapist to support while on hands and knees. If the patient can't laterally flex the trunk enough to get his/her elbow down to the mat, try providing one or two pillows or your lap to lean on. The adult patient's feet are usually left on the floor to reduce the fear of falling. However, this extra support makes it possible for the patient to place the elbow or hand on the mat table without actually putting any weight on it. Check for weightbearing by trying to move the elbow or hand around in a small circle. You'll be surprised at how many patients are just placing that extremity without actually putting any weight on it.

Gross Motor Trend III

This trend is called "Hand/Foot Preparation." Lack of hand and foot preparation is primarily a pediatric concern. The essential characteristics are listed in Table 7.8. Normal infants progress to full palmar and plantar contact because they actively seek out stimuli. They spend hours chewing on their feet and mouthing their fists to desensitize hands, feet, and mouth. This sensory input inhibits tactile defensiveness and primitive palmar and plantar reflexes. Brain-damaged children usually avoid this sensory input and often lack the motor skills needed to produce it.

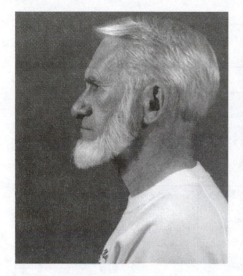

Head in Neutral Position

There is no neck flexion or extension. This position is excellent for walking, talking, and driving because it directs the gaze straight forward.

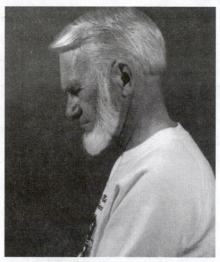

Neck Elongation

See how the neck flexes just enough to tuck the chin and make the back of the neck into a long, straight line. This position is essential for hand function because it directs the gaze slightly downward.

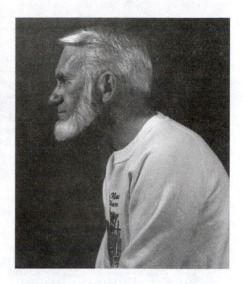

Jaw-Jutting

See how the neck extends while the jaw juts forward so the head is in front of the body. This position directs the gaze forward instead of up toward the ceiling like classic neck hyperextension does. Note the rounded posture of the upper back. Jaw-jutting does not promote mature axial extension.

Figure 7.7. Head in neutral position (*left*); neck elongation (*middle*); jaw-jutting (*right*).

Full weightbearing and hand function cannot develop normally if palmar/plantar contact is not present. Normal infants bear weight on the thenar eminence in prone for 3 months before thumb use is seen in grasp. Weightbearing stretches out physiological flexion of the hand and inhibits the grasp reflex. This sequence shows how gross motor experiences pave the way for fine motor skills. Surely, brain-damaged patients can benefit from this weight-bearing experience. Remember, while standing encourages plantar contact, sitting discourages palmar contact.

Gross Motor Trend IV

This trend is called "Mobility Superimposed on Stability." The essential characteristics are listed in Table 7.9. The primitive stage of holding a posture is NOT recommended for treatment! While normal infants work briefly on maintaining static postures, brain-damaged patients use this opportunity to rigidly fix. Static postures produce only a momentary increase in muscle excitation followed by hanging on elongated muscles in poor postural alignment. Think of how hard it is for you to sit up straight with no back support for extended periods of time.

It is much safer to go on to the transitional phase called "linear weight shift." The first characteristic of this stage is **tiny weight shifts within a posture**. The term should really be MINIATURE because these motions are initially so small that they are not visible from a distance. Even close up, you will see no movement unless you watch carefully. Miniature motions are less likely to frighten the patient and make it possible to impose movement from the very beginning of treatment.

Grady and Gilfoyle call weight shifts within a posture "bilateral linear sets" (1). They are symmetrical movements of two or four extremities whose distal segments are fixed on the support surface. The proximal segments, like the shoulders and hips, move in mid-ranges to produce a linear weight shift, like rocking on all-fours.

However, evaluation of "bilateral linear sets" cannot be done in adult patients. The combination of poor motor control and large body size makes it difficult for one therapist to safely handle an adult patient in a symmetrical position, e.g., on all-fours. Even the prone-on-elbows position is a problem because so many elderly patients cannot tolerate lying on their stomachs. For adults, I recommend asking for miniature weight shifts

Table 7.8.
Gross Motor Trend III: Hand/Foot Preparation[a]

Pediatrics	No Palm/Heel Contact	Emerging Contact	Prolonged Contact
Essential Characteristics → Test Procedures ↓	1. Weightbear on ulnar border of fisted hand; lateral border or ball of foot 2. Reflexes prevent P/H contact 3. Persistant defensive responses to P/H contact	1. Weightbear on thenar eminence of loosely fisted hand; foot intermittently flat 2. Fading reflexes permit some P/H contact 3. Brief defensive responses to P/H contact	1. Full and prolonged P/H contact 2. Palmar/plantar reflexes fully integrated 3. Easily tolerates touch/pressure on palm and heel
Weightbear on Hands	Prone on forearms: weight on *ulnar* border of fisted hands 2 mo On extended arms: weight on fisted hands 4 mo Sitting propped on extended arms: weight on *ulnar* border of fisted hands 6 mo	LFH: MPs neutral, but PIP/DIPs flex Prone on elbows: wt on *thenar* eminence of LFH 3 mo On extended arms: wt on *thenar* eminence of LFH 5 mo Sitting propped on extended arms: weight on *thenar* eminence of LFH 7 mo	On extended arms: weight on open hands with thumb extended 6 mo On all-fours: rocks over fully extended thumb and fingers 7 mo
Hand Play	Fisted hand in mouth 0–2 mo	Plays with own hands in midline 3 mo	Palm to mouth 6 mo
Grasp Reflex	Grasp reflex retains objects in hand 3–4 mo	Light touch on fingertips: drops object 5 mo	Grasp reflex fully integrated 5–7 mo
Avoidance Response	Light moving touch on back of hand/ulnar border/fingertips produces finger extension 1–2 mo	Only light touch on fingertip produces finger extension 3–4 mo	Avoidance response integrated so that voluntary release can emerge 6 mo
Feet in Supine	Feet off of floor 0–2 mo	Soles often touch each other 3 mo	Feet frequently in mouth 5 mo
Weightbear on Feet	Prone: only sides of feet contact floor 0–5 mo	Crawl: pushes with both feet 6 mo	Plays in side-lie stabilizing with the flat foot 7 mo
Positive Supporting Reflex	Tonic version of reflex prevents full plantar contact 3–5 mo	Phasic version while bouncing in standing supported 6–8 mo	No reflex while holding onto furniture 9 mo

[a]Abbreviation P/H = palmar/heel. LFH = loosely fisted hand.

over the hemiplegic elbow or extended arm in side-sitting while reaching with the sound hand (see Table 7.6).

The second characteristic of the transitional stage is **lateral weight shifts**. This side to side movement strategy is essential for freeing one limb. You must first shift the weight off one limb and transfer all the weight onto the other limb if you want to pick up an arm or leg. If a patient is still weightbearing on both arms or both legs, you will be unable to get him/her to reach for an object or take a step (see Tables 7.6 and 7.9).

The third transitional strategy is **linear transitional movements**. These movements enable us to move between postures. At this stage, transitional movements are basically linear. The ability to get up onto hands and knees, to sit up, and to stand up develops first. The ability to carefully lower oneself with graded eccentric control develops second (see Tables 7.6 and 7.9).

Locomotion using lateral weight shift is the last transitional strategy to be acquired. It can be seen in three motor milestones (see Table 7.9). One is belly-crawling like a soldier with lateral trunk. "Fish-tailing" on all-fours is another. This motion looks like true creeping, but it is performed with lateral trunk flexion instead of trunk rotation. It can be identified by the wide side-to-side swings of the pelvis, just as a trailer swings behind a car. The third milestone is walking with lateral trunk flexion and the feet wide apart. When children walk with lateral weight shifts, we call it "toddling." When adult patients walk this way, we call it a wide-based gait. See Table 7.6 for age-appropriate test items for adults.

The mature phase of mobility superimposed on stability is called "mobility with rotation." The Bobaths used **rotation** to mean rotation-counter-rotation where the shoulder and pelvic girdles rotate in opposite directions. Drop a pencil on the floor to the right of your body while sitting. If you reach for it with your left hand, you will feel your pelvis rotating backwards to keep you from falling out of your chair.

Rotation is the foundation skill that makes reciprocal limb movement possible and gives a mature gait its

Table 7.9.
Gross Motor Trend IV: Mobility Superimposed on Stability

Pediatrics	Hold a Posture: Not used in Rx!	Linear Weight Shifts	Mobility with Rotation
Essential Characteristics ⟶ Test Procedures ↓	1. Repeatedly tries to assume and hold a posture 2. Limbs rigidly fix to support body while trunk exhibits visible undulations 3. Lowers self by suddenly collapsing ↓	1. Tiny weight shifts within a posture 2. Lateral weight shifts to free one limb 3. Assumes new posture using linear weight shifts 4. Lowers self with graded control 5. Locomotion using lateral weight shifts ↓	1. Assumes new posture with axial rotation 2. Locomotion with reciprocal limb movements and axial rotation ↓
Prone on Elbow	Briefly pushes up onto ABducted elbow, then collapses 2–3 mo Reaches: falls onto trapped arm 4 mo	Reach: supporting elbow stays directly under shoulder; scap depressed 6 mo Symmetrical commando crawl 6 mo	Stable playing in side-lie 7 mo Reciprocal belly crawling with trunk rotation 7 mo
On All-Fours	Briefly pushes up onto extended arms and collapses 4 mo Briefly assumes all-4's/collapses 6 mo	Rocks on all-4's 7 mo Reach on one extended arm: doesn't elevate scap or collapse onto elbow 7 mo Creeps on all-4's: pelvis fishtails 8 mo	Bear-walks on hands and feet 8 mo Reciprocally creeps on all 4's; knees ADducted 10 mo
Sitting	Placed in sitting: —Briefly props on extended arms 6 mo —Sits erect with visible trunk undulations 7 mo —Sits erect and steady for 10+ mins 8 mo	Reaches by shifting weight onto one extended arm 7 mo Sits up by pushing with hands 7 mo Leans forward and re-erects without using hands 8 mo	Sitting: rotates to reach behind 8 mo Plays in side-sit 9 mo Pivots in a circle while sitting 10 mo
Standing	Pulls self to stand leans heavily on UE; LEs stiffly extend 9 mo	Squats smoothly holding onto support 11 mo Walks sideways while supported 11 mo Staggers alone: high arm guard; lunges at support to stop 12 mo	Walks independently and stops with advance notice 15 mo Walks with reciprocal elbow swing 21 mo Walks safely: makes sudden stops/turns 2 yr

natural beauty and confidence. Rotation is difficult to see during locomotion because it occurs in such small ranges. It is easier to see the reciprocal movements of the extremities that accompany it. Adult patients are not expected to perform mobility with rotation while weightbearing on the arms, like creeping on hands and knees. See Table 7.6 for appropriate test items for adults.

Gross Motor Trend II, Mobility Superimposed on Stability, needs to be evaluated in several postures. You will see mature strategies in lower postures like prone, while higher postures like standing will still be dominated by primitive strategies. If time does not permit you to test every position, you must not assume that the response you saw in one position is typical of other positions.

NORMAL FINE MOTOR TRENDS

The test items for the fine motor (FM) trends were pulled from developmental assessments. They are helpful for patients who are not yet able to perform adult-level fine motor tasks, like writing and buttoning. In FM Trends II and III, the cube tasks require standard 1-inch cubes. The pellet task can be done with any small object such as a bent paper clip. The spoon task can be done without food. The pencil task is restricted to drawing straight lines or a circle. The 9-Hole Pegtest can be used instead of difficult pegs like the thin brads used in the Purdue Pegtest.

Fine Motor Trend I

This trend is called "Mass to Dissociated Movement." If your adult patient can follow verbal directions, you don't need to use Fine Motor Trend I. Like the Brunnstrom procedure, it assesses independence from synergy and proximal dissociation. However, Brunnstrom's procedures are often too difficult for children and confused adults. Synergies can instead be observed by watching how patients reach for an object. The essential characteristics are listed in Table 7.10.

This trend documents only upper extremity dissociation. The few developmental milestones that focus on lower extremity dissociation include: kicks reciprocally in supine (2 months), runs one foot up and down opposite leg (4 months), and kicks with hip extension and knee flexion in prone (4 months). Reciprocal movement represents dissociation of one leg from the other. The ability to simultaneously use hip extension and knee flexion indicates freedom from pathological limb synergy.

Fine Motor Trend II

This trend is called "Static Ulnar to Radial Grasp." This trend represents distal dissociation. Initially, the

Table 7.10.
Fine Motor Trend I: Mass to Dissociated Movement

Synergy Bound: NOT USED IN TREATMENT!		Emerging Independence from Synergy		Independence from Synergy	
1. UE dominated by flexion synergy 2. Movement initiated by large, poorly graded proximal muscle groups		1. Partial freedom from synergy 2. Emerging distal timing as proximal stability emerges		1. Simultaneously performs components of flexion/extension synergies 2. Full distal dissociation	
Reach for Object	Scapula	Shoulder	Elbow	Forearm	Wrist
Unable to reach 0–2 mo	Fully elevated at rest	Arms stiffly folded next to body (arm recoil present when arm is pulled)		Stiffly pronated	Fully flexed
Unilateral ASTN swipe at side of body 3 mo	Elevation only while reaching	Wide horizontal ABduction and then fleeting shoulder flexion	More than 100° of elbow flexion	Fully pronated	Fully flexed
Bilaterally corral object 5 mo	No elevation	Some horizontal ABduction then 60° of sustained shoulder flexion	Lacks only 10°–15° of elbow extension	Partial pronation	Fully flexed
Unilateral circular reach 6 mo	No elevation	No horizon. ABduct; shoulder flexion to 90°	Full elbow extension	Forearm in neutral	Wrist in neutral
Unilateral direct reach 8 mo	No elevation	No horizon. ABduct; shoulder flexion to 90°	Full elbow extension	Forearm in neutral	Wrist in extension

hand works like a mitt, with the ulnar side of the hand being the primary contact point with objects. With maturation, the thumb, index, and middle fingers become dissociated from the hand and are able to contact objects. Grasp is initially achieved with the palm and all the fingers and later with just the tips of the radial fingers. Note that this trend only assesses static grasp. Release of objects and reaching are ignored by this trend.

The adult terms for mature prehension are listed at the bottom of Table 7.11. The adult terminology, like three-jaw chuck, only provides a present/absent scoring strategy. This can be a problem if your patient never achieves a mature type of prehension or if you need to document small changes in a short period of time. If you continue to report that a patient does not have a three-jaw chuck, it is hard to justify the need for therapy. The pediatric terms (13) identify transitional strategies and are therefore more sensitive to small changes.

Fine Motor Trend III

This trend is called "Distal Fixing to Distal Dissociation." The essential characteristics are listed in Table 7.12. It shows even more clearly than Fine Motor Trend I that the forearm, wrist, and fingers develop isolated distal movements. However, distal dissociation is preceded by rigid fixing of distal body segments. Note that during the transition phase, the patient must use a source of external support to make emerging forearm and wrist movements possible. In the mature stage, distal mobility is made possible by internal stability of proximal structures like the scapula. For a compilation of appropriate fine motor items for adults, see Table 7.13.

DECISION TREE REVISITED

An experienced therapist can perform a complete NDT evaluation in half an hour. However, even a half-hour evaluation may not be realistic. This half-hour window may be too long for an acutely ill patient. A half-hour is certainly not long enough for students who need extra time when they are first learning. When time constraints are present, use the decision tree process to decide what to test first.

A good place to start is the Brunnstrom synergy evaluation (page 1 only). This short procedure quickly enables you to grade down for the patient who is flaccid or synergy-bound and grade up for the patient who is in relative recovery. Remember, Fine Motor Trend I is the pediatric version of UE synergy evaluation.

The following clinical observations should also be done very early: sits symmetrically, active weight-shifts in sitting, shoulder subluxation, automatic reactions while rolling, and LE extension synergy during ADLs. You will have to move the patient in bed or during transfers and ADLs, so early awareness of potential dangers while moving the patient is essential.

If a patient is in Brunnstrom stages 1, 2, or 3, you must grade down by selecting tests that evaluate lower-level skills. Evaluate muscle tone. If the patient is spastic, the muscle tone results will tell you which specific motions are likely to be painful as you handle the patient during ADLs. If the patient is flaccid, the muscle tone evaluation will tell you where spasticity and contractures are emerging. Be sure to also evaluate Gross Motor Trends II and III since they measure the need for physical assistance in static postures. If the adult patient is in a coma, you need to consider evaluating tonic reflexes.

If a patient is in Brunnstrom stages 4 or 5, you can grade up. Clinical observation of the following procedures is now possible: placing reactions, eccentric control, and equilibrium in sitting and standing. Remember, only very high-functioning patients regain sufficient speed and power to perform the protective extension test. Administer Gross Motor Trends I and IV, which challenge the patient with weight shifts. To test distal dissociation, administer Fine Motor Trends II and III or the distal portion of the Brunnstrom evaluation (page 2 only).

If a patient is in Brunnstrom stage 6, coordination is near normal, which makes a manual muscle test (MMT) possible. However, irradiation makes a MMT inappropriate for lower-functioning brain-damaged patients. If a patient has spasticity, the therapist recruits more muscles as the patient tries harder and harder to resist during MMT. The test results simply prove that maximal resistance can facilitate many inappropriate muscles through irradiation. MMT is also inappropriate for brain-injured adults who have pathological limb synergies. A patient with a pathological synergy cannot perform the isolated motions required by the MMT. For example, when wrist flexion cannot be isolated from elbow flexion, where is the "maximum resistance" that the therapist feels coming from? This same patient cannot perform movements that are not a part of the pathological synergies. For example, shoulder flexion above 90° is required during a MMT, but it is never a part of the flexion synergy. Until a brain-injured patient has minimal spasticity and relative independence from synergy, a MMT is difficult to administer, and the results are not a valid test of strength.

The decision tree process allows you to wisely use brief evaluation sessions. You have a rationale for eliminating tests, for putting off tests until later sessions, and for choosing one or two essential tests for early evaluation.

CONCLUSIONS

One criticism of NDT is that it is mysterious—only certified therapists can discern changes by feeling them

Table 7.11.
Fine Motor Trend II: Static Ulnar to Radial Grasp

Pediatric	No Thumb Involvement		Thumb Flexion		Thumb Opposition	
Essential Characteristics → Test Procedures ↓	1. Ulnar side of palm contacts objects 2. Object must be stabilized by examiner 3. Thumb is flexed ACROSS PALM		1. Radial side of hand contacts object 2. No visible space between palm and object 3. Thumb contacts SIDE OF index finger/object		1. Pads of fingers or fingernails contact object 2. Visible space between palm and object 3. Thumb OPPOSITION used to contact PADS/Fingernails	
Grasp Cube	Crude grasp # 4 mo		Radial Palmar wrist flexed 6 mo		Radial Digital wrist neutral 8 mo	
	# cube handed to child Ulnar palmar grasp # 5 mo		Radial Palmar wrist exten 7 mo		Radial Digital wrist exten 9 mo	
Grasp Pellet	Raking: thumb is silent 6 mo		Scissors thumb IP is flexed 8 mo		Superior Tip Pinch 10 mo	
	Inferior Scissor: thumb fully flexed 7 mo		Inferior Tip Pinch 9 mo		Neat Pincer Grasp 12 mo	
Grasp Crayon	Palmar-supinate: shaft is ⊥ to palm; forearm may be pronated instead 1 yr		Digital-pronate: shaft diagonal in palm; index finger may flex 2 yr		Static Tripod: grasp stiffly at mid-shaft 3 yr	
Brunnstrom stages	Stage 3 = hook grasp		4 = lateral grasp 5 = palmar grasp		Stage 6 = tip pinch and 3-jaw chuck	

Table 7.12.
Fine Motor Trend III. Distal Fixing to Distal Dissociation

Pediatrics	Distal Fixing with Proximal Mobility	Distal Mobility with External Support (in italics)	Distal Mobility with Internal Proximal Stability
Essential Characteristics → Test Procedures ↓	1. All mobility comes from shoulder/elbow 2. Forearm/wrist/fingers are held stiffly in one fixed position	1. Forearm/wrist mobility emerges but fingers are still tightly flexed 2. Distal mobility possible by leaning on EXTERNAL support	1. LIGHT, PRECISE, SMALL finger motions now possible 2. Distal mobility made possible by INTERNAL proximal stability
Grasp of Objects	Grasp reflex 0–3 mo Fisted hands windmill when toy is presented 2–3 mo	Crude grasp possible if *adult hands* cube to patient 4–5 mo Cube placed on *table:* pushes cube around during grasp 4–6 mo	Grasp possible when object is placed on table top; cube doesn't move as patient lifts it 6 mo
Release of Objects	Involuntary release 0–4 mo	*Mouth* used to transfer toy hand to hand 5 mo Releases cube pressing against *table* 7 mo Releases cube into 2"-diameter box resting wrist on *rim:* 10 mo Builds tower of 3–4 cubes by *pressing* down on *tower* 18 mo	Precise release of cube into 2"-diameter box with hand in air 12 mo Places 6 1/2 inch pegs in pegboard in 25 seconds 2 yr Builds tower of 6–7 cubes: light release 2 yr
Spoon Use	Turns spoon upside down on way to mouth due to stiff wrist 15 mo Turns spoon upside down inside mouth 18 mo	Inhibits turning of spoon because of wrist mobility and scissors grasp; uses *other hand* to help fill spoon while scooping 2 yr	Holds spoon like a pencil; no spilling; scoops without using other hand because finger mobility present for fine adjustments 3 yr
Pencil Use	Whole arm moves as a single stiff unit during Palmar-Supinate grasp 1 yr Mobility of shoulder and elbow but wrist and hand stiffly flexed during Digital-Pronate grasp 2 yr	Wrist is extended and mobile, but finger movement is absent during Digital-Pronate grasp; *tightly grasps* pencil in midshaft 3 yr Copies circle and imitates drawing of cross using wrist mobility 3 yr	Dynamic tripod grasp: small finger movements present; grasps pencil near tip with middle finger extended farther than index finger 4 yr

with their hands. This chapter has attempted to make motor strategies more visible and understandable. The ability to detect small changes is also essential for therapists working with patients with short lengths of stay. This chapter should help you report those changes and develop new goals as your handling begins to succeed.

STUDY QUESTIONS

1. Define anterior versus posterior pelvic tilt, trunk elongation vs. lateral trunk flexion, placing and eccentric control, neck elongation vs. jaw-jutting, tiny weight shifts within a posture, rotation, and proximal versus distal dissociation.
2. What stereotyped movements are produced by the flexion and extension synergy of the upper and lower extremities?.
3. Why is clinical observation superior for assessing automatic reactions?
4. What landmark do you watch to observe trunk and pelvic movements?
5. What are the causes of shoulder subluxation?

Table 7.13.
Adult Fine Motor Trends

Fine Motor Trend II: Ulnar to Radial Grasp		
Grasp Cube	Cube trapped by flexed wrist/hand Ulnar-Palmar grasp with wrist flexed	Radial-Palmar grasp with wrist flexed Radial-Palmar grasp with wrist extended	Radial-Digital grasp with wrist in neutral Radial-Digital grasp with wrist extended
Grasp Paper Clip/Pellet	Raking: thumb is silent Inferior Scissor Pinch: traps object between flexed fingers and fully flexed thumb	Superior Scissors: thumb to side of index finger; thumb IP joint flexed Inferior Tip Pinch: thumb to palmar side of index finger's 2nd phalanx	Superior Tip Pinch: thumb to pulpy pad of index finger Neat Fingertip Pinch: thumbnail to fingernail of index finger
Grasp Pencil and Spoon	Palmar-Supinate grasp: shaft is perpendicular to palm; forearm may be pronated instead	Digital-Pronate grasp: shaft lies diagonally across palm; index finger may flex or extend	Static-Tripod grasp: stiffly grip tool at midshaft
Adult Grasp Terminology	Hook grasp; Gross grasp	Lateral prehension: also called key grasp	3-jaw chuck also called Digital grasp; Tip pinch

Fine Motor Trend III: Distal Fixing to Distal Dissociation		
Grasp Objects	Unable to pick up object from the table top because he/she is leaning on object which pushes it away	Grasps but pushes object across table because he/she is pushing down on object for support	Picks up object from table top without pushing the object around
Release Objects	Unable to release -or- Involuntary release	Uses exaggerated finger extension to release Releases object by pressing down on table Releases cube into 2"-diameter box by resting wrist on rim	Light, smooth hand-to-hand transfer Light, precise release to build a tower of 6–7 cubes; doesn't press down for support, so tower doesn't collapse
Spoon Use	Turns spoon upside down on way to mouth due to stiff wrist Turns spoon upside down inside mouth	Inhibits turning of spoon because of wrist mobility; uses other hand to stabilize food while scooping	No spilling due to wrist and finger mobility; scoops without using other hand to stabilize food
Pencil Use	Whole arm moves as a single stiff unit Mobility of shoulder and elbow but wrist and hand stiffly flexed	Wrist is extended and mobile, but fingers are still tightly fisted Draws circle/cross using wrist mobility	Small, precise finger movements; grasps shaft near tip; middle finger is extended further than index finger

6. Why is it important to memorize the essential characteristics of normal motor trends?
7. What gross motor test items do you have to modify for adult patients?
8. Why is pediatric terminology for grasp superior to adult terminology?

References

1. Gilfoyle EM, Grady AP, Moore JC. Children adapt. Thorofare, NJ: Charles B Slack, 1981.
2. Fiorentino MR. Reflex testing methods for evaluating C.N.S. development. 2nd ed. Springfield, IL: Charles C Thomas, 1973.
3. Milani-Comparetti B, Gidoni E. The Milani-Comparetti Motor Development Screening Test. Dev Med Child Neuro 1967;9:631.
4. Adams M. Eight week Bobath certification course. Memphis, 1982.
5. Norkin C, Levangie P. Joint structure and function. Philadelphia: FA Davis, 1983.
6. Brunnstrom S. Movement therapy in hemiplegia. Philadelphia: Harper & Row, 1970.
7. Ashton BA, Pickles B, Roll JW. Reliability of goniometric measurements of hip motion in spastic cerebral palsy. Dev Med Child Neurol 1978;20:87.
8. Harris SR, Smith LH, Krukowski L. Goniometric reliability for a child with spastic quadriplegia. J Pediatr Orthop 1985;5:348.

9. Worley JS, et al: Reliability of 3 clinical measures of muscle tone in the shoulders and wrists of poststroke patients. Am J Occup Ther 1991;45:50.

10. Bohannon RW, Smith MB. Interrater reliability of a Modified Ashworth Scale of muscle spasticity. Phys Ther 1987;67:206.

11. Broberg C, Grimby G. Measurement of torque during passive and active ankle movements in patients with muscle hypertonia. J Rehab Med 1983;9(suppl):108.

12. Boehme R. Specifics of shoulder girdle dynamics as a basis for fine motor performance. Two-day workshop, Milwaukee, 1985.

13. Erhardt RP. Developmental hand dysfunction. Laurel, MD: Ramsco Publishing, 1982.

CHAPTER 8

Neurodevelopmental Postulates Regarding Intervention

Earlier chapters discussed the need for both inhibition and facilitation techniques. However, these techniques do more than change muscle tone. They also inhibit abnormal movement and facilitate normal movement. The concepts of facilitation and inhibition are not unique to NDT, but the Bobaths made their own unique contribution to the repertoire of specific techniques that are commonly used by today's therapists.

INHIBITION TECHNIQUES

Inhibition of hypertonia is a well-accepted approach to the treatment of brain-damaged patients. Rood talked about prolonged ice, prolonged pressure, slow stroking, and slow rocking as ways to reduce spasticity (1). The Bobaths developed seven inhibition techniques that are unique to NDT. They include passive elongation, proximal dissociation, Reflex Inhibiting Patterns, inhibitory positioning devices and orthotics, weight shifting, and normal limb movements.

Passive Elongation

The first inhibition technique is called **passive elongation**. The Bobaths were convinced that it was important to look at the resting length of a muscle before asking it to contract (2). Shortened muscles lose strength because they are contracting at the end of the joint range, where muscles are weak (3). Slow, even pressure is applied to gradually elongate a shortened muscle. The fingers are gently positioned on bony areas, like either side of the elbow, or the open hand is cupped over nonspastic muscles, like the triceps. A circumferential grasp around a limb with pressure applied to the muscle belly through the fingertips is never used!

Shortened muscles keep their antagonists in very elongated positions, which gives the antagonists a mechanical disadvantage. To help you understand the mechanical disadvantage of excessively elongated mus-

cles, palpate your right pectoralis major near its origin on the humerus. Feel the strong contraction of the pectoralis major while you horizontally adduct your right arm across your chest. Keep your finger on the pectoralis major while you put your right hand in the small of your back. Now try to contract your pectoralis major without moving your right arm. You will be able to feel how difficult it is to contract a muscle that is stretched to the end of its range.

A specialized version of muscle elongation is called **proximal dissociation**. It consists of separate movements of adjacent proximal body parts (2). For example, the shoulders are depressed so the head can be rotated independently of the trunk. The shoulder girdle is rotated in the opposite direction from the pelvic girdle. The scapula is moved separately from the rib cage. One hip is flexed while the other hip is extended. In brain-damaged patients, these isolated motions are often lost. The patient moves the head and shoulders en bloc, as a solid unit. The limbs execute only symmetrical motions.

Reflex Inhibiting Patterns

Once you can passively elongate shortened spastic muscles without causing intolerable pain, you can use a complex inhibition technique called **Reflex Inhibiting Patterns** (RIPs). It isn't necessary to wait for full passive elongation to use RIPs. The patient's limb is placed in a position that is as far away as possible from flexor and extensor synergy patterns and is then asked to perform a movement (2). This makes it difficult for the spastic muscles to produce their preferred stereotyped movements. You must know specifically where pathological synergies place the limbs in order to understand RIPs.

RIPs can be facilitated using proximal key points of control or distal key points of control. **Proximal key points** include the head, trunk, pelvis, shoulder, elbow, and lower thigh. **Distal key points** include the forearm, hand, knee, and foot.

Proximal key points are used first because they influence muscle tone throughout the extremity. Proximal key points also have the advantage of leaving the distal end of the extremity free to move in space. This allows the therapist to inhibit proximal spasticity without interfering with the patient's ability to use the hand or foot for a functional movement. The whole point behind RIPs is to permit active movement (2). They are NOT USED to produce static holding of rigid postures!

RIPs by the Therapist

RIPs are used when the upper extremity and/or axial structures are dominated by flexion. To use proximal key points to inhibit arm and axial flexion, grasp the sides of the humerus to place the arm in shoulder external rotation and elbow extension while using skin traction to pull the scapula into different desired positions (see Fig. 8.1). By then placing the arm in different planes, you can inhibit flexion in different body parts (2). External rotation and elbow extension done while:

1. Raising the arm directly overhead inhibits neck and arm flexion;
2. Abducting the arm to the side inhibits trunk and arm flexion;
3. Extending the arm in front of the body inhibits scapular retraction, which is a strong component of the flexion synergy.

If inhibition of the flexion synergy does not reach the hand, distal key points of control are used. Grasp the forearm and hand to place the forearm in supination, wrist in extension, and thumb in abduction. These distal key points enable you to open the hand (see Fig. 8.1). It is important to fade your contact to just the thenar eminence as soon as possible to keep from blocking functional movement of the hand.

A different RIP is used to inhibit neck hyperextension (2). To use proximal key points to inhibit neck hyperextension, grasp the sides of the elbow to pull the shoulder into horizontal adduction and internal rotation while you protract the scapula to flex the spine. This arm position is usually more effective at inhibiting neck hyperextension than pressing on the head to flex the neck. Placing your hand on the back of the patient's head gives the patient a stable surface to push against with even greater hyperextension. Place your own arms across your chest and try to hyperextend your head. Neck hyperextension is a powerful strategy for initiating extensor thrust throughout the whole body, so it is important to be able to inhibit this pathological pattern.

Another RIP is used to inhibit the extension synergy that usually dominates the lower extremity (2). You can use proximal key points to inhibit the extension synergy

Proximal Key Points of Control

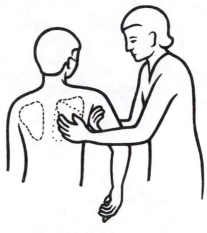

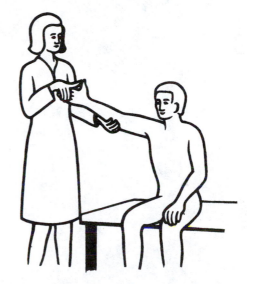

Distal Key Points of Control

Figure 8.1. RIPs used by the therapist

of the leg in sitting. Grasp the knee to pull the hip into external rotation and abduction and pull on the pelvis to produce anterior pelvic tilt. This "frog-leg" position can also be achieved using distal key points of control. Grasp the knee to abduct and externally rotate the hip and lift the outer three toes to dorsiflex the foot while the patient is sitting or standing.

RIPs by the Patient

RIPs can and should be taught to patients (4, 5). If patients do not begin to incorporate RIPs into their daily routine, the few hours in therapy will not be sufficient to inhibit spasticity, especially in patients with very high tone.

Patients can be taught to use distal key points of control to perform RIPs during ADLs. They are taught to clasp the two hands together with the hemiplegic thumb on top to open up the web space (see Fig. 8.2). Then they are taught to extend both arms in front of their bodies. This RIP position enables patients to inhibit the flexion synergy of the arm while rolling over in bed (see Fig. 8.2). This inhibits hemiplegic arm retraction, which facilitates back arching during rolling. The patient can also use this clasped hands strategy to stand up

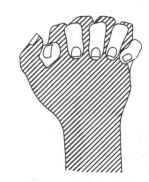

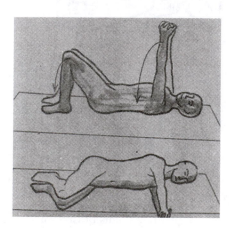

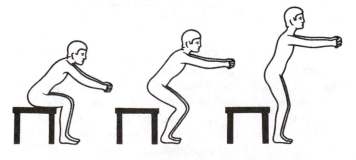

Figure 8.2.   RIPs used by the patient: distal key points of control. **A,** Clasp hands with hemiplegic thumb *(shaded)* on top to the sound thumb opens the webspace. **B,** Clasp hands, flex legs, and extend arms to facilitate log-rolling with shoulder and hip flexion rather than arching the neck and back and retracting the shoulder and hip. **C,** Clasp hands and extend arms to stand up. This inhibits the flexion synergy of the arm and posterior pelvic tilt. It also moves the center of gravity forwards over the feet.

(see Fig. 8.2). Clasping hands together brings both scapulae forward into protraction so the flexion synergy cannot retract the scapula and pull the patient back into the chair. Extending the arms in front of the body also shifts the center of gravity forward over the feet and helps to pull the pelvis into anterior tilt. Posterior tilt makes a patient very dysfunctional. It throws the patient's center of gravity backward and facilitates the LE extensor synergy, which thrusts the patient even farther back in the chair.

Patients can also be taught to use proximal key points of control to perform RIPs during ADLs. The patient can be taught to inhibit the extension synergy of the leg. The extension synergy of the leg pushes the patient backwards toward supine while sitting and prevents the knee from flexing so the patient has difficulty getting his/her foot in a pant leg opening, sock, and shoe. To inhibit the LE extension synergy, the patient can flex the hemiplegic leg by crossing it over the sound leg while dressing in sitting position (see Fig. 8.3). The patient can slide the sound foot behind the extensor-dominated knee to flex the hemiplegic leg while rolling in bed. The patient can also be taught to inhibit the flexion synergy of the arm. The patient should position the sleeve of a shirt or coat between the legs and bend forward to drop the hemiplegic arm in the dangling sleeve (see Fig. 8.3). The weight of the hemiplegic arm pulls the scapula forward into protraction. This proximal key point inhibits the flexion synergy. This position also extends the elbow so the arm will slide easily into the open sleeve.

Patients with hemiplegia are frequently taught to do RIPs during "self-range of motion," but these exercises are most helpful as a morning warm-up activity. The patient must still implement the use of RIPs during purposeful activities for maximum inhibition when spasticity is highest—when the patient is exerting him/herself.

Inhibitory Positioning and Orthotics

Passive elongation and RIPs are supplemented by **positioning devices** that maintain the elongation of shortened muscles. Figure 8.4 shows how a stroke patient can lie on the sound side with the spastic arm resting in front of him/her on a pillow at shoulder height. This keeps the scapula protracted and the elbow somewhat extended to inhibit the flexion synergy. The leg is also semi-flexed to inhibit the extension synergy of the leg. It is even more effective to lay the patient on the hemiplegic side (4). The body weight helps maintain the hemiplegic arm and leg in front of the body so they can't retract behind the body.

Positioning devices should ensure a symmetrical sitting posture. *Excessive anterior or posterior pelvic tilt can*

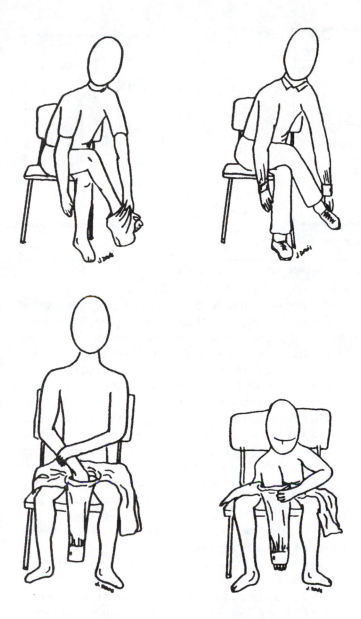

Figure 8.3. RIPs used by the patient: proximal key points of control used during ADLs. **A,** Hip and knee flexion inhibit extension synergy of leg. **B,** Scapular protraction inhibits flexion synergy in arm.

be inhibited by a hard seat insert that sits on top of the sagging Naugahyde seat that comes with every wheelchair. Excessive anterior or posterior pelvic tilt can also be inhibited by using seat belts that ensure 90° of hip flexion and position the pelvis flush against the backrest for better support. *Lateral trunk flexion* can be corrected with a hard seat, a small towel under the hip that is bearing the most weight, and an arm trough or lapboard. The arm trough and lapboard ensure symmetrical weightbearing on the elbows so the shoulders are level. More intrusive solutions to poor trunk control include lateral trunk supports and chest straps. These position-

ing devices restrict movement as well as support the trunk.

Orthotics can also supplement passive elongation and RIPs. The spasticity reduction splint, finger abduction splint, orthokinetic cuff, inflatable splint, serial casting, and dynamic sling are a few examples of orthotics that can inhibit the flexion synergy of the arm (6). Splints are usually worn after treatment to prolong the effects of handling. However, splints may be worn during treatment to provide the therapist with an extra set of hands to inhibit distal spasticity (2).

Active Movement

Weight shifting in miniature ranges is another inhibition technique that inhibits rigid fixing (2). Weight shifting includes both axial weight shifts and limb weight shifts. **Axial weight shifts** include shifting the trunk forwards, backwards, sideways, and with rotation. During **limb weight shifts**, the distal end of the extremity, such as the hand, stays in contact with the support surface while proximal joints move in small ranges. Initially, the patient needs maximal assistance to keep spasticity and "extension with retraction" under control.

Normal limb movements that are free of pathological synergies are inhibitory (2). They include distal dissociation of the forearm, wrist, fingers, and ankle. Mrs. Bobath didn't develop techniques for distal dissociation. She assumed that distal dissociation will follow once proximal control is achieved (2).

Weight shifting and normal limb movements must be used with caution! While they can inhibit abnormally high tone, they can also stimulate spasticity if the patient strains too hard. Maximum physical support, minimum resistance, and miniature speed are the keys to using these inhibition movements effectively.

FACILITATION TECHNIQUES

Facilitation is another well-accepted approach to treatment of brain-injured patients. Rood pioneered the use of quick icing, quick stretching, muscle tapping, joint compression to facilitate extensors, and joint traction to facilitate flexors (1).

The Bobaths divided facilitation into three levels (2). The lowest level is joint compression, joint traction, manual resistance, and weight shifting. Notice that weight shifting can be used as both an inhibitory and facilitory technique. Static weightbearing encourages rigid cocontraction (2), followed by hanging on stretched muscles in poor postures once the patient becomes fatigued. Active weight shifting stimulates all the muscles around the joint to contract reciprocally as the gravity line changes from flexor to extensor moment arms and back again (3).

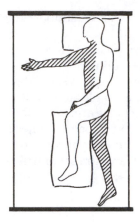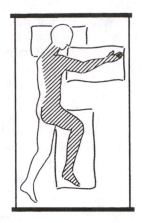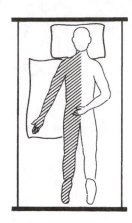

Figure 8.4. Positioning to inhibit arm and leg synergies. Hemiplegic side is shaded.

The middle level of facilitation includes pressure tapping, sweep tapping, and alternate tapping. These techniques require advanced training to be used effectively.

The highest level of facilitation is placing and eccentric lowering followed by distal dissociation. Normal limb movements require the ability to place and lower a limb with graded eccentric control rather than cocontraction of all the muscles around a joint. Distal dissociation requires the patient to move the distal body parts individually rather than as a whole unit in a stereotyped synergy.

To facilitate placing and lowering, the therapist grades his/her handling (7). The therapist places the patient's arm in the RIP to inhibit flexion and raises it overhead. The therapist can apply light joint compression to stimulate limb extension. Next, the therapist briefly lets go to see if the patient can hold the RIP position. The therapist may have to let go several times before the patient retains the sensation of this facilatory position. Once the patient can hold the posture for a few moments, the therapist uses key points of control to help the patient to slowly lower the arm in the RIP. If the therapist feels the full weight of the arm because the patient has stopped helping or begins to resist, the therapist should immediately raise the arm. Work is initially done close to a vertical position, where the patient has better control. While the arm is vertical, the gravity line is basically parallel to the line of the extremity, so gravity has little effect (3). Once the arm is parallel to the floor, it becomes a long lever arm for gravity to pull on. In this position, the patient strains more and spasticity increases.

THREE PHASES OF INHIBITION AND FACILITATION

Neurodevelopmental treatment combines inhibitory and facilatory techniques across three phases of treatment. The first phase will *give the sensation* of what normal tone and movement feels like (2). Feeling normal tone includes feeling normal elongation and body positions. The spastic patient must be passive to permit the therapist to use passive elongation, proximal dissociation, RIPs, bed and wheelchair positioning, and orthotics during this first phase of treatment.

However, "giving the sensation" means more than the patient passively allowing the therapist to move his/her body. It must quickly progress to learning what active movements feel like! The patient must also learn to track movements initiated by the therapist, such as graded weight shifts and placing and lowering. To track normal movement, the patient must keep his/her body in constant contact with the therapist's hands while the therapist moves the patient.

Purposeful activity is *not used* during this first phase of "giving the sensation." You want the patient to look at his/her body and concentrate on what normal tone and movement feels like. You don't want the patient to become distracted by cognitive challenges and emotional stress. The therapist may return to this first phase repeatedly within a single treatment session whenever abnormal tone or pathological movement patterns begin to dominate.

As soon as the patient begins to get the idea of what normal tone and movement feels like, you must quickly proceed to the second phase of treatment. This phase *lets the patient initiate movements during purposeful activity* while the therapist maintains inhibition and/or facilitation. Motor learning studies have shown that repetitive practice of foundation skills does not generalize to open tasks (8). Purposeful activity promotes motor learning during an open task in which the motor system must respond to changing conditions (9). Purposeful activities provide cognitive and emotional challenges that the patient doesn't always anticipate.

You could have a patient practice rolling over, sitting up in bed, and lying back down. But it is difficult for cognitively impaired patients to understand the purpose of abstract movement sequences. Even cognitively intact patients and their family members do not understand the purpose of repeatedly leaning forwards and backwards in sitting (10). It is easier for a patient to understand why you want him/her to initiate specific movements if you provide a purposeful activity (10). For example, you could have a patient roll over in bed to reach up for the telephone on the nightstand, then sit up slightly to reach for the TV remote control at his/her hip, and then roll over to reach at shoulder height for the nurse's call button hooked on the bed rail. When a patient engages in purposeful activity, the activity itself suggests why specific movements are necessary.

Purposeful activity naturally engages the visual system because it usually involves objects. Set up the equipment for one or two purposeful activities as soon as you get a feeling for how your patient responds to your handling. Seeing the equipment enables the patient to use visual input to plan movements, anticipate errors, and make motor corrections (9). This engages the patient in planning and initiating movement instead of passively waiting for the therapist to move his/her body (11).

Quickly choosing equipment for purposeful activities also enables the therapist to make an immediate transition to purposeful movement the instant the patient is ready. When you leave the patient to find the equipment and get it set up, the patient may no longer be ready to move when you get back. Initially, very spastic patients can maintain inhibition for only a few seconds. You must set up the equipment before you start "giving the sensation" of what normal feels like. You don't want to lose your inhibition after you've spent a strenuous 20 minutes preparing a patient for a purposeful activity.

Letting the patient initiate means *the theapist waits* for the patient to initiate the motion and plan exactly how the body part will move. Now it is the therapist's turn to track the patient's movement. When the patient takes responsibility for the movement, you continue to use key points of control to reduce pathology. Carr and Shephard refer to the therapist's responsibility in this second phase of handling as "spatial and temporal restraint" (9). The restraint provides physical support and cuts down on the degrees of freedom that the patient has to control (11). The restraint also prevents abnormal mass movements from taking over. This second phase usually lasts for several days and requires frequent return to phase one when the patient begins to use pathological movement strategies.

The final phase is *fading your control*. This allows the patient to practice normal movements with minimal assistance for controlling muscle tone and pathological movements. Fading control initially means switching from proximal to distal key points of control. Eventually, it means letting go of the patient altogether. You must risk regression to primitive behavior if you want your patient to gain independence. If your patient cannot move independently with quality movements for even a few moments, you need to rethink your long-term expectations. On the other hand, you may be surprised and find that you can fade your control much sooner than you originally thought.

EXAMPLES OF NDT POSTULATES REGARDING INTERVENTION

For an example of NDT postulates regarding intervention, see Figure 8.5. An NDT postulate regarding intervention begins with a short-term NDT goal. This NDT goal must be measurable to determine if the NDT handling and activities are producing positive change. It is essential to know the stage-specific cause. This helps you identify whether you should use inhibitory or facilitory techniques and on which muscle groups.

The three phases of inhibition and facilitation are the rationales for NDT treatment. Specific treatment techniques, like RIPs, don't need to be listed as they are in the biomechanical frame of reference. It is easy to become overwhelmed while contemplating NDT techniques. It is more helpful to list what movements the patient will feel and initiate. If you remember only three things when choosing NDT techniques, let it be GIVE THE SENSATION, LET THE PATIENT INITIATE DURING PURPOSEFUL ACTIVITY, and FADE YOUR CONTROL.

When you are ready to write in the activity description column, giving the sensation is identified as the "preparation," and letting the patient initiate is identified by a specific activity name, like tic-tac-toe. Both the preparation and activity descriptions must be specific enough to determine where the patient, the equipment, and the therapist's hands will be positioned and what the therapist will do with his/her hands. NDT is not a verbal approach. You must know what your hands are doing throughout the entire treatment session.

SUMMARY

The use of inhibition and facilitation to treat brain-damaged patients was first introduced to therapists by Margaret Rood. Many of her peers expanded this concept and made their own unique contributions to our repertoire of inhibitory and facilitory techniques. The Bobaths developed seven specific inhibition techniques. Make sure you are familiar with each of the techniques. In addition, be sure you thoroughly understand the three phases of inhibition and facilitation.

Deficit/Cause/Goal/FO	Rationale	Specific Modalities
Deficit: poor axial weight shifts in sitting *Stage-specific cause:* axial fixing *S–T NDT goal:* active axial weight shift with rotation using posterior pelvic tilt and minimal physical assistance *Functional outcome:* able to dress LE with standby supervision for sitting balance	GIVE THE SENSATION of active trunk rotation with posterior tilt	*Preparation:* Patient will sit on bench while therapist sits in back of patient with chest very close to patient's back. Passively shift patient into posterior tilt behind vertical with one hand pulling back on stomach and one hand on spine to push upper trunk forward. Rotate your own trunk while passively rotating patient's trunk by pushing the hemi-shoulder forward and keeping other hand on stomach to make sure patient maintains posterior tilt. Repeat to left side, switching hands to push sound shoulder forwards. Then have patient clasp hands and move both arms to his/her right and left to practice active trunk rotation.
	LET THE PATIENT INITIATE DURING PURPOSEFUL ACTIVITY active trunk rotation with posterior tilt	*Beanbag tic-tac-toe.* Patient is sitting on a mat table. Place beanbags slightly behind patient's trunk on mat table on patient's right side. Place game board on mat table to patient's left so half the board is behind the patient. Have patient lean back with posterior pelvic tilt and clasp hands together to pick up a beanbag on right. Return to upright position. Lean back with posterior tilt and then rotate to place beanbag on game board on left. *Handling:* same as preparation
	FADE YOUR CONTROL	*Handling:* place hands only on shoulders

Figure 8.5.   NDT Postulate Regarding Intervention

STUDY QUESTIONS

1. What do shortened spastic muscles do to their antagonists?
2. What must you know in order to understand RIPs?
3. What are proximal and distal key points of control?
4. What is the whole point behind RIPs?
5. How to the effects of the three RIP positions for the UE differ?
6. Why do patients need to learn to use RIPs?
7. Positioning and orthotic devices employ what three strategies?
8. Why is weight shifting both facilitory and inhibitory?
9. Placing and lowering are done first in what position and why?
10. What are the three phases of inhibition and facilitation?

References

1. Trombly CA. Rood approach. In: Trombly CA, ed. Occupational therapy for physical dysfunction. 3rd ed. Baltimore: Williams & Wilkins, 1989:97.
2. Adams M. Bobath certification 8 week course. Memphis, 1982.
3. Norkin CC, Levangie PK. Joint structure and function. Philadelphia: FA Davis, 1989.
4. Davis JZ. The Bobath approach to the treatment of adult hemiplegia. In: Pedretti LW, Zoltan B, eds. Occupational therapy practice skills for physical dysfunction. 3rd ed. Philadelphia: CV Mosby, 1990:351.
5. Trombly CA. Bobath neurodevelopmental approach. In: Trombly CA, ed. Occupational therapy for physical dysfunction. 3rd ed. Baltimore: Williams & Wilkins, 1989:107.
6. Trombly CA. Orthoses: purposes and types. In: Trombly CA, ed. Occupational therapy for physical dysfunction. 3rd ed. Baltimore: Williams & Wilkins, 1989:352.
7. Bobath B. Adult hemiplegia: evaluation and treatment. 2nd ed. London: William Heinemann Medical Books Limited, 1978.
8. Sabari JS. Motor learning concepts applied to activity based intervention with adults with hemiplegia. Am J Occup Ther, 1991;45:523.
9. Carr JK, Shephard RB. Movement science: foundations for physical therapy in rehabilitation. Rockville, MD: Aspen Publications, 1987.
10. Dutton R. Guidelines for using both activity and exercise. Am J Occup Ther 1989;43:576.
11. Bly L. A historical and current view of the basis of NDT. Pediatric Physical Therapy 1991;3:131.

CHAPTER / 9

Neurodevelopmental Treatment Postulates Regarding Change

Many books describe neurodevelopmental treatment (NDT) activities. This enables untrained staff to mimic Bobath treatment without knowing where to begin, how to write measurable outcome goals, and how to link NDT goals to specific functional outcomes. Chapter 8 on postulates regarding intervention provides specific "how-to" techniques, but students must grasp the concepts in this chapter to guide their treatment.

To teach students where to begin, most authors have used a "stages approach." Patients are described as being flaccid, spastic, or in relative recovery (1). This is confusing because patients can be in one stage of recovery for axial control and in a different stage for limb control or automatic reactions (see Fig. 9.1). Some authors divide NDT domains of concern into normalizing muscle tone and facilitating active movement. This encourages students to inhibit all the spastic muscles as their first goal. By the time you inhibit the last muscle, the first muscles are tight again because early inhibition doesn't last very long. Inhibition must be followed IMMEDIATELY by active movement. That is why in Memory Aid 9.1 lists passive elongation and active movement together in several boxes.

To enable students to sequence NDT treatment, I have devised a different teaching strategy. The axial control, automatic reactions, and limb control continua are given their own treatment sequence. This approach is similar to the continua for range of motion and strength in the biomechanical frame of reference. The steps in each continuum tell you where your patient is now and where he/she should go next. These NDT continua will help you write appropriate outcome goals.

In addition to being appropriate, NDT goals must also be measurable. This lends credibility to what others perceive as a magical process that can be appreciated only by certified therapists. Measurable goals also enable a therapist to observe small changes within a single treatment session. Small patient responses guide treatment because therapists can quickly modify their handling as changes occur. Progress towards measurable goals is also the best clue to the patient's prognosis.

Finally, pictures of NDT activities don't show students how to link NDT goals to *specific* functional outcomes. Preliminary research has not been able to show a link between normalizing muscle tone and independence in ADLs because these studies have been looking for a global connection. Filiatrault et al. found a correlation of only .60 between the Barthal Index for ADLs and the Fugl-Meyer Test for upper extremity freedom from synergy (2). Other factors such as emotional, visual, perceptual, and cognitive deficits can also cause a loss of independence, so the relationship between ADLs and motor function can never be a perfect correlation.

Spaulding et al. found no significant correlation between wrist spasticity and a composite ADL score (3). The results of this second study are even more misleading. First, many ADL skills can be done one-handed. Patients can gain independence using compensation regardless of whether they have flaccid or spastic muscles. Therefore, there will be a low correlation between spasticity and ADL gains achieved through compensation. Second, ADL scoring criteria are not sensitive enough to document the switch from compensation to regaining normal movement strategies. For example, a patient may graduate from cutting meat one-handed with a rocker knife to using two hands to manipulate a fork and knife, but he will still get the same ADL score. Third, even if scoring sensitivity improves, it doesn't make sense to look for a correlation between wrist spasticity and a composite ADL score. Lack of wrist dissociation is most likely to affect ADL activities that require isolated wrist movements, like flexing and extending the wrist while cutting meat. Therapists need to write and test postulates that link SPECIFIC NDT goals with SPECIFIC functional outcomes!

This chapter is organized around the three NDT continua. Each section discusses the steps in the treatment sequence that make up each continuum. The rationales

Figure 9.1

Two Patients' Recoveries: DeÆcits Are Circled

A. *Axial Extension* 1. *IF* lacking full trunk extension check passive elongation of pectorals and hamstrings 2. **CHILD ONLY**: elong. hip flexors; active axial extension prone 3. Sitting: passive ANTERIOR tilt 4. Sitting: active weight shift forwards using ANTERIOR tilt	A. *Righting Reactions:* 1. Vertical head righting: moving away from vertical 2. Rotary righting: –Log-roll with FLEXION RIPs in side-lie → into supine → from supine (neck rightg) –Segment. roll: body rightg –Segment. roll: equil. reac	A. *Limb Dissociation* 1. Arm dissociation a. Passive elonga. scapula (supine → then side-lie) b. Elongate UE into RIP 1. Leg dissociation a. Dissociation of 2 legs b. Elongate LE into RIP 2. Patient uses RIPs in ADLs
AA. *Axial Flexion* 1. Passive elongation of shortened neck and lumbar extensors 2. **CHILD ONLY**: passive elongation of hamstrings followed by active leglifts in supine 3. Sitting: passive POSTERIOR tilt 4. Sitting: active weight shift backwards using POSTERIOR tilt	B. *Equilibrium Reactions:* 1. Learn each individual component and then 2. Simultaneously perform –Head righting –Trunk ELONGATION of weightbearing side –Trunk rota/POSTERIOR tilt –Abduction uphill arm/leg	B. *Limb Weight Shifts* 1. **CHILD ONLY**: Hand/foot prep 2. MATURE extension during SMALL wt shifts over limb (e.g., on elbow → hand ×3) 3. Symmet. linear transitional movements (e.g., stand up) 4. Lateral weight shifts to locomote (e.g., transfers)
B. *Midline Symmetry* 1. Passive elongation of shortened neck and lateral trunk flexors 2. Maintain sym. sit with devices 3. Active wt shift onto hemi side with trunk elongation 4. Active wt shift side to side 5. Indepen. assume symm. sitting	C. *Protective Extension:* 1. Learn components, then 2. Simultaneously perform –Head righting –Lateral trunk FLEXION of weightbearing side –Trunk rota/ANTERIOR til –Extension downhill arm/leg	C. *Limbs Free in Space* 1. P.A. to place & lower (e.g. arm at side → on diagonal → in front of body) 2. Self-assisted place & lower (e.g., bilateral UE tasks with hands clasped) 3. Independent place & lower
C. *Advanced Axial Weight Shifts* 1. Passive elongation of neck and trunk rotators *IF* not complete 2. Active axial rotation with posterior tilt and then anterior tilt	[a]*IF* automatic react are absent check axial/limb muscle tone [b]Tonic reflexes are treated indirectly (e.g., ASTN → facilitate FLEXOR tone, symmetry, righting reacts.)	D. *Distal Skill* 1. Assumes postures and locomotes with rotation and reciprocal limb movements 2. Distal dissociation during reach/grasp/manip/release

A. *Axial Extension* 1. *IF* lacking full trunk extension check passive elongation of pectorals and hamstrings 2. **CHILD ONLY**: elongated hip flexors; active axial extension prone 3. Sitting: passive ANTERIOR tilt 4. Sitting: active weight shift forwards using ANTERIOR tilt	A. *Righting Reactions:* 1. Vertical head righting: moving away from vertical 2. Rotary righting: –Log-roll with FLEXION RIPs in side-lie → into supine → from supine (neck rightg) –Segment. roll: body rightg –Segment. roll: equil. reac	A. *Limb Dissociation* 1. Arm dissociation a. Passive elonga. scapula (supine → then side-lie) b. Elongate UE into RIP 1. Leg dissociation a. Dissociation of 2 legs b. Elongate LE into RIP 2. Patient uses RIPs in ADLs
AA. *Axial Flexion* 1. Passive elongation of shortened neck and lumbar extensors 2. **CHILD ONLY**: passive elongation of hamstrings followed by active leglifts in supine 3. Sitting: passive POSTERIOR til 4. Sitting: active weight shift backwards using POSTERIOR tilt	B. *Equilibrium Reactions:* 1. Learn each individual component and then 2. Simultaneously perform –Head righting –Trunk ELONGATION of weightbearing side –Trunk rota/POSTERIOR tilt –Abduction uphill arm/leg	B. *Limb Weight Shifts* 1. **CHILD ONLY**: Hand/foot prep 2. MATURE extension during SMALL wt shifts over limb (e.g., on elbow → hand ×3) 3. Symmet. linear transitional movements (e.g., stand up) 4. Lateral weight shifts to locomote (e.g., transfers)
B. *Midline Symmetry* 1. Passive elongation of shortened neck and lateral trunk flexors 2. Maintain sym. sit with devices 3. Active wt shift onto hemi side with trunk elongation 4. Active wt shift side to side 5. Indepen. assume symm. sitting	C. *Protective Extension:* 1. Learn components, then 2. Simultaneously perform –Head righting –Lateral trunk FLEXION of weightbearing side –Trunk rota/ANTERIOR tilt –Extension downhill arm/leg	C. *Limbs Free in Space* 1. P.A. to place & lower (e.g. arm at side → on diagonal → in front of body) 2. Self-assisted place & lower (e.g., bilateral UE tasks with hands clasped) 3. Independent place & lower
C. *Advanced Axial Weight Shifts* 1. Passive elongation of neck and trunk rotators *IF* not complete 2. Active axial rotation with posterior tilt and then anterior tilt	[a]*IF* automatic react are absent check axial/limb muscle tone [b]Tonic reflexes are treated indirectly (e.g., ASTN → facilitate FLEXOR tone, symmetry, righting reacts.)	D. *Distal Skill* 1. Assumes postures and locomotes with rotation and reciprocal limb movements 2. Distal dissociation during reach/grasp/manip/release

Memory Aid 9.1.
Neurodevelopmental Treatment Goals

I. Axial Control	II. Automatic Reactions[a, b]	III. Limb Control
A. *Axial Extension* 　1. IF lacking full trunk extension check passive elongation of pectorals and hamstrings 　2. **CHILD ONLY**: elong. hip flexors; active axial extension prone 　3. Sitting: passive ANTERIOR tilt 　4. Sitting: active weight shift forwards using ANTERIOR tilt	A. *Righting Reactions:* 　1. Vertical head righting: moving away from vertical 　2. Rotary righting: 　　—Log-roll with FLEXION and RIPs in side-lie ! into supine ! from supine (neck righting) 　　—Segment. roll: body righting 　　—Segment. roll: equil. reactions	A. *Limb Dissociation* 　1. Arm dissociation 　　a. Passive elonga. scapula (supine ! then side-lie) 　　b. Elongate UE into RIP 　1. Leg dissociation 　　a. Dissociation of 2 legs 　　b. Elongate LE into RIP 　2. Patient uses RIPs in ADLs
AA. *Axial Flexion* 　1. Passive elongation of shortened neck and lumbar extensors 　2. **CHILD ONLY**: passive elongation of hamstrings followed by active leglifts in supine 　3. Sitting: passive POSTERIOR tilt 　4. Sitting: active weight shift backwards using POSTERIOR tilt	B. *Equilibrium Reactions:* 　1. Learn each individual component and then 　2. Simultaneously perform 　　—Head righting 　　—Trunk ELONGATION of weightbearing side 　　—Trunk rota/POSTERIOR tilt 　　—Abduction uphill arm/leg	B. *Limb Weight Shifts* 　1. **CHILD ONLY**: Hand/foot prep 　2. MATURE extension during SMALL wt shifts over limb (e.g., on elbow ! hand ×3) 　3. Symmet. linear transitional movements (e.g., stand up) 　4. Lateral weight shifts to locomote (e.g., transfers)
B. *Midline Symmetry* 　1. Passive elongation of shortened neck and lateral trunk flexors 　2. Maintain sym. sit with devices 　3. Active weight shift onto hemi-side with trunk elongation 　4. Active wt shift side to side 　5. Indepen. assume symm. sitting	C. *Protective Extension:* 　1. Learn components, then 　2. Simultaneously perform 　　—Head righting 　　—Lateral trunk FLEXION of weight-bearing side 　　—Trunk rota/ANTERIOR tilt 　　—Extension downhill arm/leg	C. *Limbs Free in Space* 　1. P.A. to place & lower (e.g. arm at side ! on diagonal ! in front of body) 　2. Self-assisted place & lower (e.g., bilateral UE tasks with hands clasped) 　3. Independent place & lower
C. *Advanced Axial Weight Shifts* 　1. Passive elongation of neck and trunk rotators IF not complete 　2. Active axial rotation with posterior tilt and then anterior tilt	[a]IF automatic react are absent check axial/limb muscle tone [b]Tonic reflexes are treated indirectly (e.g., ASTN ! facilitate FLEXOR tone, symmetry, righting reacts.)	D. *Distal Skill* 　1. Assumes postures and locomotes with rotation and reciprocal limb movements 　2. Distal dissociation during reach/grasp/manipulation/release

for sequencing will help you understand and remember the sequence. Note that some of the steps in the sequence apply only to children. Each section also provides strategies for making NDT goals measurable and for linking NDT goals to specific functional outcomes. The chapter ends with situational thinking about time lines and chunking, which tells you how to move patients with individual differences through the three continua.

AXIAL CONTROL POSTULATES

Sequencing Treatment

Axial control is divided into four levels, shown in boxes in Memory Aid 9.1:

1. Axial extension;
2. Axial flexion;
3. Midline symmetry; and
4. Advanced axial weight shifts.

The first two steps are listed as A. and AA. on Memory Aid 9.1 to signify that this is not a treatment sequence. Patients can lack either axial flexion or axial extension.

Axial Extension

This box involves voluntary control of neck and trunk extensors. *If* axial extension is incomplete, you need to check the passive elongation of the antagonists. The neck flexors and oblique abdominals rarely become shortened. However, active axial extension can be delayed by shortening of shoulder and knee flexors (4). If the pectoralis major is severely shortened, it pulls the clavicle and scapula forward. This rounds the upper back and stretches out the thoracic extensors so they are at the end of their range, where they have little power. Similarly, tight hamstrings cause patients to posterior-tilt and round their back while sitting to get relief from the painful stretch of these tight leg muscles. While normal adults often demonstrate posterior tilting for relief in LONG-LEG sitting, some brain-damaged patients exhibit posterior tilt while sitting in a regular chair with knees flexed. Such patients try to stay flexed when the therapist tries to pull the pelvis into neutral and extend the back. The first step towards axial extension is elongation of the pectoralis and hamstrings, BUT ONLY IF they are shortened severely enough to pull the trunk into flexion.

The second step is for children only because most adult patients cannot tolerate the prone position. Prone on elbows is used to develop axial extension in children who cannot sit up. Before you work on axial extension in prone, you may need to passively elongate shortened hip flexors that keep the buttocks up in the air (5). The child will never be able to lift his/her head in prone if the buttocks are up in the air at the same time. Wedges and bolsters are used to facilitate neck and trunk extension in prone. Yet, you must be careful when you use this equipment. It must be high enough to lift the chest off the floor to ensure neck elongation. It should force the child to depress and protract the scapula in order to keep the elbows on the ground. These scapular motions will permit the neck to elongate. This equipment is safe only when it is big enough to inhibit the transition strategy of extension with retraction. The wedge must also be long enough to accommodate the length of the trunk and thighs so that the hips are in zero degrees of flexion while the knees flex, which inhibits both leg synergies.

The third step for axial extension focuses on full passive anterior pelvic tilt in sitting. While you may have stretched out the tight hamstrings enough to get the pelvis into neutral tilt, additional elongation may be needed to permit full anterior tilt. Make sure the patient's feet are supported on a firm surface and provide maximal physical contact to reassure the patient that he/she will not fall forward onto the floor. Some patients are so used to posterior tilting that anterior tilt frightens them badly, so at first they use their motor return to rigidly fix.

For both children and adults, the last step is to work on active axial extension while leaning forwards in sitting (3). Remember, static weightbearing produces only momentary excitation of flaccid trunk extensors, so static sitting is skipped. Make sure that forward weight shift is achieved using anterior tilt and low back extension instead of using posterior tilt and excessive thoracic and cervical flexion to get the head in front of the feet. Patients are often afraid to lean forwards because they misperceive where vertical is and experience a terrifying sense of falling towards the floor. You will need to ask for miniature amounts of movement and make sure that their feet are flat on the floor to give them a stable base. Sometimes this means putting a board under their feet so they are not leaning forward with their feet dangling. It is common to have the patient clasp hands with the hemiplegic thumb on top and lift both arms in front of the body to shoulder height (see Fig. 8.2) to facilitate

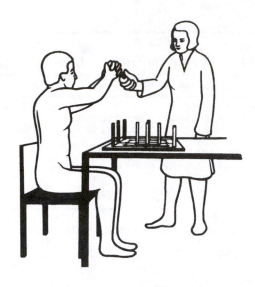

Figure 9.2.   Clasping hands to encourage axial rotation.

the forward weight shift (6). This arm position moves the center of gravity forward and inhibits the flexor synergy in the hemiplegic arm.

Axial Flexion

This box in Memory Aid 9.1 refers to the voluntary control of neck flexors and abdominals. Like axial extension, axial flexion may be delayed due to shortened antagonists. Recovery of cervical and lumbar extensors often precedes recovery of axial flexors (4). This leaves the axial extensors unopposed. Eventually the axial extensors become shortened, and the axial flexors become long and lax.

The first step is elongation of shortened neck and low back extensors. If these axial extensors show moderate to maximal resistance to elongation, facilitation of floppy axial flexors will fail. When elongation of neck and lumbar extensors is really needed, it is usually done in supine (5). The support surface stabilizes the spastic shoulder girdle and low back while the therapist places traction on the head and pelvis to elongate the neck and low back. The supine position also gives patients maximum physical support so they won't feel like they're falling as you pull the cervical and lumbar extensors into an elongated position.

The second step is for children only. Shortened hamstrings will interfere with leg raises while supine with knees extended (5). Leg raises are a typical activity for strengthening abdominals in children. Once you have elongated neck and lumbar extensors and hamstrings, the child is ready for abdominal work in supine position. This includes lifting the head to look at objects, lifting the legs to play with the feet, and pulling up to sit from supine.

In step three, you must make sure that the patient has full passive posterior tilt in sitting. Tight hip flexors may keep the pelvis in anterior tilt (5). This makes it difficult to lean backwards in sitting to strengthen the abdominals. If passive posterior tilt is already present, you can proceed directly to active axial weight shifts backwards.

Step four strengthens the flaccid abdominals by leaning behind vertical in sitting with posterior tilt and neck flexion (5). Sitting upright is a **light work position** for the neck and trunk because the gravity line passes directly down through the center of the spine and therefore has minimal effect on the trunk (7). Axial flexion in supine is a **heavy work position** because gravity has the full length of the trunk to act on as you try to sit up. Think of how much harder it is to start a sit-up in supine than it is to finish it once you are almost upright. The patient can control the light work position with less effort and therefore with less pathological tone. Check to make sure the patient is not fixing in neutral tilt or arching the back as he/she leans back.

Midline Symmetry

This box in Memory Aid 9.1 refers to symmetry of both sides of the body around the midline. It is treated immediately after axial flexion and extension are normalized because symmetry relies on a balance of these two muscle groups.

The first step is to elongate shortened neck and trunk lateral flexors (5). In children, the shortening may be quite pronounced, especially if the ASTN Reflex is present. In adults, the shortening may not be felt until the end of range. If passive elongation is present, proceed to the next step.

The second step is to find out which devices help the patient maintain a symmetrical posture after the patient is placed in a correct sitting position. Even if you remove the devices for treatment, make sure you end every treatment session with symmetrical positioning! This step should be part of every short-term treatment plan for patients who sit asymmetrically. Whether you leave your patient at bedside or send him/her on to the next treatment in a wheelchair, the patient should look like a normal, symmetrically positioned person. With low-functioning patients, this second step of maintaining midline symmetry with positioning devices may be all that can be achieved.

The third step is to achieve weight shifts onto the hemiplegic side (5). Unlike weight shifts backwards and forwards, lateral weight shifts require the patient to lift one hip off of the support surface (called **hip-hiking**). This loss of support is frightening when the patient is accustomed to rigidly fixing, so start with gentle assisted movement. Initially, you may be able to get only one or two very slow weight shifts onto the hemiplegic hip with minimal hip-hiking. Be sure to start with an unmoving surface, like a mat table. Moving patients and moving support surfaces initially don't mix. One therapist doesn't have enough hands to control a frightened patient and an out-of-control ball or bolster.

The fourth step is to achieve axial weight shift from side to side (5). This involves moving onto the hemiplegic side, back into the midline, onto the sound hip where the patient usually likes to stay, and then back onto the hemiplegic hip. This lateral weight shift prepares the patient for rotation because small amounts of rotation occur as the facets of the spine bend from side to side (7). Begin with active assistive movement to facilitate both trunk elongation of the weightbearing side and hiking of the non-weightbearing hip.

The fifth step is to independently assume a symmetrical position. Some patients may still need positioning devices, but at this level, they can straighten up to make themselves more comfortable and presentable without the help of an attendant. Not every patient achieves this fifth step. While waiting to see if the patient can achieve this last step, proceed to advanced axial weight shifts as soon as the patient can perform a weight shift side to side with minimal physical assistance.

Advanced Axial Weight Shifts

This is the last box (in Memory Aid 9.1) in the axial domain. Axial weight shifts were used throughout this continuum except for weight shift with full rotation. Some passive elongation of axial muscles should already be present, so the first step is to check to see if passive elongation of neck and trunk rotators is complete.

Once passive elongation is present, you can begin to facilitate active axial rotation. Start in prone or sitting on an unmoving surface. The surface stabilizes the pelvic girdle while you counter-rotate the shoulder girdle or vice versa. If you try this in standing, the whole body just rotates as a stiff log. Therapists often sit behind the patient on a mat table or bench to facilitate rotation of the shoulder girdle and pelvic tilt. Start with axial rotation with posterior tilt if your patient has too much anterior tilt. Make sure the patient has to lean slightly behind vertical if you want rotation with posterior pelvic tilt. Conversely, start with axial rotation with anterior tilt if your patient has too much posterior tilt. It is common to have the patient clasp hands and move the arms in an arc side to side to facilitate axial rotation (see Fig. 9.2).

Making Axial Goals Measurable

Short-term axial goals may initially describe gains in passive elongation (see Table 7.4). Use the muscle tone baseline to help you describe the behavior the patient will exhibit. For example, you could say that the patient will exhibit moderate resistance to passive trunk elongation at the end of range.

Axial goals may also describe the active movement that is achieved at the end of each axial box in Memory Aid 9.1. **High-quality axial weight shifts backwards** include: (1) active weight shifts initiated independently with (2) posterior pelvic tilt and (3) graded control. **High-quality axial weight shifts forward** include: (1) active weight shifts initiated independently with (2) anterior pelvic tilt and (3) graded control. **High-quality midline symmetry** includes maintaining: (1) the head erect and in the midline, (2) the shoulders level, (3) the pelvis in neutral tilt, (4) equal weight on both hips, (5) symmetrical hip abduction, and (6) both feet flat on the floor. **High-quality axial weight shifts from side to side** include: (1) active elongation of the weightbearing side and (2) hip-hiking on the non-weightbearing side, (3) initiated independently with (4) a smooth transition across the midline in both directions. **High-quality axial rotation** includes: (1) active rotation initiated independently with (2) elongation on the weightbearing side, (3) pelvic mobility, and (4) graded control.

Measurable goals DO NOT have to include an exhaustive description of quality movement like the ones just listed!! If a patient already sits with symmetrical hip abduction, you do not need to include this behavior in your measurable goal. You need only list the behaviors you expect to change. However, measurable axial goals MUST include specific positioning equipment needed and specific amounts of physical assistance provided to achieve the above behaviors. For example, a seat belt and moderate physical assistance to properly position the patient specifies the conditions needed to achieve the goal.

Functional Outcomes for Axial Goals

Even if hand function and independent ambulation do not return, gains in axial control can have a profound effect on discharge placement. Axial control gives the patient's sound arm and leg the ability to interact with the environment. If a patient does not regain head and trunk control, he/she essentially becomes a "functional quadriplegic." Hand and foot function of the sound side is sacrificed because the patient must use the intact limbs to prop up the trunk to prevent falling. Poor trunk control also makes the patient fight the caregiver because the patient feels so helpless about falling. If your patient cannot regain some head and trunk control, he/she is a poor candidate for discharge to the home!

If the patient can regain normal axial flexion and extension, including axial weight shifts forwards and backwards, he/she can begin to help the caregiver.

Leaning forward with anterior pelvic tilt is essential for standing up. It enables the patient to put his/her weight over the feet and inhibits backward thrusting when standing up. Backward thrusting significantly increases the amount of physical assistance needed to help the patient stand up. Transfers may require only minimal physical assistance if the patient can lean forward with anterior pelvic tilt. Weight shifts forward also permit the patient to use the sound hand to reach forward for objects out of reach. The ability to lean backward with posterior pelvic tilt makes it easier for the caregiver to lift the patient's legs during lower extremity dressing and hygiene and during car and tub transfers.

If the patient can regain midline symmetry, including axial weight shifts from side to side, he/she may require only minimal physical assistance for ADLs in sitting. Assistance is still needed for balance, but the fear of falling is less severe. Weight shifts side to side make it easier to lift either leg during lower extremity dressing and hygiene and during car and tub transfers. The patient can now shift onto either hip to hike the opposite hip to bathe the buttocks while sitting on a tub seat and to wipe after toileting. Finally, weight shifts side to side permit the patient to use the sound hand to reach on either side of the midline. If the patient reaches across the midline with the sound hand to get the toilet paper, a weight shift sideways will prevent falling once the sound hand comes off of the grab bar.

Advanced axial weight shifts with rotation and posterior pelvic tilt give the patient the potential to perform equilibrium reactions. This reduces the likelihood of falling because the patient can regain his/her balance if righting reactions fail. This makes it easier for the family to leave the patient unattended for short periods of time (like running to the store).

AUTOMATIC REACTIONS POSTULATES

Sequencing Treatment

Automatic reactions cannot truly be separated from the other deficits addressed by the NDT frame of reference. The axial continuum uses vertical righting reactions to facilitate normal trunk tone. Normal limb movements are needed to perform full-blown equilibrium reactions and protective extension. However, automatic reactions do have their own treatment sequence:

1. righting reactions;
2. equilibrium reactions; and
3. protective extension.

Righting Reactions

Righting reactions are in the first box in Memory Aid 9.1 because they develop first in normal infants. Righting reactions are used in the very first treatment session (5). They enable the therapist to safely move the patient within a posture. Even if patients are sitting supported or lying down, they feel threatened if they cannot return to an upright orientation or symmetrical body alignment.

Vertical righting reactions are facilitated first in the upright position. This is the light work position for the neck and trunk. Start in vertical and slowly move away from it (5). If your patient cannot sit up, support his/her back and concentrate on facilitating head control. If neck muscles are flaccid, the slight movement away from vertical will stimulate these muscles. If the ATNR is present, you must help the patient maintain a midline head position. Once head righting in vertical is present, it is easier to facilitate rotary righting reactions, which require head righting to protect the head while rolling.

Rotary righting reactions can be facilitated in several ways (5). Adult patients start by learning to log-roll from supine to side-lying using neck righting and FLEXION. The patient is taught to clasp hands together, place the sound leg under the hemiplegic leg to flex and lift it, and then use the momentum of arms and legs to roll (see Fig. 8.2). However, if a patient has too much axial extension and retraction of the hemiplegic arm and leg for the therapist to control while rolling from supine to side-lying, grade down. Instead, work on miniature rolling motions on either side of midline while in side-lying position. Once you can control some of the patient's excessive extensor thrust, grade up to rolling from side-lying back into supine. Extensor thrust doesn't have a chance to get started because the patient initiates the roll backwards from side-lying with shoulder and hip flexion. Next, the patient is ready to initiate rolling from supine to side-lying using FLEXION. Only advanced-level patients can learn to roll segmentally using body-righting or equilibrium reactions. Body righting is a chain reaction, so the patient must be taught to stop the rolling motion with his/her sound arm and leg. Equilibrium reactions allow patients to stop rolling anywhere they want to.

Equilibrium Reactions/Protective Extension

Some therapists place protective extension next in the treatment sequence for automatic reactions because normal infants develop protective extension when tipped forwards in sitting 1 month earlier than equilibrium reactions in sitting. Nevertheless, I have placed equilibrium reactions next in the sequence for three reasons. First, you could argue that equilibrium reactions come first because they develop in prone position 1 month before protective extension forward emerges in sitting. Yet, normal infants frequently deviate from the age norms by a month or two. These 1-month differences

do not provide compelling evidence that a strict developmental model should be used. Second, equilibrium reactions are our first line of defense when our righting reactions fail us. How many times a year do you fall on a outstretched arm? It's a strategy that is used only as a last resort. If healthy people use equilibrium reactions more often than protective extension, I think equilibrium should be emphasized early in treatment. Third, protective extension is the hardest automatic reaction to teach. It requires speed combined with strength, which many patients never regain in their hemiplegic arm. Equilibrium reactions can be facilitated with slower movement and depend more on recovery of axial control, which more patients can achieve.

Equilibrium reactions and protective extension are taught in two stages. First, the individual components of the automatic reaction, like elongation of the trunk, are facilitated. The second stage involves learning to coordinate all the components. Make sure your patient has at least a crude form of each of the individual components before going on to the second stage.

Making Automatic Reaction Goals Measurable

You can make automatic reactions measurable by listing the high-quality movements you expect to emerge after treatment. **High-quality vertical righting reactions** include: (1) an immediate response as soon as movement away from vertical begins, which is (2) consistently present. **Segmental rolling** includes: (1) shoulder flexion of the weightbearing arm to keep it from being trapped underneath the body, (2) trunk rotation, and (3) lateral head righting and trunk elongation of the weightbearing side when approaching side-lie. Segmental rolling is ideal, but **log-rolling** is functional as long as the patient initiates the roll with neck and limb flexion instead of arching and retracting the limbs.

High-quality equilibrium reactions include: (1) head righting, (2) trunk elongation on the weight bearing side, (3) trunk rotation with POSTERIOR pelvic tilt as abdominals are recruited, and (4) abduction of the uphill arm and leg. Abduction of the arm and leg on the side the patient is falling away from (uphill side) is not seen until the patient can tolerate being tipped quite a distance from vertical. **High-quality protective extension** includes: (1) lateral head righting, (2) trunk lateral flexion of the weightbearing side, (3) trunk rotation with ANTERIOR pelvic tilt, and (4) swift, forceful extension of the downhill arm and leg. Again, it is not necessary to list every one of the movement components discussed involved. Your automatic reactions goal should include only those movements you expect to see change.

Functional Outcomes for Automatic Reactions

Head righting maintains the head in a vertical position with the patient's eyes parallel to the ground. This is a normal facial orientation that facilitates social interaction and makes the patient appear more intelligent. Head righting also enables the patient to lift his/her head off of the bed. This frees the caregiver from physically supporting the head during bed care. Rotary righting reactions are also needed to ease handling during bed mobility. It is easy for the caregiver to injure his/her back while leaning over the bed and struggling with a patient who is using neck righting to arch backwards. Equilibrium in sitting makes it safer to leave the patient unattended for short periods of time. If a patient leans over, he/she will be able to re-erect himself instead of waiting for someone to come back to straighten him/her up. If patients have good standing balance, they are less likely to struggle against the caregiver with a "death grip" when being transferred and more likely to respond to sudden changes when walking in a crowded environment like a shopping mall.

LIMB CONTROL POSTULATES

Sequencing Treatment

The limb control sequence is designed for patients with brain damage. It is different from the biomechanical sequence that addresses passive range of motion, strength, and endurance. Limb control is divided into four boxes, shown in Memory Aid 9.1: (*1*) limb dissociation, (*2*) limb weight shift, (*3*) limbs free in space, and (*4*) distal skill. They are labeled *A–D* in Memory Aid 9.1 to denote a treatment sequence.

Limb Dissociation

This box refers to elongation of the limb into antisynergy positions. Severe shortening of limb muscles can occur in children with cerebral palsy who go untreated in the first year of life, in adults with traumatic head injury who are not properly positioned during the coma stage, and adults with strokes who quickly become synergy-bound. Patients who remain flaccid for several weeks don't need limb dissociation.

Shoulder dissociation begins with elongation of scapular muscles (5). The scapula usually needs to be protracted and depressed. Elongation is started in supine if the scapular muscles offer maximal resistance. Both hands will be needed to mobilize the patient's scapula. One hand may be pulling on the scapula while the other hand is pulling on the clavicle or humerus of the same shoulder (see Fig. 8.1). Another common position to elongate severely spastic scapular muscles is to roll the patient into side-lying so that weightbearing on the involved, protracted scapula will inhibit spasticity.

Once SCAPULAR tone can be controlled, the therapist is free to move his/her second hand more distally to elongate the entire upper extremity into a **Reflex Inhibiting Pattern** (RIP). Initially, the therapist uses proximal "key points of control" such as the scapula and elbow to inhibit early proximal movement. Remember, normal limb movement is characterized by proximal stability and distal movement in the early part of the range. Brain-damaged patients often reverse this pattern by moving the proximal joints first and never moving the stiffly cocontracting distal muscles. While using proximal key points, the therapist may not be able to facilitate the distal components of this RIP. As proximal tone normalizes, relaxation cacades down the limb, and the therapist can move his/her hands to distal key points of control, such as the forearm and hand, which brings in more of the distal components. Review Chapter 8 to help you choose a specific RIP.

Leg dissociation begins with separation of the two legs (5). In severe cases, both legs may flex together and extend together. Most lower extremity activities require separation of the legs. For example, during lower extremity dressing, one leg lifts to put on the garment while the other foot stays on the floor for balance. For adult patients who can usually separate the two legs, you can elongate each leg into a total RIP. This includes mid-range of hip flexion, hip abduction and external rotation, knee flexion, and ankle dorsiflexion to inhibit the extensor synergy. Unlike the arm, the leg is sometimes more easily handled first with distal key points of control, such as the big toe and calf.

As soon as you can passively elongate an extremity into an RIP, you need to IMMEDIATELY teach the patient to use the RIP during daily activities. By immediate, I mean within the same treatment session. Elongation by the therapist prepares the muscles for new positions and makes it easier for the patient to accept new ways of doing familiar activities. However, if the patient doesn't learn how to incorporate RIPs into daily activities, the effects of handling will be lost as soon as the patient goes home. See the chapter on NDT techniques for several examples on how to teach a patient to use RIPs in ADLs. On the other hand, if your patient has potential for recovery of limb movements, you can skip this step and go on to limb weight shifts and use of the limb in space.

Limb Weight Shifts

This box refers to the ability to move within a posture while weightbearing on the extremities. Remember, static weightbearing promotes fixing, so it is never used in NDT (5). Miniature movements are used in early treatment because they inhibit fixing. It is feasible to impose early weight shifts on even weak or frightened patients because the therapist provides FULL physical support and asks for MINIATURE motions.

The first step in limb weight shifts is primarily for children. Hand and foot preparation are needed for children who cannot tolerate any weightbearing on their hands or feet (5). Some patients are so tactually defensive on the palms of their hands and soles of their feet that contact with the supporting surface produces severe discomfort. Preparation begins with a non-weightbearing position. Firm, static, manual pressure is applied to the palm or heel. The hand and foot can also be placed firmly on a surface with no weight on the extremity. It can take several weeks for a severely impaired patient to tolerate weightbearing. However, you can introduce weightbearing with transitional behaviors while you wait for full palmar/plantar contact to develop.

The second step in limb weight shifts is weight shifts within a posture (5). Brief weightbearing is done to make sure that extension is performed without retraction. This is followed IMMEDIATELY by miniature movements of proximal joints in mid-ranges with the distal end of the extremity fixed on the support surface. For example, the weightbearing hemiplegic shoulder shifts over the hemiplegic elbow while the patient reaches for an object with the sound hand.

For children, weight shifts within a posture usually involve bilateral limb activities. For example, the therapist can completely support the child's body to prevent extension with retraction while the child rocks forward and backward on hands and knees over a bolster.

An adult may be too large for the therapist to support and shift the patient's weight onto both legs or both arms, so asymmetrical activities are used (1). The majority of the weight is supported by the sound arm or the therapist, so the involved extremity bears only partial body weight. For example, an adult can be asked to shift partial weight onto the involved arm in sitting or in **modified plantigrade** (standing while leaning slightly forwards to lean on hands or elbows on a table top).

Weight shifts within a posture for the arm are broken down into a four-part mini-sequence (5). Treatment begins with shifting weight over the elbow with as much external rotation as possible to inhibit the flexor synergy. Second, the arm is extended behind the trunk with the fingers pointing backward for maximal external rotation to inhibit the extension synergy. Third, the arm is extended at the patient's side with the fingers pointing out to the side (see Fig. 9.3). Fourth, the arm is extended in front of the body with the fingers pointing forward for moderate internal rotation. This last position is safe only if the patient has relative independence from synergy.

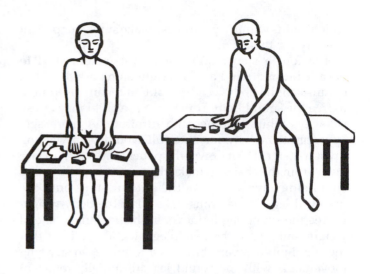

Figure 9.3. Partial weightbearing on an extended arm.

When asking for weight shifts over an extended arm, beware! To avoid falling on their face, patients often lean away from the weightbearing arm to take pressure off of it. For example, it is common to see children in quadruped sit back on their heels with minimal weight on their arms. An adult can place a hand on the table and put no weight on it when flexing and extending the elbow. When you graduate to weight shifting on extended arms, provide maximal support to make sure that the patient is not just placing to prevent a fall. Initially, position objects very close to the body so the patient only has to perform a miniature weight shift in order to reach the objects with the sound hand.

Leg weight shifts within a posture are also broken down into a mini-sequence that requires increasing amounts of leg extension (5). The physical therapist will start weight shifts on a flexed leg because this inhibits the extension synergy. For example, children can straddle a bolster with knees bent and hips externally rotated and abducted in order to rock side to side. Once weight shifts can be done in standing with minimal physical support, the occupational therapist needs to design purposeful activities that require miniature LE weight shifts while the patient is cognitively and emotionally challenged.

The third step under limb weight shifts is **linear transitional movements**. These movements enable a person to move from one position to another, like pushing up to sitting in bed using the involved arm or putting equal weight on both legs to stand up. The distal end of the extremity is still fixed on the support surface, but the proximal movements must be large enough to move the body through space to a new position. These larger movements are more frightening than the miniature weight shifts within a posture, so make sure your patient is ready for them.

The fourth step requires a **lateral weight shift to permit locomotion**. Lateral weight shifts are done last because all the body weight is put on the involved limb to free the sound limb. For example, a child may cruise sideways while holding onto furniture. A more age-appropriate activity for an adult would be a walking pivot transfer. To sit down, the patient must turn to face away from the chair. To make the turn, the patient takes small sideways steps. As the patient steps onto the involved leg, this leg must take all of the body weight to free the sound leg to move. In the beginning, lateral weight shifts onto the hemiplegic leg are so brief that the free limb has very little time to move, so stepping movements with the sound leg are initially reluctant and limited to a few inches at a time.

Limbs Free in Space

This box refers to the ability to move an extremity through space because proximal stability and freedom from synergy are emerging. The limb eventually feels light and moves with graded control. When this limb skill matures, movements are no longer stereotyped, and the patient can respond to varying demands in the environment. However, this box requires patients who can follow verbal directions.

The first step in this box is placing and lowering the limb with physical assistance from the therapist (1). Review Chapter 8 for instructions on how to grade amounts of physical assistance. Placing and lowering the arm are broken down into a four-part mini-sequence that gradually moves the arm closer to the extensor synergy position (1). It begins in supine with 90° of shoulder flexion and the arm in an RIP. This is a light work position and is easy for the patient to control. Gravity helps the patient eccentrically lower the arm towards his/her lap and lower it back over the head. Second in the mini-sequence is placing and lowering with the arm out to side while sitting. Sitting demands greater anti-gravity work and less support for the scapula. When the arm is out to the side, it is as far from both synergy trajectories as possible. As independence from synergies emerges, you can proceed to the third step, which is placing and lowering on the diagonal while sitting. Fourth, the patient places and lowers directly in front of his/her own body while sitting. This is the most dangerous position because it is closest to both synergy patterns.

Once the patient can place and lower with physical assistance from the therapist, he/she is ready for the second step of limbs free in space. This is self-assisted placing and lowering. The patient can maintain elbow and wrist extension with partial external rotation by clasping the involved hand with the sound hand. Many bilateral UE tasks are done with hands clasped to help the involved arm place and lower while keeping it in an RIP (see Fig. 9.4). A patient can also lift, place and lower the hemiplegic leg with assistance from the sound hand.

The third step of limbs free in space is independent, unilateral placing and lowering. Ideally, the patient will place and lower the involved limbs without assistance.

Distal Skill

This box refers to the ability to move with rotation and distal dissociation (5). Movement with rotation enables the patient to locomote with reciprocal limb movements and move efficiently between postures. **Distal dissociation** enables the patient to move the forearm, wrist, thumb, fingers, ankle, and foot independently from each other and from proximal body parts.

The physical therapist will work on rotation during transitional movements and locomotion. For example, the therapist can support the patient in standing as he/she takes one step forward and then one step backward while keeping the stance leg in the same place (1, 5).

NDT does not provide much information about the treatment sequence for distal dissociation of the upper extremity. Mrs. Bobath talked about practicing isolated elbow movements such as bending the elbow to touch the opposite shoulder or the top of the head (1). She said that facilitating skilled hand movements is difficult because of their complexity. See Figure 9.5 for two activities recommended by Eggers that encourage distal dissociation during supination, gross grasp, and release (8). Therapists instinctively stabilize objects for patients who lack distal dissociation so they can grasp the objects without chasing them all over the table. Maybe it is time to consciously use this transitional strategy of external support in treatment.

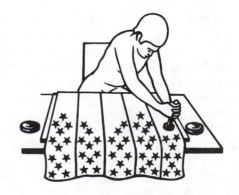

Figure 9.4. Bilateral tasks for placing and lowering.

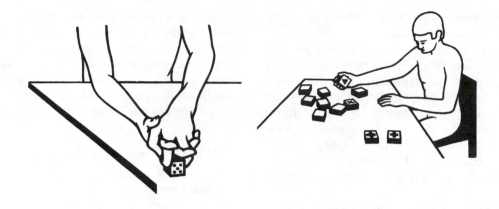

Figure 9.5. Activities that encourage supination/gross grasp/release.

Making Limb Goals Measurable

Limb dissociation goals can be made measurable by first documenting gains in passive elongation (see Table 7.4) or the use of RIPs during ADLs. For example, the goal for the biceps may be to achieve minimal resistance during passive elongation at mid-range. As the patient learns to use RIPs during ADLs, you should document the decreased need for physical assistance and increased consistency of use of RIPs without reminders.

Limb weight-shift goals should document gains in mature extension and mobility within a posture (see Tables 7.6 and 7.9). These **high-quality movements** include: (1) exhibiting graded movements with (2) scapular depression and protraction, (3) hip extension and adduction, and (4) an open hand and flat foot. Limb weight-shift goals should also document the **difficulty level** of weight shifts: (1) miniature weight shifts within a posture, (2) lateral weight shifts to free one limb, (3) linear transition movements to assume a new posture, (4) lowering self with graded linear control, and finally (5) locomotion with lateral weight shift. Remember, a limb weight-shift goal includes only the specific components of quality movement and difficulty level you expect your patient to achieve after treatment.

Limb free in space goals should document independence from synergy (see Tables 7.3A and 7.10). Choose goals slightly above the Brunnstrom evaluation results and placing and lowering baseline. For example, one goal might be to have the patient place and hold the involved arm at shoulder height while putting on a shirt or to hold up the involved leg while bathing.

Distal dissociation of the hand can be documented by:

1. Naming the new static grasp that will be acquired;
2. Independent movement of the wrist, thumb, index, and middle fingers while manipulating objects; and

3. Light, precise movements of the forearm, wrist, and fingers during reach and release, which shows a decreased need for external support.

For example, a hand dissociation goal might be to pick up a spoon with a lateral pinch by pushing lightly down on the table for external stability and scooping up food using wrist mobility (see Tables 7.3C, 7.11, 7.12, and 7.13).

Functional Outcomes for NDT Limb Goals

Lack of limb dissociation has serious functional consequences. If the patient does not regain passive elongation of the involved arm, he/she is at risk for shoulder-hand syndrome and hand deformities. Both conditions can be very painful and make it difficult for the patient or caretaker to perform activities of daily living. The arm has to be raised to wash the armpit. The hand has to open so it can be washed and the fingernails cut. Proximal dissociation of the legs is needed as well. Separation of the two legs is essential for diapering and toileting. Putting shoes on a patient is impossible with an ankle that is frozen in plantarflexion by the extensor synergy.

Limb weight shifts within a posture produce many functional gains. Many safety features put in patients' homes rely on weight shifting onto the involved arm. If the patient can lean the involved forearm on the grab bar in the bathroom, it will give him/her better balance while using the sound hand to manipulate the toilet paper and flush the toilet. Shifting onto the involved forearm on the wheelchair armrest makes the patient safer while reaching down with the sound hand to lock brakes, pick up objects, and put on shoes. Even everyday furniture makes the patient safer if he/she can lean on the involved arm. The ambulatory patient may be able to extend the involved arm to lean on the kitchen countertop for better balance while taking food out of the refrigerator with the sound hand.

Linear transitional movements reduce the amount of physical assistance needed during transfers and bed mobility. The patient can lift more of his/her own weight during transfers if equal weight is placed on both legs than if he/she were to put all the weight on the sound leg. Linear transitional movement of the arms allows the patient to push with the hemiplegic arm to sit in bed. Ease of transfers and bed mobility can make the difference between going home and going to a nursing home.

Lateral weight shifts enable the patient to perform a walking transfer with minimal assistance. This is the easiest type of transfer for a family member to perform. If the patient can lead with either side, it also makes him/her less vulnerable to architectural barriers. Many patients can lead with their sound leg and drag the involved leg to meet it. However, leading with the sound side doesn't meet the needs of every situation. Sometimes there isn't room to turn the wheelchair around so the patient can lead with the sound side. Bathrooms and parking spaces are notorious for being cramped. When it is difficult to make the patient lead with the involved side, trips to small spaces may have to be avoided.

Placing and lowering combined with a gross grasp enable the patient to use the involved hand as a gross assister to hold down an object while the sound hand manipulates the object. Bilateral activities that require object stabilization include zipping, writing, cutting food, spreading butter on bread, putting toothpaste on a toothbrush, cutting with scissors, and soaping up a washcloth. If the patient can use his/her involved hand to hold down these objects, he/she will need fewer assistive devices.

Unfortunately, a mature static grasp does not give a patient a functional, dominant hand. For example, one adult patient had a mature three-jaw-chuck grasp of the cube, superior tip pinch of the paper clip, and tripod grasp of the pencil. Yet, she spilled while using a spoon and was not able to write because she had a total lack of wrist mobility. She also had to chase the spoon, pencil, and paper clip around the table because she was trying to press on them for external support. Distal dissociation of the arm enables the patient to use the involved fingers to manipulate objects, like writing with a pencil. It also allows the patient to place either hand in a variety of orientations in space to grasp objects of different sizes in different positions.

Distal dissociation of the leg provides the small adjustments in ankle and foot positions needed to walk on irregular surfaces like shag carpeting, throw rugs, and gravel. Distal dissociation also includes locomotion with rotation and reciprocal limb movements. These mature gait strategies produce a faster gait with a greater ability to adjust to the unexpected movements of others and to rooms stuffed with furniture. Many patients can walk in a fire width hallway without people and furniture in it. Rotation helps the patient safely and quickly turn in small spaces to avoid bumping into furniture and people in stores, movie theaters, and restaurants.

SITUATIONAL THINKING

Time Lines

The treatment goals for axial control, automatic reactions, and limb control listed in Memory Aid 9.1 are intended to address the needs of a wide variety of patients. A single patient will not need to work on every one of them. If your patient has already achieved a specific goal, you can skip to the next appropriate one in the sequence.

Unlike the biomechanical frame of reference, which lists all the data for a single goal on one test sheet, you have to disassemble the formally organized NDT test sheets. For example, evaluation of muscle tone is relevant to numerous treatment boxes in Memory Aid 9.1. Table 9.1 tells you where to find the baseline data so you can identify where the patient is in each of the three treatment sequences. Your job is to predict how far down the three continua your patient will get in 1 week based on his/her initial amount of abnormal muscle tone.

At one extreme, you may feel maximal resistance to passive elongation early in the range. You will need several minutes to slowly elongate the spastic, stiff, painful muscles. There will be LESS time to work on active motion. However, it is not helpful to passively elongate the entire body and then wait to ask for active movement during a later session (5). You must ask for active movement of a body part AS SOON AS it is elongated so the patient won't forget this new sensation. You will spend proportionately more treatment time on inhibition than on facilitating active movement in the severely spastic patient. Therefore, shorter practice periods of active movement will slow down progress toward active movement goals.

The severely spastic patient needs active movements that are as far away as possible from the positions where abnormal movement strategies occur (1). You will not be able to speed up treatment by skipping over the safer positions that are listed first in the "mini-treatment sequences." For example, the patient with profound flexion synergy should weightbear on an extended arm with fingers pointed backwards instead of in front of the trunk, where the pathological synergies are strongest.

Since it is difficult for the highly spastic patient to maintain normal tone during transitional movements,

Table 9.1.
Partitioning the NDT Evaluation Results

I. Axial Control	II. Automatic Reactions	III. Limb Control

A. *Axial Extension*
  1. GM II: axial extension items
  2. Muscle Tone Sheet: pectorals and hamstrings, passive anterior tilt
  3. Clinical Observations: axial weight shift forward
	A. *Righting Reactions*
	  1. Clinical Observations: righting while rolling and lateral head righting during sitting balance
	  2. GM I: head righting when leaning backward
		A. *Limb Preparation*
		  1. Muscle Tone Sheet: scapular, shoulder, and hip items
		  2. Clinical Observations: LE synergy; shoulder subluxation

AA. *Axial Flexion*
  1. Muscle Tone Sheet: axial extensors; hip and knee flexors; passive posterior tilt
  2. GM I: all test items
  3. Clinical Observations: axial weight shift backwards
	B. *Equilibrium Reactions*
	  1. Clinical Observations: Equilibrium in sitting
		B. *Limb Weight Shifts*
		  1. GM III: Hand/Foot Preparation
		  2. GM II: limb items
		  3. GM IV: Transitional stage only = linear weight shift

B. *Midline Symmetry*
  1. Muscle Tone Sheet: axial items
  2. Clinical Observations: sits symmetrically; axial weight shift sideways in sitting
  3. Evaluate sitting with positioning devices during early Rx sessions
	C. *Protective Extension*
	  1. Clinical Observations: Protective extension
		C. *Limbs Free in Space*
		  1. Brunnstrom Evaluation, Page 1 *OR* FM I if patient can't follow complex commands
		  2. Clinical Observations: Placing and Eccentric Control

C. *Advanced Axial Weight Shifts*
  1. Muscle Tone Sheet: passive neck and trunk rotation
  2. Clinical Observations: axial weight shifts with rotation sitting
	D. *Tonic Reflexs*
	  1. Fiorentino's *Reflex Testing*
		D. *Distal Skill*
		  1. Brunnstrom Evaluation, Page 2
		  2. GM IV: Mature stage only = mobility with rotation
		  3. FM II: Ulnar to Radial Grasp
		  4. FM III: Distal Mobility

you will need to provide maximal manual inhibition. If you lose your inhibition while moving this patient to a new position, you will lose treatment time and may have to start all over again. Spastic diplegics in particular need to spend a lot of treatment time working on transitional movements. They should be graduated quickly from weight shifts within a posture to transitional movements. Transitional movements require larger movements that will inhibit persistent fixing seen in spastic diplegia (5).

At the other extreme, you may feel minimal resistance to passive elongation in the last half of the range. You will be able to passively elongate several muscle groups from adjacent boxes from Memory Aid 9.1 in a few minutes. For example, a therapist may passively posterior tilt, anterior tilt, and elongate the trunk on the weight-bearing side in rapid succession. Quick elongation gives you time to ask for several active movements early in the treatment session. It is common to see a therapist work on axial weight shifts forward, backward, and sideways in the same session with a high-level patient. This speeds up progress towards active movement goals.

Low spasticity also enables you to work the patient in positions where abnormal movements are stronger (e.g., leg extension with adduction is in the extension synergy position). This speeds up treatment since you can skip the lower level mini-steps. Finally, it will be easier to maintain normal tone during transitional

movements in a patient with minimal spasticity. You're not as likely to lose treatment time when you move your patient to a new position. Table 9.2 summarizes these guidelines for situational thinking about time-lines for the severely and minimally spastic patient.

Of course, there are patients who are in between minimal and maximal levels of spasticity, so it is impossible to say what will work until you try it. Remember, experienced therapists just get their estimates in the ballpark.

Abnormal tone also includes the flaccid and athetoid patient. These types of patients do not need passive elongation of most muscles, so you can skip directly to facilitation of active movement. Athetoid patients particularly need to work on small graded movements in mid-ranges within a posture because they exhibit explosive motions in large ranges as tone fluctuates wildly (5). Rather than facilitating movement, the therapist uses his/her hands to provide proximal stability of shoulder and hip girdles while the patient tries to move his/her limbs in mid-ranges.

There comes a time when a patient's muscle tone is close to normal. If you feel minimal resistance to passive elongation at the end of range, it is time to take the risk of OMITTING DIRECT TREATMENT. Sometimes minor deficits can be resolved indirectly by remediating something else. Use periodic reevaluation to track these minor deficits to see if treatment is still needed.

Table 9.2.
Situational Thinking About Time-Lines

Maximum Resistance at Beginning of Range	Minimum Resistance at End of Range
1. Need several minutes to slowly elongate 1 or 2 muscles in one box of Memory Aid 9.1	1. Only need 1–2 minutes to elongate several muscles from several boxes of Memory Aid 9.1
2. Brief time left to practice active movements later in the session slows down progress toward active movement goals	2. Can ask for early active movements from several boxes and achieve active movement goals quickly
3. Must work in positions that are as far as possible from pathological patterns; these additional steps in the mini-sequences take more time	3. Can save time by skipping ahead to work in the positions that are close to the pathological patterns observed in this patient
4. Can lose inhibition during transitional movements and may have to start inhibition over	4. Can easily maintain normal tone with minimal handling during transitional movements

Figure 9.6
Chunking NDT Goals

I. Axial Control	II. Automatic Reactions[a, b]	III. Limb Control

A. *Axial Extension*
  1. IF lacking full trunk extension check passive elongation of pectorals and hamstrings
  2. **CHILD ONLY**: elong. hip flexors; active axial extension prone
  3. Sitting: passive ANTERIOR tilt
  4. Sitting: active weight shift forwards using ANTERIOR tilt
	A. *Righting Reactions:*
	  1. Vertical head righting: moving away from vertical
	  2. Rotary righting:
	  —Log-roll with FLEXION RIPs in side-lie ! into supine ! from supine (neck rightg)
	  —Segment. roll: body rightg
	  —Segment. roll: equil. reac
		A. *Limb Dissociation*
		  1. Arm dissociation
		   a. Passive elonga. scapula (supine ! then sidelie)
		   b. Elongate UE into RIP
		  1. Leg dissociation
		   a. Dissociation of 2 legs
		   b. Elongate LE into RIP
		  2. Patient uses RIPs in ADLs

AA. *Axial Flexion*
  1. Passive elongation of shortened neck and lumbar extensors
  2. **CHILD ONLY**: passive elongation of hamstrings followed by active leglifts in supine
  3. Sitting: passive POSTERIOR tilt
  4. Sitting: active weight shift backwards using POSTERIOR tilt
	B. *Equilibrium Reactions:*
	  1. Learn each individual component and then
	  2. Simultaneously perform
	  —Head righting
	  —Trunk ELONGATION of weightbearing side
	  —Trunk rota/POSTERIOR tilt
	  —Abduction uphill arm/leg
		B. *Limb Weight Shifts*
		  1. **CHILD ONLY**: Hand/foot prep
		  2. MATURE extension during SMALL wt shifts over limb (e.g., on elbow ! hand ×3)
		  3. Symmet. linear transitional movements (e.g., stand up)
		  4. Lateral weight shifts to locomote (e.g., transfers)

B. *Midline Symmetry*
  1. Passive elongation of shortened neck and lateral trunk flexors
  2. Maintain sym. sit with devices
  3. Active weight shift onto hemi-side with trunk elongation
  4. Active wt shift side to side
  5. Indepen. assume symm. sitting
	C. *Protective Extension:*
	  1. Learn components, then
	  2. Simultaneously perform
	  —Head righting
	  —Lateral trunk FLEXION of weightbearing side
	  —Trunk rota/ANTERIOR tilt
	  —Extension downhill arm/leg
		C. *Limbs Free in Space*
		  1. P.A. to place & lower (e.g., arm at side ! on diagonal ! in front of body)
		  2. Self-assisted place & lower (e.g., bilateral UE tasks with hands clasped)
		  3. Independent place & lower

C. *Advanced Axial Weight Shifts*
  1. Passive elongation of neck and trunk rotators IF not complete
  2. Active axial rotation with posterior tilt and then anterior tilt
	[a]IF automatic react are absent check axial/limb muscle tone
	[b]Tonic reflexes are treated indirectly (e.g., ASTN ! facilitate FLEXOR tone, symmetry, righting reacts.)
		D. *Distal Skill*
		  1. Assumes postures and locomotes with rotation and reciprocal limb movements
		  2. Distal dissociation during reach/grasp/manip/release

ok = able to do
circle = possible in one week

Chunking

Chunking NDT goals helps you reduce the minutiae of the evaluation down to the "bigger picture" of a few goals. Start by identifying NDT goals that are already achieved (see "OK" in Fig. 9.6). This reduces your anxiety by elimi-nating goals that don't have to be considered. Then, circle goals that are possible in 1 week using the time-line suggestions just listed (see goals circled in Fig. 9.6).

The easiest way to label a short-term NDT goal is to chunk the steps from a single box in Memory Aid 9.1.

The name of the box becomes the name of the goal. Circle the total number of behaviors in the box that you think the patient will achieve in a week. For example, in the midline symmetry box, a very spastic patient may exhibit less resistance to passive elongation of lateral trunk flexors and be able to sit symmetrically with maximum assistance and seating devices in 1 week.

With a high-level patient, one short-term chunk may come from adjacent boxes from one continuum in Memory Aid 9.1. For example, the therapist may be able to elongate the arm into an RIP (limb box *A*), weight shift on an extended arm (limb box *B*), and practice placing and lowering (limb box *C*) in 1 week.

Sometimes a short-term chunk is created by combining goals from two different NDT continua. For example, an axial/limb goal might consist of passive elongation of hamstrings to permit active axial weight shift forward in sitting from the axial extension box (axial box *A*), which leads directly to standing up symmetrically from the limb weight shifts box (limb box *C*). Whenever you combine boxes from two continua, you have to make up your own name for the chunk. The axial/limb chunk just listed could simply be called "standing up symmetrically." Circle all the steps you think the patient will achieve and connect them with straight lines.

With a large chunk, it is not necessary to list all the steps in your treatment sequence in the medical chart! While all these steps will be included in a single treatment session, you only need to document progress toward the last step in the chunk that you think the patient will achieve in 1 week.

There are many correct ways to chunk short-term NDT goals. Experienced therapists would not agree on how to chunk short-term NDT goals for a specific patient. What an experienced therapist would not do is to take one box from Memory Aid 9.1 and blow the three or four steps listed in one box into an entire treatment plan for the week.

ONE NDT POSTULATE REGARDING CHANGE

A postulate regarding change links an NDT deficit to a functional outcome in a specific format. For example:

General deficit: Poor midline symmetry
Stage-specific cause: spastic trunk muscles on hemiplegic side
Measurable short-term NDT goal: patient will shift her weight onto the hemiplegic hip with trunk elongation and hip-hiking with minimal physical assistance
Functional outcome: spouse will be able to wash bottom of sound hip while patient sits on a bathtub stool

A simple way to identify the NDT deficit is to name a box in Memory Aid 9.1. The deficit can be general since the NDT goal is measurable. Notice that the NDT goal describes the movement strategies the patient will use. A patient may already be able to independently shift onto his/her hemiplegic hip using lateral trunk flexion, which does not hike the hip and elongate the trunk. A descriptive NDT goal makes it possible to justify why treatment of axial weight shifts is still needed. The NDT goal should also relate specifically to the functional outcome. The patient and family members should be able to see a direct connection.

It is essential to identify the stage-specific cause of the NDT deficit. During the early stage of recovery, flaccidity (cause #1) is usually present. As muscle tone emerges, the patient usually develops voluntary axial fixing (#2) to keep from falling, especially if head righting is absent (#3). With time, spasticity (#4) and pathological limb synergies (#5) emerge. Eventually, untreated spasticity can cause overutilized spastic muscles to shorten and become contractured (#6). Children with brain damage may exhibit tonic reflexes (#7) and severe tactile defensiveness (#8) of hands and feet, which makes weightbearing difficult. The mildly involved patient may make the transition from flaccidity to spasticity with minimal excess tone and axial fixing, but he/she may have forgotten how to initiate active axial and limb movements (#9). The patient may continue to use neck righting (#10) during rolling out of habit. Even if a patient can perform the individual components of a normal equilibrium reaction, the patient may still need to practice coordinating all the components at once (#11).

SUMMARY

NDT goals can be sequenced with the three continua for axial control, automatic reactions, and limb control. These continua enable you to identify where your patient is now and what he/she should be able to do next. There is no general rule for which continuum should be listed first on a particular treatment plan. Some patients need limb dissociation first, so the therapist can use RIPs to facilitate axial movements. Other patients need vertical righting reactions and axial elongation first to make it possible for the therapist to move the patient. When one of the three continua is a prerequisite for the others, a definite priority emerges. Sometimes the three continua can be addressed in any order.

NDT goals can and must be measurable. This is usually accomplished with descriptive goals that state which movement strategies the patient will exhibit, like sitting with shoulders level and head in midline, rather than quantitative goals, like how many minutes a patient can sit.

SPECIFIC NDT goals must be linked to SPECIFIC functional outcomes. Physicians do not claim there is a connection between gallbladder surgery and a composite index of health. They claim there is a connection between gallbladder surgery and a specific digestive function. The connection between NDT goals and functional outcomes should be just as specific.

STUDY QUESTIONS

1. What are the mini-treatment sequences for axial flexion, axial extension, midline symmetry, and advanced axial weight shifts?
2. What is the two-step treatment sequence for automatic reactions?
3. What are the mini-treatment sequences for limb dissociation, limb weight shifts, and limbs free in space?
4. How does treatment progress differently for patients with maximal spasticity, minimal spasticity, and flaccidity?
5. What two general strategies make NDT goals measurable?
6. What specific strategies are recommended for making limbs free in space goals and distal dissociation goals measurable?
7. Why is it important to make specific connections between NDT goals and functional outcomes?

References

1. Bobath B. Adult hemiplegia: evaluation and treatment. 2nd ed. London: William Heinemann Medical Books Limited, 1978.
2. Filiatrault J, et al. Motor function and activities of daily living assessments: a study of three tests for persons with hemiplegia. Am J Occup Ther 1991;45:806.
3. Spaulding SJ, et al. Wrist muscle tone and self-care skill in persons with hemiparesis. Am J Occup Ther 1989;43:11.
4. Boehme R. The specifics of shoulder girdle dynamics as a basis for fine motor development. Workshop in Milwaukee, 1985.
5. Adams M. Bobath Certification (8-week course). Memphis, 1982.
6. Davis JZ. Neurodevelopmental treatment. In: Pedretti WP, Zoltan B, eds. Occupational therapy practice skills for physical dysfunction. 3rd ed. Philadelphia: CV Mosby, 1990: 351.
7. Norkin C, Levangie P. Joint structure and function. Philadelphia: FA Davis, 1983.
8. Eggers O. Occupational therapy in the treatment of adult hemiplegia. Rockville, MD: Aspen Publications, 1984.

Neurodevelopmental Treatment Case Simulation

CREATING NARRATIVE HYPOTHESES AND AN EVALUATION PLAN

> Odessa is a 70-year-old black retired social worker who had a right cerebral vascular accident (CVA) 1 month ago. She is a widow with one daughter and two grandsons. She will be discharged to live with her daughter. Her daughter has a three-story house with six steps up to the front door and a bathroom on the second and third story. When her husband was alive, she cleaned and did the laundry, but did not cook.

Student's Narrative Hypotheses

Use this space to write your narrative hypotheses. Restrict yourself to ± 7 hypotheses by chunking related concerns. Read an entry-level chapter on hemiplegia before you start. Use Memory Aid 2.2 to guide you.

Suggested Narrative Hypotheses

Based on the diagnosis of right CVA, date of onset, and brief social history, I would expect:

1. Somatosensory loss of the LUE and LLE;
2. Mixed muscle tone with emerging synergies of the LUE and LLE;
3. Poor bilateral trunk control with posterior pelvic tilt and midline asymmetry;
4. Impaired automatic reactions;
5. Perceptual-cognitive deficits such as unilateral neglect and apraxia;
6. Emotional lability which sometimes accompanies stroke;
7. More information is needed about her family and architectural barriers; and
8. Loss of independence in ADLs

Student's Evaluation Plan

Use this space to design an evaluation package. Identify the domains of concern you would test. Name the tests you would use and justify why you would choose these tests. In-depth testing is not indicated all the time.

Concern	*Name of Test*	*What the Data Will Be Used for*

Suggested Evaluation Plan

Based on the narrative hypotheses, I would recommend the following tests for the initial evaluation:

Concern	Name of Tests	What the Data Will Be Used for
Sensory loss	Kinesthesia	This primitive skill returns first. If present, continue sensory testing.
Mixed muscle tone	Complete evaluation	I must know specifically which muscles to inhibit and which to facilitate.
Independence from synergy	Brunnstrom eval.: p.1; GM Trend II and IV; LE synergy during ADLs and transfers	Emerging synergy may require RIPs now. It's too early to expect distal dissociation. Evaluate UE weightbearing ONLY if UE tone is emerging. I must know about LE synegy during ADLs and transfer for discharge planning.
Axial control	GM Trend I and II; sit symmetrically; axial weight shifts in sitting	Posterior pelvic tilt will make transfers extremely difficult. Midline asymmetry may require immediate prescription of positioning devices.
Automatic reactions	Vertical and rotary righting; sitting balance	I need to know how easy or difficult it will be to move the patient during treatment sessions.
Cognitive	Comprehensive OT Evaluation (COTE)	Need to decide if further testing is possible or necessary.
Psychosocial	COTE	Need information about her emotional response to her illness without invasive interviewing at first.
Environment	Talk to social worker	Same as psychosocial concerns.
ADLs	Bed mobility; transfers; toileting; feeding; put on pants; ambulation	Functional skills should be returning after 1 month of treatment if prognosis is good. Skills listed are vital to discharge to home. Putting pants on is safer way to eval LE than bathing for now.

EVALUATION RESULTS

Physical assets and deficits are listed on the muscle tone form, the clinical observation sheet, and Gross Motor Trends I, II, and IV (see Figs 10.1–10.3) Odessa is right-hand dominant. Her LUE is in Brunnstrom stage 2 with minimal active shoulder movements that include shoulder abduction. She is unable to open and close her left hand. She can detect light touch with her LUE, but kinesthesia and stereognosis are absent. She ignores her LLE during transfers and stands with minimal weight on her left foot.

Name: _____ Odessa _____   Date: _____

SLOWLY move body part passively from zero position. *STOP* as soon as you feel resistance. Estimate where in the range you stopped (e.g., about 90°). Estimate how much resistance you feel by going beyond where resistance started.

> Minimal = therapist easily moved body part beyond point of resistance
>
> Moderate= therapist moved body part past initial resistance by moving slowly and with effort; patient may experience discomfort
>
> Maximal = therapist is unwilling to use the full force needed to break through resistance; patient will deÆnitely experience discomfort

CIRCLE RESISTED MOTION	*Where Resistance First Felt*	*Min/Mod/Max*
lateral flex R (0°±45°)		
lateral flex L (0±45°)		
(Neck flexion (0°±45°))	End of range	Bony block
R (0°±60°)		
(Neck rotation L (0°±60°))	At 30°	Bony block
posterior		
(Pelvic tilt anterior)	Beginning of range	Maximum
®		
(Trunk elongation L)	Mid-range	Moderate
®		
Trunk rotation L	Mid-range	Moderate
depression (3 cm)		
(Scapular elevation (4"))	Mid-range	Maximum
(Scapular protraction (4"))	Beginning of range	Maximum
Shoulder flexion (0°±170°)	Just past 145°	Moderate
(Shoulder abduction (0°±170°)	Only when scapula held down	Moderate
Scap upward rota. starts at 30°)	Immediate lateral winging	None
horz. ADduction (0°±40°)		
(Sh. horz. ABduction (0°±130°))	At 0°	Moderate
internal (0°±90°)		
(Sh. rota. external (0°±90°))	Mid-range	Maximum
flexion (0°±135°)		
Elbow extension (0°±135°)	OK	
pronation (0°±90°)		
Forearm supination (0°±90°)	OK	
flexion (0°±80°)		
(Wrist extension (0°±70°))	End of range	Minimum
CMC Abduct (0°±50°)		
Thumb CMC exten (0°±50°)	OK	
MP flexion (0°±90°)		
Finger IP flexion (0°±110°)	OK	
knees bent	Just before 90°	
(Hip flexion (0°±120°))	Moderate	Moderate
internal (0°±45°)		
(Hip rota. external (0°±45°))	Beginning of range	Maximum
flexion (0°±135°)		
Knee extension (0°±135°)	OK	
plantar flexion (0°±50°)		
(Ankle dorsi flexion (0°±15°))	At −10°	Bony block

Figure 10.1   Muscle Tone Evaluation

Yes = patient is able to perform
PA = physical assistance (max/mod/min)
± = partial performance

No = patient is not able to perform
I = independent
NT = Not Tested

Sits Symmetrically:
Yes Head in midline & erect
_No_ Shoulder height is even: R > ? (< L)(circle 1)
Yes Neutral pelvic tilt
_No_ Equal weight on both hips (R >)? < L
_No_ Symmetrical hip abduction: R > ? (< L)
_No_ Both feet ∅at on ∅oor

SUBLUXATION: _No_ Ængers wide on____ side
____ Scapula downwardly rotated
____ Lateral trunk ∅exion____ side
____ Arm internally rotated/pronated

AUTOMATIC REACTIONS WHILE ROLLING: Choose only one!
____ No log-roll during LE Derotative procedure (trunk is ∅accid)
____ Log-rolls upper body during LE Derotative procedure
Yes Log-rolls using unsafe arching and limb retraction (Neck Righting)
____ Log-rolls safely with neck, shoulder, and hip ∅exion (Neck Righting)
____ Segmentally rolls but can't stop roll, even at edge (Body Righting)
____ Can stop segmental roll at any point in space (Equilibrium Reactions)

LE EXTENSION SYNERGY DURING ADLs IN SITTING: P = Present   A = Absent
_P_ Resists external rotation when legs cross or foot rests on opposite knee
_A_ Resists knee ∅exion when crossing hemiplegic leg over sound leg
_A_ Knee extends so hemiplegic foot rests in front of sound foot on ∅oor
_P_ Resists hip ∅exion when patient tries to touch hemiplegic foot on ∅oor
_P_ Resists ankle dorsi∅exion when trying to put shoes on

PLACING REACTION of _L_ arm:
_NT_ Arm in RIP at side
_NT_ Arm in RIP diagonally
_NT_ Arm in front of body

ACTIVE WEIGHT SHIFT IN SITTING:
_I_ Lean forward with
    (circle 1)
    anterior/(neutral)/posterior tilt
_I_ Lean 1/3 way back towards supine with
    (circle 1)
    (posterior)/neutral/anterior tilt
    Higher functioning patients:
_No_ Sideways to R/trunk elong
_No_ Sideways to L/trunk elong
_No_ Active trunk rotation to R
_No_ Active trunk rotation to L

ECCENTRIC CONTROL of _L_ arm:
_NT_ Lower arm at side of body
_NT_ Lower arm diagonally
_NT_ Lower arm in front of body

EQUILIBRIUM IN SITTING: tilt to

Left		Right
Yes	Vertical head righting	_Yes_
_No_	Trunk elongation of weightbearing side	_No_
_No_	Rotation w/posterior tilt	_No_
_No_	Abduct uphill arm/leg	_No_

PROTECTIVE EXTENSION IN SITTING:

Left		Right
_NT_	Vertical head righting	_NT_
_NT_	Lateral trunk ∅exion of weightbearing side	_NT_
_NT_	Rotation w/anterior tilt	_NT_
_NT_	Extend downhill arm/leg	_NT_

Figure 10.2. Muscle Tone Evaluation

Psychosocial and cognitive skills are listed on the COTE form (see Fig. 10.4). Memory appears to be good, and she is alert and oriented. She appears to have left-sided neglect, but intermittently scans to her left. She is impulsive during ADLs. Being a grandmother is "very important to her."

She feeds herself with a rocker knife and set-up assistance. She requires only minimal physical assistance for bed mobility and UE dressing, but needs moderate assistance for transfers and LE dressing. She is dependent with fastenings and with hair care because she wears her hair twisted and pinned.

Gross Motor Trend I: Hypotonic to Strong Axial Flexion			
Neck Flexors Activate	Lower-to-Supine: brief or no head control	Lower-to-Supine: head held in a line with elevated shoulders	Lower-to-Supine: head flexed in front of depressed shldrs _YES_
Abdominals Activate	Lower-to-Supine: loss of trunk control during 1/3 way back	Lower-to-Supine: _YES_ controls trunk for 1/3 way back with _posterior_ tilt	Lower-to-Supine: _NO_ controls trunk for 2/3's way back; posterior tilt

Gross Motor Trend II: Flexor to Extensor Tone			
Lean on One Elbow	Places elbow on mat but arm is easily moved in a circle by the OT; hand is fisted	Puts full weight on _YES_ elbow with cues but scapula elevates/retracts; hand is loosely fisted	Spontaneously puts _NO_ full weight on elbow; scap. depressed/protracted; hand is open
Lean on One Extended Arm	Places hand on mat but arm is easily moved in a circle by the OT; hand fisted _YES_	Puts full weight on _NO_ hand with cues but scap. elevates/retracts; hand is loosely fisted	Spontaneously puts full weight on hand; scap. depressed/protracted; hand is open
Sitting to Test Axial Extension	Sits supported: head completely sags forward; rounded back; hand is fisted	Sits unsupported: head forward but steady; only upper trunk extended; scap. elevated; hand loosely fisted	Sits unsupported: _YES_ head erect/steady; full trunk extension; scap. depressed; hand is open
Standing to Test LE Extension	Stands supported: hips & knees flexed; takes most of weight; hand is fisted	Stands supported: knees extend BUT hips flex; trunk leans forward; hand loosely fisted	Stands supported: _YES_ BLE fully extend _more wt_ so feet are directly _on LLE_ under trunk; hand open

Gross Motor Trend IV: Mobility Superimposed on Stability			
Reach on One Elbow	Reach on elbow: _YES_ collapses onto trapped arm	Reach: scap. _NT_ elevates/retracts; elbow is not directly under shoulder	Reach: scap. is depressed/ protracted; elbow is directly under shldr
Reach on Extended Arm	Reach on extended arm: _NT_ collapses onto elbow	Reach: scap. elevates/retracts; hand is not directly under shldr	Reach: scap. is depressed/ protracted; hand directly under shldr
Sitting	See Clinical Observations for Axial Weight Shifts in Sitting		
Walking	Pulls self up to _YES_ standing with _moderate_ P.A.; leans heavily on UE's and puts more weight on LLE	Sits down smoothly _YES_ holding onto support Steps sideways during walking pivot transfer _NT_ Walks with _not able_ P.A. & _____ aids; leg circumduction; foot drop; wide base	Walks independently _NT_ with _____ aids; stops; only with advance notice Walks with reciprocal elbow swing Walks safely: makes sudden stops/ turns

Figure 10.3 Adult Modifications of Gross Motor Trends for Odessa

INTERPRETING THE TEST RSULTS

On the blank page, list each hypothesis, *but* leave a generous space under each hypothesis to list the evaluation results that you believe are relevant to each hypothesis. In front of each cue, write one of the following symbols. A plus means a cue confirms and a minus means the cue disconfirms a hypothesis. A ± means a cue partially confirms and partially disconfirms a hypothesis. A question mark means the cue's relevance is unclear. Remember, these symbols are feedback to you about the accuracy of your hypotheses! They do not indicate the patient's assets and deficits! At the bottom of each list, conclude that each hypothesis was confirmed as written, *OR* write a revised hypothesis. Cues that are completely unrelated to your hypotheses should be preceded by a capital N for New and added to the end of the list.

A. ENGAGEMENT
- ⓪-Needs no encouragement to begin task
- 1 -Encourage once to begin activity
- 2 -Encourage two or three times to engage in activity
- 3 -Engages in activity only after much encouragement
- 4 -Does not engage in activity

B. CONCENTRATION
- 0 -No difficulty concentrating during full session
- ①-Off task less than one-fourth time
- 2 -Off task half the time
- 3 -Off task three-fourths time
- 4 -Loses concentration in less than 1 minute

C. RESPONSIBILITY
- 0 -Takes responsibility for own actions
- ①-Denies responsibility for 1 or 2 actions
- 2 -Denies responsibility for several actions
- 3 -Denies responsibility for most actions
- 4 -Denial of responsibility; messes up project and blames therapist or others

D. FOLLOW DIRECTIONS
- 0 -Carries out directions without problems
- ①-Occasional trouble with more than three step directions
- 2 -Carries out simple directions; has trouble with two-step directions
- 3--Can carry out only very simple one step directions (demonstrated, written, or oral)
- 4 -Unable to carry out any directions

E. ACTIVITY NEATNESS
- 0 -Activity done neatly
- ①-Occasionally ignores fine detail
- 2 -Often ignores fine detail; materials are scattered
- 3 -Ignores fine detail; work habits disturbing to those around
- 4 -Unaware of fine detail; so sloppy that therapist has to intervene

F. PROBLEM SOLVING
- 0 -Solves problems without assistance
- ①-Solves problems after assistance given once
- 2 -Can solve only after repeated instructions
- 3 -Recognizes a problem but cannot solve it
- 4 -Unable to recognize or solve a problem

G. SOCIABILITY
- ⓪-Socializes with staff and patients
- 1 -Socializes with staff and occasionally with other patients or vice-versa
- 2 -Socializes only with staff or with patients
- 3 -Socializes only if approached
- 4 -Does not join others in activities

H. COMPLEXITY AND ORGANIZATION OF TASK
- 0 -Organizes and performs all tasks given
- 1 -Occasional trouble organizing complex tasks he should be able to do
- ②-Organizes simple but not complex tasks
- 3 -Can do only very simple activities with organization imposed by therapist
- 4 -Unable to organize or carry out task when materials/directions available

I. INITIAL LEARNING
- 0 -Learns new activity quickly and easily
- 1 -Occasionally has difficulty learning a complex activity
- ②-Frequent difficulty learning complex activity but can learn simple one
- 3 -Unable to learn complex activities; occasional difficulty learning
- 4 -Unable to learn a new activity

K. INTEREST IN ACCOMPLISHMENT
- ⓪-Interested in finishing activities
- 1 -Occasional lack of interest or pleasure in finishing a long-term activity
- 2 -Interest or pleasure in accomplishment of short-term activity; lack of interest in a long-term activity
- 3 -Only occasional interest in finishing
- 4 -No interest or pleasure in finishing

L. DECISION MAKING
- ⓪-Makes own decisions
- 1 -Makes decisions but occasionally seeks therapist approval
- 2 -Makes decisions but often seeks therapist approval
- 3 -Makes decision when given two choices
- 4 -Refuses to or cannot make any decisions

M. FRUSTRATION TOLERANCE
- 0 -Handles all tasks without becoming overly frustrated
- ①-Occasionally becomes frustrated with complex tasks; can handle simple ones
- 2 -Often becomes frustrated with complex tasks; can handle simple ones
- 3 -Often becomes frustrated with any task but attempts to continue
- 4 -Becomes so frustrated with simple tasks that refuses or is unable to function

N. EXPRESSION
- ⓪-Expression consistent with situation and setting
- 1 -Occasionally inappropriate
- 2 -Inapropriate several times during session
- 3 -Expression inconsistent with situation
- 4 -Extremes of expression: bizarre, uncontrolled or no expression

Figure 10.4.   Excerpts from COTE: ODESSA

Student's Cue Interpretation List

1.

Student's Problem List

The cue interpretation list and hypothesis evaluation represents an inner dialogue that is too lengthy to put in a medical chart. A facility will want you to write a Problem List that consists of general deficits and dysfunction. On this page, convert your confirmed hypotheses into a Problem List. By definition, a Problem List does not include assets and function, so delete them. Feel free to change the numbers and descriptions from the ones used in the hypotheses. Remember, working memory is limited to ± 7 pieces of information, so eliminate unconfirmed hypotheses and chunk related problems. Don't forget to add new problems not anticipated by your hypotheses!

1.

2.

3.

4.

5.

6.

7.

8.

Suggested Cue Interpretation List

1. *SOMATOSENSORY LOSS OF LUE/LLE*
   - −   Detection of light touch present
   - +   Kinesthesia and stereognosis are absent in LUE
   - +   Ignores LLE during transfers

   Confirmed as written

2. *MIXED MUSCLE TONE WITH EMERGING SYNERGY/WEIGHT SHIFTS OF LUE/LLE*
   - +   Moderate/Maximal resistance of scapula/shoulder/hip BUT No/Min resistance of elbow/forearm/fingers/thumb/knee/ankle
   - ±   LUE Stage 2: minimal shoulder motions (abduction version) and unable to open/close hand
   - +   Unable to place or lower LUE
   - +   LE extension synergy interferes with LE ADLs
   - +   Weightbears on elbow with retraction; collapses during weight shift
   - −   Minimal weightbearing on LLE in standing

Confirmed: mixed muscle tone with emerging synergy in LUE and LLE
Revision: weightbearing emerging in UE, but absent in LE

3. *POOR BILATERAL TRUNK CONTROL/MIDLINE ASYMMETRY/POSTERIOR PELVIC TILT*
   - −   Moderate resistance ONLY during trunk elongation/rotation to her right
   - +   No active axial weight shifts to left AND right in sitting
   - +   Sits asymmetrically with lateral trunk flexion of right side
   - +   Maximum resistance to anterior tilt starting in neutral tilt
   - −   No resistance to passive hamstring elongation
   - ±   Axial weight shifts forward done independently with neutral pelvic tilt

Revision: Bilateral axial fixing with midline asymmetry

4. *IMPAIRED AUTOMATIC REACTIONS*
   - −   Vertical head righting present
   - +   Log-rolls with extension
   - +   No equilibrium in sitting

Confirmed as written

5. *PERCEPTUAL-COGNITIVE IMPAIRMENT*
   - +   Impulsive during ADLs
   - +   Unilateral neglect to her left
   - +   Difficulty learning/organizing complex tasks
   - +   Occasional trouble with more than three-step directions
   - −   Oriented, alert, and attentive
   - −   Initiates and completes tasks

Unilateral neglect, but unclear perceptual-cognitive deficits

6. *EMOTIONAL LABILITY*
   - −   Socially appropriate
   - −   Socializes with others

Disconfirmed

7. *SUPPORTIVE FAMILY BUT ARCHITECTURAL BARRIERS*
   - +   Architectural barriers at daughter's house where she'll be D/C
   - ?   Family's emotional and financial resources

Partially confirmed: architectural barriers present, but environmental resources are still unclear

8. *LOSS OF INDEPENDENCE IN ADLs*
   - +   Moderate assistance needed for dressing/bed mobility/transfers
   - +   Dependent in hair care and fastenings
   - +   Nonambulatory 1 month postonset
   - ±   Set-up assistance for eating

Confirmed as written

N. *BONY BLOCK OF NECK/ANKLE*

Suggested Problem List

1. Significant somatosensory loss
2. UE has severe proximal spasticity with emerging flexion synergy
3. Bony block of neck and ankle

4. Nonambulatory; More information needed about LLE during transfers
5. Bilateral axial fixing with midline asymmetry
6. Impaired automatic reactions
7. Unilateral neglect, but unclear perceptual-cognitive deficits
8. Architectural barriers with unknown financial and social resources
9. Needs moderate/maximum assistance in self-care except for eating

Reflection on the Problem List

Note that some numbers have changed from the hypothesis list to the Problem List. This is customary since test results often redefine the therapist's focus. Feel free to chunk the problems differently. Chunking is a personal strategy that helps an individual remember the main treatment issues.

1. *Somatosensory loss.* Detection of light touch is present, but it is so primitive that it has minimal significance for motor return and safety. Lack of kinesthesia and stereognosis still represent a significant sensory loss.

2. *UE has severe proximal spasticity with emerging flexion synergy.* She has almost no synergy activity, which is unexpected for 1 month postonset.

3. *Bony block.* Note the addition of new data which had no hypothesis number.

4. *More information needed about LLE.* Her ability to transfer with only moderate assistance when she is unable to weightbear on her LLE is a major discrepancy. Her quadriceps have minimal spasticity, which could make her knee unstable. She may lack confidence in her LLE because she can't feel where it is and can't get her foot flat due to the bony block. More information is needed about her LLE during transfers.

5. *Bilateral axial fixing with midline asymmetry.* Resistance to passive trunk elongation was felt only to her right, which conflicts with her inability to initiate active weight shifts to either side. Another discrepancy is maximum resistance to passive anterior tilt, even though she doesn't resist passive hamstring elongation and is able to actively weight-shift forward in sitting with neutral tilt. She is probably using axial fixing during passive tilt because she doesn't feel comfortable giving up voluntary control.

6. *Impaired automatic reactions.* Vertical head righting is present, but all other automatic reactions are absent. This make her unsafe when unattended and will dramatically affect discharge planning if not remediated.

NOTE: Hypothesis #6 concerning emotional lability was disconfirmed. She acts appropriately and interacts well with others. Problem Lists ignore assets.

7. *Unilateral neglect but unclear perceptual-cognitive deficits.* Several conflicting cues require further evaluation. She has unilateral neglect, but good attention. She is impulsive and has poor organization with complex tasks, yet she has some executive functions such as initiating a task. Impulsiveness during ADLs may be due to unilateral neglect or to complex visual perception deficits. Frequent difficulty with organizing and learning complex tasks may be due to cognitive deficits or stress reactions.

IDENTIFYING DEFICITS NOT ADDRESSED BY NDT

Before you design NDT treatment activities, it is important to identify the blind spots that will be present in your treatment plan because NDT concerns are restricted to axial control, automatic reactions, and limb control. You don't need to divert your energy by solving all these problems now, but you do need to identify these unaddressed concerns before you get too involved in the minutiae of NDT evaluation data. Make sure you list BOTH the name of the concern and the specific evaluation results to prove that each specific concern exists. For example, ignoring all the letters on the left side of the page (behavior observed during initial evaluation) might indicate visual neglect (specific perceptual-cognitive concern).

Student's List of Deficits Not Addressed by NDT

Use this space to identify three MOHO assets or deficits. Name each MOHO concern. Then substantiate each one with specifics from the evaluation results. Use Memory Aid 14.1 to guide you.

1.

2.

3.

Use this space to identify two psychosocial assets or deficits that are ignored by the MOHO frame of reference. Name each psychosocial concern. Substantiate each one with specifics from the evaluation results, or write reasonable questions regarding this concern. Use Memory Aid 14.1 to guide you.

1.

2.

Use this space to identify one biomechanical deficit. Name the biomechanical concern. Then substantiate it with specifics from the evaluation results. Use Memory Aid 4.1 to guide you.

Use this space to identify three perceptual-cognitive assets or deficits. Name the perceptual-cognitive concern. Then substantiate each concern with specifics from the evaluation results. Use Memory Aid 15.1 to guide you.

1.

2.

3.

Use this space to identify two sensory-motor assets or deficits. Name the sensory-motor concern. Then substantiate each concern with specifics from the evaluation results. Use Memory Aid 16.1 to guide you.

1.

2.

Use this space to identify one homeostatic deficit. Name the specific concern, not just the homeostatic system. If you can't substantiate this concern with evaluation results, suggest a reasonable concern and explain why it is a realistic concern given the diagnosis and date of onset. Use Memory Aid 17.1 to guide you.

Use this space to list current rehabilitation concerns with specifics from the evaluation results. Use Memory Aid 2.2 to guide you.

Suggested List of Deficits Not Addressed by NDT

MOHO assets and deficits. Notice the use of quotation marks to indicate patient report.

External locus of control: she denies responsibility for one to two actions
Roles: grandmother role is "very important" to her
Habits: when husband was alive, she cleaned and did laundry, but didn't cook
Social appropriateness: emotional expression is consistent with her situation and setting
Social group: widow with one daughter and two grandsons; will be discharged to her daughter's house
Objects: daughter's home is a three-story house with six steps up to front door and bathrooms on the second and third floor

Psychosocial assets and deficits that are ignored by MOHO. Note the use of question marks to indicate reasonable questions about issues not specifically mentioned in the report.

Frustration tolerance: she occasionally becomes frustrated with more complex tasks; can readily handle simple tasks
Sexuality: how is she responding to her lack of feminine appearance? Did she have male significant others after her husband died?
Stress reactions: is she depressed or showing other stress reactions?
"needs encouragement to begin tasks" = stress reaction?
"occasionally not interested in new activities" = a stress reaction?
Sociability: socializes readily with staff and other patients

Biomechanical deficits. Bony block of neck and ankle.

Perceptual-cognitive assets and deficits. Note the use of quotation marks to indicate that some of the data were available only in the form of vaguely stated quotes. Any concept under higher cognitive processes is acceptable since consensus about what to call them does not yet exist.

Arousal/Orientation: "she is alert and oriented"
Attention: off-task less than 1/4 of the time
Unilateral neglect: only intermittently scans to her left side
Memory: "appears to be good"
Encoding: occasionally has trouble with more than three-step directions
Executive functions:
Problem solving: solves problems after assistance given once; makes her own decisions
Learning: has frequent difficulty learning complex activities
Organization: can organize simple but not complex activities
Self-regulation: impulsiveness during ADLs

Sensory-motor assets and deficits.
Manual dexterity of her dominant hand should be intact
Detection of light touch is present
Kinesthesia and stereognosis are absent
Bilateral limb coordination is absent due to nonfunctional LUE

Homeostatic deficits. Notice the use of reasonable questions because substantiating data were not present in the initial evaluation.
Was her stroke caused by high blood pressure or diabetes?
Does she have heart disease that requires cardiac precautions?
Does she have osteoporosis, which is common in elderly women?

Rehabilitation chunks.   Two strategies are listed. Both are correct.

Strategy #1.
  Setup/minimum assistance: feeding, UE dressing, bed mobility
  Moderate assistance: LE dressing, transfers
  Dependent: hair care, fastenings, ambulation

Strategy #2.
  Self-care: needs only minimum to moderate assistance in most tasks, but
    dependent in hair care, fastenings, and ambulation
  Home care: never cooked when her husband was alive
  Work: retired social worker. How did she structure her retirement time?

GENERATING TREATMENT GOALS

Use the next page to generate an NDT goal spreadsheet. Look at the NDT deficits from the Problem List. Use Memory Aid 9.1 to help you chunk NDT goals into short-term (possible in 1 week) and long-term. Identify short-term goals by thinking about what is safe, functionally significant, possible in one week, and goals that must be treated directly. Prioritize within short-term by asking if one goal is a prerequisite for another goal. Make NDT goals measurable!! Finish with suggested functional outcomes. Be sure to include compensatory devices and procedures in the functional outcomes if your long-term goals indicate that full recovery is not possible.

Student's Goal Spreadsheet

Dysfunction.

To help you write functional outcomes for every S-T NDT goal, BRIEFLY list Odessa's current dysfunction.

Short-term NDT Goals (in 1 week seen twice a day): Name the NDT goal (chunk), and list all the steps in each mini-treatment sequence.

Long-term NDT Goals (if patient gets as much therapy as she needs):

Suggested NDT Goal Spreadsheet

Dysfunction

Minimal physical assistance for feeding, bed mobility, UE dressing
Moderate physical assistance for LE dressing, transfers
Dependent in hair care and fastenings
Impulsive during ADLs (unilateral neglect?)

Short-term NDT Goals (in 1 week seen twice daily):

1. *Improve normal axial extension*
   a. moderate resistance to passive anterior tilt at mid-range
   b. active axial weight shift forward in sitting using anterior tilt and moderate physical assistance
   FO: to reduce physical assistance for transfers to minimal
2. *Achieve midline symmetry*
   a. minimum resistance at mid-range during passive trunk elongation to R
   b. active axial weight shift onto hemiplegic hip with elongation of the weight-bearing side and hip-hiking using moderate physical assistance
   c. maintain sit symmetrically with shoulders level, equal weight on both hips, hips symmetrically abducted, feet flat with positioning devices
   FO: to reduce physical assistance for LE dressing/bathing to minimal
3. *Develop shoulder dissociation/rotary righting*
   a. moderate resistance at mid-range to passive protraction, elevation, horizontal ABduction without lateral winging, and external rotation
   b. active weight shifting onto scapula in side-lie with scapula protracted
   c. elongate UE into hands clasped in anti-flexion RIP while log-rolling
   FO: to reduce assistance for UE dressing/bed mobility to distant supervision
4. *Utilize LE RIPs*
   a. moderate resistance to passive hip flexion at 100°
   b. maximal resistance to passive hip external rotation at 30°
   c. elongate LE into an anti-extension RIP in sitting
   FO: to reduce physical assistance for LE dressing/bathing to minimal

Long-term NDT Goals (if patient gets as much therapy as she needs):
1. Learn to use RIPs during ADLs with supervision
2. Weight shift onto hemiplegic elbow with scapular depression
3. Brief lateral weight shift onto hemiplegic leg during pivot transfers
4. Vertical head righting while log-rolling with neck righting

Reflection on the Goal Spreadsheet

Short-term goals were selected on the basis of functional significance and what was unsafe to leave untreated. Normal axial extension was placed in short-term because hip extensor spasticity during transfers is very dysfunctional. It is difficult to lean Odessa forward before having her stand up. The spastic hip extensors also need to be addressed in short-term because hip flexion is needed during LE dressing and bathing training. Midline asymmetry is functionally significant because the absence of axial weight shifts side to side require moderate assistance during LE ADLs. It is not safe to place shoulder dissociation in long-term goals because it can result in shoulder-hand syndrome. Early, aggressive treatment of the arm is needed.

Situational thinking about chunking and time-lines was used. Several short-term concerns were chunked into four major NDT goals. Axial extension (#1) and midline symmetry (#2) came from two boxes in the axial column. Chunking by the box is a recommended strategy for condensing related goals. Shoulder dissociation (#3) and LE RIPs (#4) came from a single box in the limb column. They were listed separately because several minutes will be needed to implement each limb goal for this severely spastic patient. Rather than make a separate righting reaction goal, rolling was chunked together with the UE limb goal. Easier, more pain-free rolling should be one of the natural consequences of increased scapular dissociation. It is not wrong to make a separate righting reaction goal, and many therapists would choose to do so.

"Mini-goals" are listed under each short-term goal. These mini-goals constitute a treatment sequence. You need only document the connection between each short-term goal and functional outcomes in progress notes. For example, shoulder dissociation and rotary righting will reduce the physical assistance needed for bed mobility.

The order of some short-term goals in this list could be reversed. Axial extension (#1) and midline symmetry (#2) could be reversed. Some patients respond better to trunk elongation sideways than weight shift forwards, which gives the sensation of falling toward the floor. Shoulder dissociation (#3) and LE RIPs (#4) could also be reversed. It is hard to predict what she will tolerate first, arm or leg elongation. The axial goals (#1 and #2) were placed first because proximal relaxation should overflow into the limbs. This should make her severely spastic limbs (#3 and #4) easier to elongate second. Notice that shoulder dissociation is a prerequisite for rolling onto the hemiplegic arm (#3). Rolling onto a painful tight arm that becomes trapped underneath the body does not make for a successful treatment session.

Limbs free in space, distal dissociation, and protective extension are probably not possible. The severe spasticity just 1 month postonset, bony block of the ankle, and continued absence of kinesthesia are not good prognostic signs for high-level limb recovery. Regaining equilibrium reactions are also doubtful. Odessa's resistance to axial movements will make balance reactions difficult to achieve.

Suggested functional outcomes include skills that I think *can* change. The next step is to talk with Odessa to determine which ones *should* be achieved.

DESIGNING TREATMENT ACTIVITIES

Use the next two pages to design two NDT treatment activities (see Figs 10.5 and 10.6). Choose any two short-term NDT goals from your spreadsheet to generate postulates regarding change and postulates regarding intervention. List all of the mini-goals under each short-term goal. This will help you visualize the entire treatment sequence from preparation to purposeful activity.

I encourage you to draw stick figures in the Rationale column. Verbal descriptions of NDT activities can be difficult to understand without visual aids.

Try to use the same purposeful activity for both NDT short-term goals. If serendipity strikes and you are able to use the same activity again, you don't need to describe the entire activity a second time. You need only describe the modifications that make the second NDT goal possible. Remember, there are many advantages to using the same activity more than once, such as cutting down on set-up and clean-up time.

I chose low-level activities to start with because I am still unsure about her level of perceptual-cognitive impairment. I would rather start with an activity that is too easy than have the first treatment session end in failure (see Figs 10.7–10.10).

Remember, the functional outcomes and specific activities that are actually implemented must be selected in concert with the patient's input. The postulates shown on the following pages are only a preliminary draft. They are useful only as an introduction to help elicit concrete ideas from the patient about her treatment plan. They should be presented as examples of what could be done. Concrete examples can empower the patient if the student remains flexible and respects the patient's right to actively participate in her own treatment story.

Deficit/Cause/Goal/FO	Rationale	Specific Modality: Name, Description, Precautions

Figure 10.5. Student's Activity #1

Deficit/Cause/Goal/FO	Rationale	Specific Modality: Name, Description, Precautions

Figure 10.6. Student's Activity #2

Deficit/Cause/Goal/FO	Rationale	Specific Modality: Name, Description, Precautions

Deficit #1:
  poor axial extension
 	
Stage Specific Cause:
  spastic hamstrings
 	
S–T NDT Goal:
—moderate resistance to
  passive anterior pelvic tilt
  at midrange
	GIVE THE SENSATION of
	1. passive anterior tilt
	2. active weight shifts
	   forward with anterior
	   pelvic tilt
	
		Preparation: Sit patient on a bench. Therapist stands in front of patient with hands on back of patient's pelvis. Therapist steps backward to passively move patient's trunk SLIGHTLY forward while pulling pelvis forward. Have patient look up at ceiling and inhale when you shift her forward. Re-erect. Gradually move farther away from vertical until pelvis reaches mid-range for anterior tilt. Once patient follows your handling a few times, help her initiate active weight shifts forward.

—active weight shift forward
  in sitting using anterior
  pelvic tilt and moderate
  physical assistance
 	
Functional Outcome:
  patient will stand up with
  minimal physical assistance
	DURING PURPOSEFUL TASK, LET THE PATIENT INITIATE active axial weight shifts with anterior tilt
	
		Activity: Pegboard game. Patient sitting on same bench as above. Place bucket with large pegs on knee-height bench on patient's sound side. Place an upright pegboard on table in front of patient out of arm's reach. Patient reaches for peg with sound hand and then leans forwards with anterior tilt to place peg in board following a sample design.
		
		Handling: therapist stands on hemiplegic side with one hand on back of pelvis and one on hemiplegic elbow to facilitate forward weight shift with anterior tilt. WAIT for patient to initiate movement.

	FADE CONTROL	*Handling:* move hands to forearm and thenar eminence. Keep hemiplegic arm to about 30° of shoulder flexion until proximal dissociation begins to loosen shoulder. Use tactile prompt on pelvis if necessary.

Figure 10.7. NDT Postulates for Odessa

Deficit/Cause/Goal/FO	Rationale	Specific Modality: Name, Description, Precautions
Deficit #2: midline asymmetry *Stage Specific Cause:* axial fixing *S–T NDT Goal:* —minimum resistance at mid-range to passive trunk elongation to her right —active weight shift onto right hip using trunk elongation, hip hiking, and moderate physical assistance —sit with both shoulders level, hips symmetrically abducted, equal weight on both hips, and feet flat using positioning devices and minimal physical assistance *Functional Outcome:* patient will look socially presentable when her grandchildren visit	GIVE THE SENSATION of 1. passive trunk elongation 2. active weight shift onto right side 3. symmetrical sitting	*Preparation:* Sit patient on a bench. Therapist stands very close behind patient on her right. Passively elongate right side through a miniature range by lifting her sound shoulder with OT's arm under her abducted right arm while OT's other hand pushes up on hemiplegic waist. Once patient follows your movement, help her initiate weight shift onto right hip. Gradually add hip-hiking with hand under hemiplegic buttock. Finally, place in symmetrical position described in goal while sitting with a small towel underneath her sound hip that takes too much weight. Therapist gives the sensation of sitting symmetrically for a few seconds by pulling down on high hemiplegic shoulder and adducting hemiplegic leg.
	DURING PURPOSEFUL TASK, LET THE PATIENT INITIATE 1. active weight shift onto right side and 2. symmetrical sitting 	*Pegboard modifications.* Place upright pegboard on her right on a shelf at shoulder height and beyond arm's reach. Place bucket with large pegs on table slightly to her left but within arm's reach. Help patient assume symmetrical sitting while getting a peg from the bucket with sound hand. Prompt her to look left because of unilateral neglect. Ask her to initiate weight shift with trunk elongation onto right hip while placing peg with sound hand. *Handling:* Therapist stands behind patient with hands under sound arm and hemiplegic buttock. WAIT for her to initiate.
	FADE CONTROL	*Handling:* one hand on sound elbow.

Figure 10.8. NDT Postulates for Odessa

Deficit/Cause/Goal/FO	Rationale	Specific Modality: Name, Description, Precautions
Deficit #3: poor shoulder dissociation while rolling *Stage-Specific Cause:* spastic scapular retractors/ depressors and axial fixing *S–T NDT Goal:* —moderate resistance at mid-range to passive protraction/ elevation, horz. aBduction without lateral winging, and external rotation —active weight shift onto protracting scapula —elongate LUE into anti-flexion RIP with hands clasped while log rolling with minimal physical assistance	GIVE THE SENSATION of 1. passive elongation of scapular muscles 2. active weight shift on scapula 3. log-rolling with flexion	*Preparation:* Place patient in supine in middle of mat table with head on a pillow. Standing on patient's left side, place hands on scapula and clavicle. Imperceptibly move scapula into and out of protraction/elevation. Move hands to scapular and humerus. Slowly horizontally abduct shoulder while compressing scapula to separate scapulo-humeral block. Then slowly extend hemiplegic arm in front of chest while applying traction to protract scapula. Ask patient to roll over onto protracted scapula to side-lie. Passively elongate shoulder to 45° of external rotation. Once shoulder is relaxed, have patient actively roll between side-lie and halfway back to supine with clasped hands with hemiplegic thumb on top while therapist maintains traction on hemiplegic arm. Repeat until you feel whole hemiplegic arm relax.
Functional Outcome: bed mobility with distant supervision	DURING PURPOSEFUL TASK, LET THE PATIENT INITIATE log-rolling with flexion 	*Activity:* Ring Drop. Patient rolls onto hemiplegic side on mat table with scapula protracted; shoulder externally rotated/flexed to 90°. Light plastic rings are placed behind patient at hip level. Pole is in front of patient on a short stool; top of pole is slightly below mat table height. Patient rolls back to clasp ring with sound hand and then rolls forward to drop it on pole. *Handling:* hands on hemiplegic scapula and forearm for compression during horizontal abduction when rolling onto back; traction to protract when rolling onto side.
	FADE YOUR CONTROL	*Handling:* hand just above hemiplegic wrist.

Figure 10.9. NDT Postulates for Odessa

Deficit/Cause/Goal/FO	Rationale	Specific Modality: Name, Description, Precautions
Deficit #4: poor LE dissociation *Stage-Specific Cause:* spastic hip extensors and internal rotators *S–T NDT Goal:* —moderate resistance to passive hip flexion at 110° —maximal resistance to external rota. at 30° —elongate LE into anti-extension RIP in sitting *Functional Outcome:* LE dressing and bathing with minimal physical assistance	GIVE THE SENSATION of 1. LE passive elongation 2. LE anti-extension RIP	*Preparation:* Place patient in supine perpendicular to edge of mat table with calves hanging off edge. Have sound foot resting on footstool. Slowly passively elongate hemiplegic leg into 110° of hip flexion with hands on hemi knee and heel. Once patient relaxes, slowly passively elongate hip into 30° of external rotation with knee bent. Remove footstool and help the patient sit up with one hand around patient's shoulders and one hand on hemiplegic knee. Place board under feet if feet do not rest flat on floor. Have patient clasp hands with hemiplegic thumb on top. Patient then clasps hemiplegic knee between clasped hands while therapist maintains hip flexion and external rotation with hands on hemiplegic knee and foot. Therapist helps patient use clasped hands to cross hemiplegic leg on top of sound leg.
	DURING PURPOSEFUL TASK, LET THE PATIENT INITIATE a LE anti-extension RIP	*Activity:* Put on pants. Patient sits on mat table with hemiplegic leg crossed over sound leg. Patient maneuvers pantleg over hemiplegic foot with long-handled reacher held in sound hand (additional hip flexion while leaning over is not possible now). Once pantleg is over knee, patient places sound hand under pantleg and knee to uncross leg. Patient continues to work pantleg up over thigh using lateral weight shift with trunk elongation to R (see Goal #2 for details). Patient anterior tilts (see Goal #1 for details) and stands up with moderate physical assistance to get pants up to waist. Therapist helps patient with fastenings. *Handling:* hands on hemiplegic knee and ankle maintaining hip flexion and external rotation while sitting.
	FADE YOUR CONTROL	*Handling:* tactile prompts on hemiplegic knee and ankle

Figure 10.10.   NDT Postulates for Odessa

SECTION IV

REHABILITATION FRAME OF REFERENCE

CHAPTER / 11

Introduction to the Rehabilitation Frame of Reference

The rehabilitation frame of reference teaches compensation when remediation of underlying deficits is not possible. One man with hemiplegia wrote a manual on self-help devices as early as 1822 (1). Compensatory techniques became a formal part of patient treatment when occupational and physical therapy aides were established by the Medical Department of the Army in January of 1918 (2). By 1919, Dr. Dunton had published *Reconstruction Therapy*, which included some devices for dressing and principles of work simplification (3). The interest in compensation grew when soldiers returned home after World War II. The first rehabilitation center in the U.S. was established at New York University Hospital in 1946. Thanks to Dr. Rusk at NYU, the concept of rehabilitation altered the philosophy of medical care. A patient's care was not complete until the patient had learned to "work with what he had left" (4). By 1949, university professors were publishing pamphlets on handicapped homemaking techniques (5–7). By 1956, Dr. Rusk and his staff at NYU were publishing pamphlets on compensatory self-care and homemaking equipment and procedures (8–10).

The philosophy of rehabilitation became a national reality through legislation. Funds for medical and psychiatric services during vocational rehabilitation were mandated for the first time by the Vocational Rehabilitation Amendment Act of 1954 (11). This act, however, did not permit medical and psychiatric personnel to charge for treatment of activities of daily living (ADLs), leisure skills, and family roles such as parenting during vocational training (11). The Social Rehabilitation Act of 1963 corrected this error by redefining the goal of rehabilitation. This goal is to "restore a person to maximum usefulness to himself, his family, and his community" (12). A patient can now receive reimbursement for rehabilitation even if he/she doesn't have employment potential. Accessibility to new buildings built with federal funds was mandated by the Architectural Barriers Act of 1968 (13). In 1984, the uniform federal access standards stated that old public buildings must eventually meet the new standards for accessibility (14). However, this 1968 law on architectural barriers does not apply to the private sector.

The latest legislation is the 1990 Americans with Disabilities Act (ADA). The ADA prohibits discrimination against people with disabilities in employment, transportation, public accommodations operated by private entities, such as restaurants, stores, and hotels, state and local government, and communications (15). This list addresses many of the gaps left by previous bills. A "**person with a disability**" is anyone who has a physical or mental impairment that substantially limits one or more major life activity; who has a history of such impairment (but is not disabled now), or is regarded as having such an impairment (even though no real impairment exists). The bill does not cover a "direct threat," such as someone who has a contagious disease or illegally uses drugs or alcohol. A "**qualified individual with a disability**" is any person with a disability who can perform what an employer considers to be the essential functions of a job, with or without reasonable accommodations. "**Reasonable accommodation**" may include: (*a*) modifying existing facilities, such as adding wheelchair ramps, and (*b*) job restructuring, such as modifying work schedules. Accommodation must be made unless there is undue hardship. "**Undue hardship**" is any action that requires significant difficulty or expense given the type and overall financial resources of the operation.

Despite this 75-year history of legislation, rehabilitation was not identified as a specific frame of reference in an entry-level textbook for occupational therapists until 1985 (16). Javetz and Katz suggested that rehabilitation is seen as a group of techniques rather than as a theoretical approach (17). This chapter identifies the assumptions and critiques the evaluation tools of the rehabilitation frame of reference.

ASSUMPTIONS

The first assumption of the rehabilitation frame of reference is the belief that a patient can regain independence using compensation when underlying deficits cannot be remediated. While some patients may regain independence, they will not do things the way they did before their illness. For example, they may use a built-up spoon to substitute for poor grasp. Once patients finally allow themselves to hear the word "substitution," they are understandably upset and often go through a grieving process.

How much independence a patient actually regains depends on his/her motivation. Therefore, the second assumption is the belief that motivation for independence cannot be separated from the volitional and habituation subsystems (18). Motivation can be influenced by **life-long values** that sustain a commitment to action. If taking care of loved ones and being taken care of by them in return is a life-long value, independence may never be valued. Motivation can be influenced by **new roles**. If an outpatient perceives the patient role as the primary role, he/she may ask friends to help dress him/her so he/she won't be late late for doctor visits and therapy sessions. Motivation can be influenced by **preferences** for certain functional tasks. If a patient did not associate pleasure with a functional task before the illness, it is not likely that he/she will want to do it after the illness. Motivation can be influenced by **a sense of purpose** (18). When life is no longer full of pleasurable and successful experiences, a sense of purpose may become paramount in the patient's mind. A patient may ask, "What is the purpose of learning to comb my hair when I am too embarrassed to go out in public?"

Rogers talks about the ethical reasoning a therapist must use to decide what ought to be done in therapy (20). The therapist has the training to determine what tasks the patient CAN DO independently. However, the patient must participate in choosing what he/she SHOULD DO independently. The reason for telling patients what is possible is to empower them to be their own moral agents. As Rogers states: "The therapist is privileged to help the patient select from the available opportunities those that are to be brought to fruition. As the patient executes and fulfills his or her choice, the therapist learns about the healing power of occupation. Occupational choice rekindles the will to live and mobilizes the mind to discipline the body" (20, p. 610).

The third assumption states that motivation for independence cannot be separated from the environmental context (19). You must consider the discharge placement (e.g., nursing home), the patient's previous life-style (i.e., did he/she do it before?), the family's financial and emotional resources, and the family's cultural heritage.

In one case study, a hemiplegic patient was sent home to a 150-year-old brick row house with attached houses on either side (21). The narrow floor plan and fixed income of $18,000 a year did not permit substantial environmental modification. Her family was not a do-it-yourself group. The neighborhood was closely knit, and relatives lived two doors away and around the corner. This patient had others do all of her home care, including cooking all her meals. Environmental context strongly affects motivation for independence.

Cohen suggests that total independence may not be as appropriate as reciprocity with environmental resources such as family, friends, and outside vendors (22). For example, I can mow the lawn, take out the garbage, and fill out my tax forms, but I don't choose to do any of these things. I have negotiated with my husband to do some of them. I pay outside vendors to do some of them. Reciprocity is a reality for all of us in some area of our life.

Therapists usually don't require reciprocity in self-care, but therapists are not the appropriate normative group for physically challenged individuals. If it takes a person with a spinal cord injury 3 hours to bathe and dress, full-time employment is out of the question. Similarly, what good is it to be able to do all of your own self-care if you are too tired to spend time with your children after breakfast or have sex with your husband after dinner? All of the environmental demands must be considered to decide if reciprocity is required. Reciprocity may be the only way to perform the MOST VALUED tasks.

The fourth assumption of the rehabilitation frame of reference states that a minimum level of emotional and cognitive prerequisite skill must be present to make independence possible. For example, clinically significant depression is a strong predictor of rehabilitation failure (19). Severely depressed patients are poorly motivated, easily fatigued, and have impaired retention. Some life-long personality traits are also strong predictors of rehabilitation failure (19). For example, dependency does not foster the initiative that is needed to fully participate in therapy.

An attitude of assertiveness is helpful. An assertive patient asks questions, wants to understand the therapy plan, sticks up for his/her rights, and takes responsibility for his/her decisions. Assertive patients may not be appreciated by the staff as much as passive, compliant patients, but "experience dictates that these persons have better outcomes" (19, p. 54). Another emotional prerequisite is a high frustration tolerance. Compensatory strategies impose changes that many people find very frustrating. Frustration tolerance may be related to a person's ability to risk failure while learning something new. Some adult learners cannot tolerate making the errors that are an essential part of learning a new skill. An adult learner may see one error as total failure.

A minimum level of cognitive prerequisite skills must also be present to achieve independence. Compensation requires learning new ways to do things. Older patients may learn in a different manner and may take longer to learn than younger patients (19). Brain-damaged patients of all ages may have cognitive deficits that interfere with the teaching-learning process. For example, poor judgment and other executive functions can make the patient unaware of safety precautions.

Allen describes six cognitive levels and how well each level uses compensatory techniques (23). It is easiest to understand these detailed cognitive levels in list form (see Table 11.1). Patients at cognitive level 4 and below cannot be trained in short periods of time, so it is crucial to train caregivers. Patients at cognitive level 5 are unable to implement abstract procedures like joint protection. Even for a level 6 patient with intact cognition, short lengths of stay require training to stress active problem solving by the patient rather than teaching every possible compensation by rote practice (24).

The fifth and final assumption of the rehabilitation frame of reference is the belief that clinical reasoning should take a top-down approach. It is easy to use a bottom-up approach by thinking first about the adaptive devices and procedures that you learned about in school and then thinking about the patient afterwards. A graduate student in rehabilitation engineering said that at first he wanted to give a computerized phone system to every physically involved patient that he saw. After he spent time with an occupational therapist, he learned to first ask what component of the task the patient was unable to perform. If the patient is unable to pick up the telephone receiver, a clip holder might be all the patient needs. Unfortunately, formal ADL assessments don't guide students through a top-down approach. ADL forms focus on the patient's functional capabilities without looking at environmental demands and what prerequisite skills each task demands (25).

The *first step* in the top-down hierarchy is identifying environmental demands and resources. For example, one survey found that only 5% of the patients in a rehabilitation unit performed full meal preparation at home (26). The majority of patients in this study did self-service (eating in a restaurant or with the family), cold food preparation (e.g., making a sandwich), or hot food preparation (reheating; cooking microwave dinners;

Table 11.1.
Cognitive Prerequisites for ADL by Claudia Allen

Level 1 exhibits automatic actions that briefly arouse patient

- Supervision: cannot be left unattended
- Resists caregiver when physical assistance is given during ADLs
- Performs reflex actions like swallowing food placed in mouth

Level 2 exhibits familiar, repetitive gross motor actions that "feel good"

- Supervision: cannot be left unattended
- May cooperate with caregiver when physical assistance is given in ADLs
- W/C: patient is unable to steer around obstacles; may attempt to get up and walk with seatbelt on

Level 3 exhibits manual actions that are recognizable but perseverative

- Supervision: one-to-one supervision needed during ADLs.
  Attendant must make selection, break activity down into one-step actions, hand supplies to patient one at a time, and check for errors.
- Adaptive devices: unable to use equipment requiring new motor patterns
- W/C or walker: patient can maneuver around a room but may get lost on the way to another room and lacks safety awareness (e.g., locks W/C brakes)

Level 4 exhibits goal-directed actions that enables patient to imitate others

- Supervision: performs ADLs with intermittent supervision (e.g., can feed self but needs supervision to share food eaten family style; to season food)
- Supervision: still lacks error detection (e.g., forgets to rinse shampoo off back of head; puts clothes on inside out)
- Adaptive devices: can be used only if actions are familiar, requires no more than three steps, or the effect is obvious (e.g., can use rocker knife)
- Adapted procedures (e.g., one-handed dressing) and home exercises (e.g., self-ROM) are mastered only after WEEKS OF PRACTICE!

Level 5 exhibits exploratory actions that use overt trial and error learning

- Supervision: independent in eating, grooming, dressing
- Supervision: set-up assistance is required for complex tasks that require abstract reasoning to anticipate hazards (e.g., cooking)
- Adapted procedures (e.g., one-handed techniques) and home exercises: can learn simple techniques in two to four sessions
- Adapted procedures: work simplification, energy conservation, joint protection, and hip precautions may be too abstract for patient to apply

Level 6 has all cognitive prerequisites for ADLs

cooking simple stove-top meals like spaghetti in a can). Environmental demands and resources can be evaluated by talking to the patient, family, and social worker. This first step should cause "Not Applicable" to appear several times on the ADL form.

The *second step* is asking about the volition and habituation subsystems. For example, if a patient has always hated doing a particular task, he/she is not likely to want to learn how to do it when he/she is ill. Additional "Not Applicable" notations should appear on the ADL form as a result of this second step.

The *third step* in the top-down hierarchy is determining functional capability. What functional tasks can the patient perform independently? ADL evaluation forms always ask for this information.

The *fourth step* is identifying which prerequisite skills the functional task demands and the patient lacks. How do specific prerequisite deficits relate to a specific dysfunction? Is the patient dependent in dressing because he/she lacks sufficient grip strength or because he/she has a cognitive deficit? ADL assessment forms are not designed to elicit this information. You must add clinical observations to the ADL evaluation form to explain why the patient can't perform a particular function. If you don't identify missing prerequisite skills, it is difficult to recommend devices and procedures appropriately. If the patient has a weak grip, a heavy long-handled reacher will only make the patient more dysfunctional!

The *fifth step* in the top-down hierarchy is selecting the type of method used. Rehabilitation methods include adaptive devices, UE orthotics, environmental modification, wheelchair modification, ambulatory devices, adapted procedures, and safety education. Selection is achieved by matching the rationale for using each method to the prerequisite skills that the patient lacks. These rationales are discussed in detail in Chapter 12. Patient input at step five is important since a negative reaction to one rehabilitation method should signal the therapist to search for alternative methods that achieve the same goal.

The *sixth step* is choosing the specific device or procedure. Once you know what prerequisite skills the patient lacks and the methods the patient prefers, you can suggest the use of a plate guard and tenodesis grasp to substitute for a lost motion.

FUNCTION/DYSFUNCTION ADDRESSED

There are three function-dysfunction continua for the rehabilitation frame of reference (27). The first continuum is activities of daily living (ADLs). **ADLs** include **self-care** activities such as eating, grooming, bathing, dressing, toileting, bowel and bladder control, skin care, bed mobility, transfers, wheelchair propulsion, and walking with ambulatory devices. ADLs also include

taking medications, use of environmental hardware such as light switches and doorknobs, socialization, communication, and sexual expression. Therefore, self-care and ADLs are not synonymous. The second continuum is **work**. Work includes taking care of others such as children, educational activities, vocational activities, and home management. Home management includes meal preparation, meal service (setting the table and doing dishes), light house cleaning (e.g., dusting), heavy house cleaning (e.g., mopping), laundry, shopping, budgeting, and simple home repair. The third continuum is **leisure activities**. Since the possibilities for leisure activities are endless, examples are usually not given.

EVALUATION CRITIQUED

ADL Evaluation

ADL evaluation forms list the levels of physical assistance as minimal, moderate, or maximal. Medicare guidelines have been revised to include levels of supervisory assistance (28). Table 11.2 shows how both types of assistance have been incorporated into a single scale. Both types of assistance must be documented for all Medicare patients. The supervisory levels were developed for cognitively impaired patients, but they can also be used to document the learning curve for cognitively intact patients.

Therapists are sensitive to the burden imposed on caregivers by physical assistance because they have to lift patients many times each day. Supervision is a more subtle demand for therapists to appreciate because they never take care of a patient for 24 hours at a time.

The heaviest burden on the caregiver is **constant one-to-one cuing**. This level of supervision requires significant sacrifice. It does not permit the caregiver to do any other activity, such as cook dinner, as long as the patient is awake. Doors may have to be locked to prevent wandering. It's unrealistic for families to sustain this level of supervision without respite care.

The next level of supervision is **intermittent cuing** while in the immediate vicinity. The caregiver can engage in his/her own activity, but he/she must be within arm's reach. Leaving the room to go to the bathroom or to talk to a friend at the front door would not be possible. Some local clinics call this close supervision.

Even **minimum supervision** does not enable the caregiver to leave the house to go the store or to pick up children after school. The caregiver can engage in his/her own activity elsewhere in the same room, but must remember to repeatedly check on the family member. The caregiver must check for compliance with safety precautions, like leaving a coffee pot burning on the stove, and for stopping errors, like putting clothes on

Table 11.2.
Levels of Assistance[a]

D	= Dependent	Unable to do any part of the task = 100% assistance needed *Two to three people needed to lift patient
Max	= Maximum assist	Maximum physical assistance = 75% assistance from one person Maximum effort of one person to safely lift patient Constant one-to-one cuing needed to complete tasks
Mod	= Moderate assist	Moderate physical assistance = 50% assistance from one person Moderate effort of one person to safely lift patient Intermittent cuing with caretaker in immediate vicinity throughout entire activity (*close supervision = within arm's reach) *Contact guarding with hands on patient at all times ready to give assistance whenever needed

Min	= Minimum assist	Minimum physical assistance = 25% assistance from one person
		Minimum effort of one person to safely to lift patient
		Set-up assistance to get activity started
		Minimum supervision with caregiver in same room to check patient who cannot be trusted to correct mistakes or
		    follow safety precautions
		    (*distant supervision = within eyesight)

SB	= Standby	Initial supervision to modify environment and teach new procedures that have safety modifications built in, allowing caregiver to leave patient unattended (patient cannot detect errors or anticipate safety precautions, so the caregiver must design a safe environment and teach safety procedures to patient in every *NEW* situation with potential danger)
I	= Independent	No physical assistance needed *May use adaptive equipment or procedures No supervision needed

[a]*Asterisks* indicate criteria NOT included in the Medicare guidelines for levels of assistance but commonly used in the clinic.

backwards. Some local clinics call this distant supervision.

The level of supervision that puts the least burden on the caregiver is **standby supervision**. The caregiver must modify the environment to remove potential hazards and then teach the patient to perform new tasks that have safety precautions built in to them. Parents give standby supervision when they remove breakable objects from a play area and then show their children that the trucks can be run on the carpet but not on the walls while parents are engaged in another activity close by, such as working in the garden. When a family member is truly ready for standby supervision, the caregiver can leave once the safety instructions are learned. However, every new situation must be assessed by the caregiver for potential danger.

Most OT departments have their own self-care evaluation form. In recent years there has been a push to adopt one form that would standardize ADL ratings from one facility to the next. Attempts to standardize ADL evaluations have produced little consensus. The five evaluations listed in Table 11.3 show that the skills tested vary considerably. The most frequently omitted skills are bed mobility, bowel and bladder control, skin care, communication, and use of environmental hardware like doorknobs. Scoring can vary from a 2-point scale to a 7-point scale.

Tests that award different scores for several different levels of independence are more sensitive to small changes than tests that only give a score of independent or dependent. When the Kenny, Barthel, and Katz scales were given to the same 100 rehabilitation patients, the Kenny 5-point scale was the most sensitive to small changes (29). This sensitivity helps justify the need for therapy when the patient does not achieve complete independence by discharge time. It is especially helpful when patients have a short length of stay or show only small changes.

Most ADL evaluations lack reliability data. Minimal, moderate, and maximal physical assistance have always been defined subjectively. This subjectivity lowers reliability. Even the FIM (see Table 11.3) does not provide clear definitions of physical assistance. The FIM doesn't define what 50 to 74% assistance means for a particular task. It is more reliable for a single therapist to administer both the baseline and discharge ADL evaluation for a particular patient.

Patients' variable performance adds to reliability problems. It is common for therapists to give a double score such as "min/mod" assistance to indicate a range of performance over the full day. The greater amount of assistance should be weighed more heavily when making discharge plans. The potential caregiver must be able to provide the highest rather than the lowest level of assistance needed. Subjective grading criteria and patient variability makes inter-rater reliability difficult to achieve for ADL evaluations.

Table 11.3.
Comparison of ADL Evaluation Tools

Name of Test	Skills Assessed	Sensitivity[a]	Reliability	Validity
Katz Index of ADL[a]	feeding/ /toileting dressing/transfers/bathing incontinence	2-point scale: Independent and dependent	Differences between raters occurred less than one out of 20 evaluations	Scores correlate with house confinement after discharge
Barthel Index[a]	feeding/grooming/toileting /bathing / WC locomotion walking/stairs/incontinence	3-point scale		Score below 40 has poor prognosis for discharge to home
Kenny Self-care Evaluation[a]	feeding/ dressing/transfers/bathing bed mobility/ WC locomotion walking/stairs	5-point scale: Minimal assist includes supervision		Learning curve predicts total rehabilitation time
Functional Independence Measure (FIM)	feeding/grooming/toileting dressing/transfers/bathing bed mobility/ WC locomotion walking/stairs environmental hardware are included under each individual task comprehension/expression	7-point scale: Assistance includes use of adaptive devices, set-up assistance, and supervision	Inter-rater reliability = .86 to .88, but physical assistance defined as does 75%–100% of task (min), 50–74% of task (mod), 25–49% of task (max), and 24–0% of task (depen)	
Extended Routine Task Inventory (ERTI)	feeding/grooming/toileting dressing/ /bathing walking/ using adaptive equipment listening/talking/ reading/writing	6-point scale based on cognitive demands of the task	On shorter version inter-rater reliability = .98 and test-retest reliability = .91.	

[a]When the Kenny, Barthel, and Katz scales were given to the same 100 rehabilitation patients, the Kenny 5-point scale was the most sensitive to small changes. This sensitivity can help justify the need for therapy when patients do not achieve complete independence by discharge time.

Although most experts agree that ADL evaluations have good face validity (see Appendix), predictive validity data are rarely available. One study concluded that a score of 40 or below out of 100 possible points on the Barthel Index indicates a poor prognosis for discharge to the home (30). Yet, two patients with Barthel scores of 10 and 15 were living at home in another study (31). Eggert et al. found that three factors predicted discharge placement: (a) the patient's level of ADL function; (b) the family's willingness and ability to provide physical assistance; and (c) the family's financial resources to cover home care costs (32). More studies of the predictive validity of ADL evaluations need to be done.

Home Management Evaluation

Home management evaluations usually consist of departmental evaluation forms. These forms list skills that are associated with different home management tasks such as sorting, folding, ironing, and using the washing machine for doing the laundry. The levels of assistance that were discussed under ADL can be used to score homemaking skills.

One formal assessment of home management skills looks only at the levels of supervision needed. This is the community scale of the Extended Routine Task Inventory (33). It is a six-point scale that assesses housekeeping, preparing food, spending money, doing laundry, traveling (inside the home and out in the community), telephoning, and child care. The therapist chooses descriptions that best fit the patient's behavior. For example, supervision may be needed because the patient does not consider care instructions when laundering new garments, may leave a child unattended if distracted by another interesting stimulus, or may not anticipate monthly shopping needs.

The home management evaluation sheets list only what the patient can or cannot do. They do not ask about the environmental demands the patient must meet when he/she is discharged! One way to identify the environmental demands is to ask what the patient did before the illness. You can then mark all tasks that are inappropriate with NA (not applicable) BEFORE you begin the evaluation. If a patient has a family member prepare hot food, this home management skill should be marked NA. Home management forms also do not ask the examiner to determine what underlying deficit is causing the dysfunction. They may not even leave room on the form to record poor attention, poor balance, unilateral disregard, and other deficits that emerge as you observe the patient. You must discipline yourself to make these clinical observations. When you don't identify underlying deficits that must be compensated for, you have no rationale for choosing a particular adaptive device, modification, or procedure.

Work Evaluations

Work evaluations assess four types of work abilities:

1. Work behaviors;
2. Work tolerance;
3. General work traits; and
4. Specific work skills.

Work behaviors are general habits that make a person employable. They include the acceptance of supervision, personal hygiene, punctuality, organized work habits, and neatness. However, personality traits like poor judgment or quick temper are not considered to be symptoms of a mental disorder and, therefore, are not covered by the ADA (34). Work behaviors are usually evaluated with clinical observation. For example, The Expanded Routine Task Inventory has a work scale that evaluates the ability to follow directions, perform simple to complex tasks, maintain an appropriate work pace, get along with coworkers, follow safety precautions, and plan a work task for self and others (33).

Work tolerance is the ability to: (a) sustain effort for prolonged periods of time; (b) maintain an acceptable work pace; (c) maintain an acceptable quality of workmanship; and (d) handle work pressures (35). Some clinical procedures, like a work conditioning circuit, only assess the ability to sustain physical effort (component a). A work tolerance evaluation is not valid (testing what it says it tests) unless realistic work pace, acceptable workmanship, and appropriate stress are included in the test procedure. All four components of work tolerance are legitimate concerns for an employer of a qualified individual with a disability.

General work traits are abilities that are common to several jobs (36). They can be evaluated with one test that measures a single work trait or by batteries that evaluate several work traits. One work trait called fine motor coordination is evaluated with the Purdue Pegboard Test, the Crawford Small Parts Test, and the Minnesota Rate of Manipulation Test. Batteries like the Valpar test a variety of work traits like upper extremity range of motion (ROM), whole body ROM, eye-hand-foot coordination, size discrimination, numerical sorting, and problem solving.

General work-trait evaluations lack content validity (see Appendix) because they evaluate skills in an oversimplified work environment. It isn't enough to know if the patient can lift 45 pounds. The worker must deal with real-time scheduling demands, attend to what is in the boxes he/she is lifting to know where each one goes, and mentally shift gears when a supervisor interrupts him/her to do something else. General work-trait evaluations don't tell us how much a patient's physical skills deteriorate when he/she is distracted by cognitive challenges and emotional stress.

Here is an example of how tests for general work traits can oversimplify the work environment. Stooping and lifting can be evaluated by the Valpar Test #19 and the West 2 Body Mechanics Evaluation. Carlton found that cafeteria workers who received body mechanics training improved on the West 2, but they did not generalize good body mechanics to their work environment (37). Two reasons cited were the extremely fast pace of the cafeteria line environment and the awkward layout of machines and storage units, which made it difficult to use good body mechanics.

Tests that evaluate general work traits also lack predictive validity. An OT department that works with seamen with hand injuries learned about the importance of predictive validity (38). Their tests of general work traits indicated that the seamen were ready to go back to active duty when, in fact, they could not safely perform all of their duties. For example, general grip strength on a dynamometer turned out to be different from using a heavy pipe wrench to open a valve placed overhead in a submarine. Seamen were returning from duty with reinjured hands. This OT department got the Navy to donate parts of old ships to build a realistic environment to evaluate hand injuries. This mock ship requires the patient to ascend 45°- stairs, open a hatch cover, cross the top, descend a 90°- vertical ladder, and manipulate various valves and levers securely fastened and placed in awkward positions as they would be on a Navy vessel.

Finally, tests for general work traits do not comply with ADA regulations. The ADA prohibits preemployment medical inquiries about physical skills and function unless this information is required for all other employees (15). However, before the job begins the employer can: (a) ask a therapist to evaluate if an applicant can perform essential job tasks, and (b) make the job offer conditional based on the results of job-specific testing (15). For example, the employer can ask if the person can carry files that weigh 25 pounds or deal with the constant pressure of weekly deadlines. Tests that evaluate nonessential job functions are prohibited. For example, a test battery cannot include an eye-hand coordination test if this is not an essential skill for a receptionist. Tests for general work traits also do not identify whether an individual can perform specific skills *if* reasonable accommodations are made. For example, the person might be functional if he/she uses a cart for transporting 25-pound files. Failure to restrict testing to essential job skills and to identify reasonable accommodations are serious weaknesses of tests for general work traits. It is better to use tests for general work traits to document gains from therapy than to determine who is ready for a specific job.

Specific work skills are tasks that are part of an actual job (39). Work skills can be tested with standardized job samples or simulated job samples. Standardized job samples require the patient to perform specific tasks related to jewelry making, welding, engraving, and sewing machine operation. Tests that assess these types of job skills include the TOWER system, COATS, and subtests from the Valpar for clerical aptitude, soldering, electric circuitry, and drafting. There are no standardized tests for professional and executive-level job samples (35). There aren't even standardized tests for computer skills.

To fill the gap left by standardized tests, a therapist may design a simulated work sample for an individual patient. The therapist selects factors essential to the patient's job that he/she cannot perform. The therapist then sets up a task that includes these factors in a format that is as close as possible to the actual job (40). The Baltimore Therapeutic Equipment (BTE) Work Simulator has a variety of attachments that simulate different jobs like shoveling (39). The BTE can be adjusted to different angles and heights, depending on job demands.

However, simulated work samples are highly dependent on an intimate knowledge of the work environment. The first step in setting up a simulated work sample is to do a job analysis. **Job analysis** includes assessment of: (*a*) the worker's capacity for job-specific positions, force, and speed of movement; (*b*) the workstation environment provided by the employer; and (*c*) the tools provided for a particular job (35). After a job analysis, the therapist can identify the essential factors that the patient cannot perform and design an INDIVIDUALIZED simulated work sample. Without this level of individualized analysis, a simulated work sample is not in compliance with the ADA. The expertise that a therapist brings to work simulation is the ability to test what the job requires, not what the work simulation equipment can demand.

Vocational tests were first developed in the 1940s before rigorous standards for test construction were established in occupational therapy. Many standardized tests for work abilities lack reliability data. Inconsistent patient performance is a legitimate concern, but what causes it? It is essential to know that every therapist is consistently administering and scoring work evaluations in exactly the same way every time (36). Test-retest and inter-rater reliability data could help us determine how much of the variability in a patient's score is created by the therapist's administration and scoring. Work simulation machines must also be recalibrated on a regular basis to ensure reliability.

Despite the high-tech appearance of work simulators and standardized work evaluations, validity still has not been established for many of the tests used today. This is a source of major concern because physicians rely heavily on job evaluation results to make job impairment determinations (40). We must know that a test measures what it says it measures before we use test scores to decide if someone can go back to a specific job.

Therapists working in general rehabilitation settings are more likely to evaluate general work traits and do **work conditioning,** which focuses on general physical conditioning (41). The majority of these therapists do not evaluate specific work skills because of cost considerations. Tests like the Valpar cost from $1,000 to $4,000 per subtest (39). The TOWER system requires you to provide all your own equipment for testing jobs like electronics assembly. This test equipment requires frequent patient use to justify their expense.

Therapists in work-hardening programs are more likely to have expensive tests or to build their own work environments. **Work-hardening** programs focus on the physical, emotional-social, and cognitive demands of a job (41). Work-hardening programs are accredited by the Commission on Accreditation of Rehabilitation Facilities (CARF) only when they address all three types of demands of a specific job. Employers need employees who can perform the physical, psychosocial, and cognitive demands of a job.

POSTULATES REGARDING CHANGE

Postulates regarding change identify the connection between general dysfunction and functional outcomes in a specific format:

1. *General dysfunction:* dependence in toileting;
2. *Stage-specific cause:* flaccid hemiplegia, hemianopsia, hemianesthesia, and shoulder pain;
3. *Short-term functional outcome:* toileting with maximal physical assistance and constant verbal cuing by the therapist; and
4. *Long-term functional outcome:* toileting with minimal physical assistance and minimal verbal cuing by the patient's spouse at home.

Postulates regarding change in the rehabilitation frame of reference begin with a statement about dysfunction, like dependence in toileting, rather than a statement about a deficit, like loss of range of motion. This frame of reference is used when remediation of existing deficits is not possible, so compensation to correct dysfunction is the focus of both short-and long-term goals.

It is essential to identify the stage-specific cause of the dysfunction. Since the patient just described is in the flaccid stage of stroke recovery, adapted procedures that inhibit spasticity are NOT appropriate. One-handed procedures for the sound arm will have to be used until motor return emerges in the involved upper extremity. Shoulder pain can make the patient uncooperative. Hemianopsia and hemianesthesia can make the patient dangerous to him/herself and the caregiver. While one-handed devices and procedures may be necessary, they are rarely sufficient when used in isolation in complex conditions such as hemiplegia. Independence may not be achieved if all the deficits that cause dysfunction are not identified and remediated or compensated for.

The functional outcome must have all three components of a measurable goal. It must have behavior, criterion, and condition statements (42). The following example has all three statements.

The patient will feed himself (behavior) with minimum supervision and refusal 1 in 5 times (criteria = what level of independence) with a rocker-knife at bedside (condition = with what and where).

Since the level of assistance may never improve, condition statements and additional criteria statements may be the only way to document change. For example, a patient with arthritis may already be independent in ADLs, so the therapist's goal is to change the conditions under which ADLs take place. Conditions, like using joint protection procedures, will be what changes, instead of the level of independence. Additional changes in the criteria statement are reimbursable even when the level of assistance does not change (43). Reimbursable changes include performing with decreased refusals, decreased cuing, increased safety, increased consistency, and increased generalization (e.g., eating in the dining room in addition to eating at bedside).

SUMMARY

The five assumptions of the rehabilitation frame of reference provide a philosophical screen that influences your decisions about compensation. Independence may mean performing tasks in a new way when underlying deficits cannot be remediated. Motivation for independence cannot be separated from volition and habituation or from environmental context. Realistic goals for independence are possible only when you take into account emotional and cognitive prerequisite skills. Cognitive deficits are especially important because they interfere with the teaching-learning process required to learn new methods. The ideal way to select rehabilitation methods is with a top-down approach that begins with environmental demands and resources.

Considerable reliability and validity data need to be collected on ADL, home management, and work evaluations. Inter-rater reliability is needed to rule out therapist-induced inconsistency in patient scores. Predictive validity is needed to enable therapists to use hospital- or clinic-based data to predict performance in real-life situations. Additional evaluation procedures need to be developed for leisure interests. Currently, leisure skills are assessed only by an interest checklist for adult patients.

It is crucial to include all stage specific causes of dysfunction in postulates regarding change for the rehabilitation frame of reference. Without them, correct solutions that lead to functional gains may not be prescribed. Functional outcomes should include both criterion and condition statements. These descriptive statements enable the therapist to justify the need for therapy even when the levels of assistance do not change.

STUDY QUESTIONS

1. Motivation for independence cannot be separated from what concerns?
2. What is reciprocity and why is it important?
3. Why do cognitive deficits interfere with compensation?
4. What are the six steps in the top-down hierarchy?
5. What are the three domains of concern for the rehabilitation frame of reference?
6. Differentiate between supervision given at the standby, minimum, moderate, and maximum-assistance level.
7. What increases sensitivity of an ADL evaluation?
8. What steps should be taken BEFORE home management or ADL activities are evaluated?
9. Define the four types of work abilities. How are they assessed?
10. Work evaluations lack validity when they ignore what conditions and job demands?
11. Independence may not be achieved if the therapist ignores what important link in the postulate regarding change?
12. T or F: Postulates regarding change need only name the behavior and level of assistance required.

References

1. DeRenzy GW. Enchiridion: or a handbook for the one-handed. London: 1822, reprinted by Elizabeth Litch, publisher, New Haven:1962.
2. Hopkins HL. An historical perspective on occupational therapy. In: Hopkins HL, Smith HD, eds. Willard and Spackman's occupational therapy. 7th ed. Philadelphia: JB Lippincott, 1988:23.
3. Spackman CS. A history of the practice of occupational therapy for restoration of physical function: 1917–1967. Am J Occup Ther 1968;22:67.
4. Rusk HA. Rehabilitation medicine. 3rd ed. St. Louis: CV Mosby, 1971:1.
5. McCullough H. Cabinet space for the kitchen. Small Homes Council Bulletin 5, University of Illinois, 1949.

6. Muse M. Seating housewives at their ironing. Agricultural Experiment Station Bulletin 559. University of Vermont and State Agricultural College, 1951.

7. Heiner MK, Steidl RE. Let your kitchen arrangement work for you. Extension Bulletin 814. Cornell University, 1953.

8. Lawton EB. Rehabilitation Monograph X: activities of daily living, testing, training and equipment. New York: Institute of Physical Medicine and Rehabilitation, 1956.

9. Rusk HA, et al. A functional home for easier living. Institute of Physical Medicine and Rehabilitation, New York, 1960.

10. Cookman H, Zimmerman ME. Functional fashions for the physically handicapped. New York: Institute of Physical Medicine and Rehabilitation, 1961.

11. Reed KL. Models of practice in occupational therapy. Baltimore: Williams & Wilkins, 1984.

12. US House of Representatives, 87th Congress, 1st session. Special Education and Rehabilitation. Hearings before the Subcommittee on Education of the Committee on Education and Labor, August, 1961:128.

13. Zimmerman ME. Homemaking training units for rehabilitation centers. Am J Occup Ther 1966;20:226.

14. General Services Administration: Uniform Federal Standards. Department of Defense, 1984.

15. Americans with Disabilities Act (1990). P.L. 101-336, 42 U.S.C. 12101.

16. Pedretti LW, Pasquinelli-Estrada S. A frame of reference for occupational therapy in physical dysfunction. In: Pedretti LW, ed. Occupational therapy practice skills for physical dysfunction. 2nd ed. Philadelphia: CV Mosby, 1985:5.

17. Javetz R, Katz N. Knowledgeability of theories of occupational therapy practitioners in Israel. Am J Occup Ther 1989;43:664.

18. Kielhofner G. A model of human occupation. Baltimore: Williams & Wilkins.

19. Kemp B. The psychosocial context of geriatric rehabilitation. In: Kemp B, Brummel-Smith K, Ramsdell JW, eds. Geriatric rehabilitation. Boston: Little, Brown & Co., 1990.

20. Rogers JC. Eleanor Clarke Slagle Lectureship—1983; Clinical reasoning: the ethics, science, and art. Am J Occup Ther 1983:37:601, 610.

21. Levine RE. Community home health. In: Hopkins HL, Smith HD, eds. Willard and Spackman's occupational therapy. 7th ed. Philadelphia: JB Lippincott, 1988:772.

22. Cohen ES. The elderly mystique: constraints on the autonomy of the elderly with disabilities. Gerontologist 1988;28(suppl):29.

23. Levy LL. Activity adaptation in rehabilitation of the physically and cognitively disabled aged. Topics in Geriatric Rehabilitation 1989;4:53.

24. Pendelton HM. Occupational therapists' current use of independent living skills training for adult patients who are physically disabled. Occupational Therapy and Health Care 1990;6:93.

25. Rogers JC. Improving the ability to perform daily tasks. In: Kemp B, Brummel-Smith K, Ramsdell JW, eds. Geriatric rehabilitation. Boston: Little, Brown & Company, 1990:139.

26. Reigle-Ganzars D. Therapist satisfaction with unstructured and structured kitchen environments. Unpublished thesis, Temple University, 1991.

27. American Occupational Therapy Association. Uniform terminology for occupational therapy. 2nd ed. Am J Occup Ther 1989;43:808.

28. Health Care Financing Administration. Outpatient Occupational Therapy Medicare Part B Guidelines (DHHS Transmittal No. 55). In: Health Insurance Manual, Baltimore, 1989.

29. Donaldson WE, Wagner CC, Gresham GE. A unified ADL form. Arch Phys Med Rehabil 1973;54:175.

30. Granger C, Dewis L, Peters N, Sherwood C, Barrett J. Stroke rehabilitation: analysis of repeated Barthel index measures. Arch Phys Med Rehabil 1979;60:14.

31. Hasselkus BR. Barthel self-care index and geriatric home care patients. Physical and Occupational Therapy in Geriatrics 1982;1:11.

32. Eggert G, Granger C, Morris R, Pendleton S. Caring for the patient with long-term disability. Geriatrics 1977;32:102.

33. Allen CA, Earhart CA. Cognitive disabilities: expanded activity analysis. Workbook introduced at the Institute on Cognitive Disabilities. AOTA National Conference, Phoenix, AZ, 1988.

34. U.S. Deparment of Justice, Civil Rights Division. ADA—Title II—Technical Assistance Manual, 1990.

35. Trombly CA. Employment for the physically disabled. In: Trombly CA, ed. Occupational therapy for physical dysfunction. 3rd ed. Baltimore: Williams & Wilkins, 1989:441.

36. Bryan TH. Overview of standardized worksamples and norms for injured workers. Occupational Therapy and Practice 1990;1:1.

37. Carlton RS. The effects of body mechanics instruction on work performance. Am J Occup Ther 1987;41:16.

38. Zila RC. Navy ship—a popular clinic. Advance for Occupational Therapy 1990;6:1.

39. Jacobs K. Occupational therapy for the workplace. In: Hopkins HL, Smith HD, eds. Willard and Spackman's occupational therapy. 7th ed. Philadelphia: JB Lippincott, 1988:272.

40. Taylor SE. Occupational therapy in industrial rehabilitation. In: Hopkins HL, Smith HD, eds. Willard and Spackman's occupational therapy. 7th ed. Philadelphia: JB Lippincott, 1988:299.

41. Egan M. Focus: work hardening. Programs use different means to achieve same goal. Occupational Therapy Week 1992;30:16.

42. Denton PL. Psychiatric occupational therapy: a workbook of practical skills. Boston: Little, Brown & Co. 1987.

43. Gillard M. Money and reimbursement versus OT practice. Pennsylvania Occupational Therapy Association workshop. Philadelphia, 1990.

CHAPTER / 12

Rehabilitation Postulates Regarding Intervention

The information in this chapter is not new material. The information is organized differently to help students think about compensatory techniques in a systematic and unbiased way. Unfortunately, many techniques are associated only with specific diagnoses. For example, energy conservation was developed for patients with rheumatoid arthritis. Yet, patients with spinal cord injuries can benefit from these techniques since they have fewer muscles to do the same task as healthy persons. Some techniques were initially developed for specific ADL tasks. For example, work simplification was first applied to cooking and other home-care tasks. At the same time, this adaptive procedure is helpful during bathing, like remembering to get all your bathing supplies and clean clothes before transferring onto a tubseat. It is time to stop teaching the use of rehabilitation methods only in a diagnosis-specific and task-specific context.

There are seven methods used in the rehabilitation frame of reference. They include:

1. Adaptive devices;
2. Upper extremity orthotics;
3. Environmental modifications;
4. Wheelchair modifications;
5. Ambulatory devices;
6. Adapted procedures; and
7. Safety education.

Several rehabilitation methods can compensate for the same prerequisite skill, like reaching. This redundancy is needed because a method can work beautifully with one patient and backfire with the next. This chapter will help you choose methods intelligently by being aware of the advantages and disadvantages of each method.

This chapter will also make you more aware of the rationales for rehabilitation methods. Rationales for adaptive devices and procedures are well established. For example, entry-level textbooks clearly state that long-handled shoehorns are used when a patient lacks sufficient reach (1–3). Unfortunately, other rehabilitation methods, like wheelchair and environmental modifications, are presented with a "catalog-ordering approach" (e.g., how to order wheelchair armrests). The rationales for choosing among three different armrests or choosing between wheelchair vs. environmental modifications are not emphasized.

Rationales are important for many reasons. Rationales identify the prerequisite skill that the patient cannot perform. Once you know that your patient lacks full hand closure, you have significantly narrowed down the type of adaptive device you can use. This makes selecting a compensatory device less overwhelming. It is also important for students to be able to verbalize their rationale for choosing specific devices and procedures. You can't respond intelligently to challenges like "I did it my way for 40 years" if you don't know why you are suggesting a particular change. Once the patient knows the rationale for a therapist's suggestions, he/she can understand and participate in the decision-making process. Otherwise, the patient has to use the device or procedure just because "you said so." Some patients don't react well to this type of explanation. Finally, rationales provide the justification for reimbursement that third-party payers require. Without this justification, insurance coverage may be denied.

ADAPTIVE DEVICES

Adaptive devices offer one of the largest number of rationales for compensation. Twelve rationales have been identified (see Tables 12.1 and 12.2). You must use clinical observation during ADL evaluations to identify which prerequisite deficits are affecting function before you can choose the appropriate adaptive device. The majority of rationales for adaptive devices address a loss of range of motion and/or strength. A moderate number of devices are available for the loss of one arm due to hemiplegia, severe hand injury, or amputation.

Table 12.1.
Adaptive Devices and Orthotics

Goal	Method	Rationale	Examples
1. Independence in ADLs will be maximized by using	A. ADAPTIVE DEVICES and ORTHOTICS, which:	Compensate for lack of full reach	Bathing: long-handled sponge Dressing: dressing stick; stocking aid; elastic shoelaces Environmental control: long-handled reacher for light switches, etc. Feeding: long-handled utensils; long straw with clip Grooming: long-handled comb; aerosol deodorant Toileting: wiping tongs; suppository inserter Cooking: reacher tongs for lighweight objects Cleaning: vacuum cleaner wand attachments; long-handled dustpan
		Compensate for lack of UE strength	Communication: mouthstick for typewriter; speaker phone Feeding: mobile arm support; overhead suspension sling; raised lapboard Cleaning: put laundry in bag and carry it on lap in wheelchair
		Compensate for lack of supination	Feeding: swivel spoon; curved handles on utensils
		Compensate for lack of full hand closure	Communication: lightweight built-up handle on pencil; flexor hinge split Environmental control: built-up doorknobs, dresser knobs, etc. Feeding: lightweight built-up handles on utensils Grooming: lightweight built-up handles on comb, toothbrush; wash mitt Cooking: built-up handles on pots and pans Cleaning: built-up handles on brooms, irons, etc.
		Compensate for lack of power grip or pinch	Communication: telephone clip holder Feeding: universal cuff; flexor hinge splint; lightweight built-up handles on utensils Grooming: electric razor with hand cuff; universal cuff on toothbrush; deodorant and hair spray can adapter Bathing: bath mitt; soap-on-a-rope Dressing: fastening aides (e.g., button-hook; elastic shoelaces) thumb hooks (e.g., zipper pull; loops on pants; belt loop) clothing (e.g., Velcro closures; front openings; one size larger) Cooking: loop handle on spatula; electric scissors to open cooking pouches
		Eliminate spills	Feeding: non-skid matt; plate guard; scoop bowl; long straw with clip Grooming: articles on a rope, like a shaver or soap
		Eliminate cuts	Feeding: plastisol-coated utensils Shaving: electric razor
		Compensate for lack of internal stability (ataxia)	Feeding: friction-feeder; heavy-handled utensils Grooming: heavy electric shaver Weights: weighted vest; 1 1/2-lb. wrist cuff; 3/4-lb. ankle cuff Cooking: heavy pots and pans; non-skid matts Cleaning: put dish towel in bottom of sink to wash dishes
		Compensate for lack of a hand to stabilize objects (e.g., cerebral vascular accident; amputee)	Communication: writing frame; book holder Fastenings: zipper pull; elastic shoelaces Feeding: rocker knife; plate guard Grooming: suction-cup nail brush and denture holder Cooking: suction cup for bowls; spike cutting board; Zim jar opener; one-handed sifter; electric can opener; chef's egg cracker; salad tongs; grater with suction feet; rocker knife Cleaning: bottle brush on suction base for glasses; mop with mechanism to wring sponge one-handed
		Ensure joint protection	1. No fingers (use strongest joint): loops on pants to pull them up 2. Use a loose grip: large handles on pots, pencils, tools, etc. 3. Avoid ulnar deviation: folding knife; rubber grip aid to open jar 4. Avoid lateral pressure on fingers: adaptive key holder; hoop scissors 5. Avoid static postures: book holder to prop up book; stand for mixing bowl
		Ensure hip precautions	1. Avoid hip flexion beyond 90°: long-handled reacher; sock donner; removable plastic raised toilet seat
		Compensate for lack of vision	Communication: page magnifier; prism glasses for reading in bed Bathing: long-handled skin inspection mirror

Table 12.2.
Environmental Modifications

Goal	Method	Rationale	Examples
1. Independence in ADLs will be maximized by using	B. ENVIRONMENTAL MODIFICATIONS, which	Provide access to housing, public and private facilities, recreation, and transportation	Handicapped transport system: paratransit will not take you out of the house; kneeling bus; buses with lifts; tie-downs in buses/trains Private transportation: modified driver controls; vans with lifts Parking spaces: located near entrances; 16 ft wide for side-exit vans Ramps: with rise of 1″ for every 12″; 5 sq. ft at top for turning W/C Doorways: Minimum 32″ wide; electric doors with 13-second closure delay Elevator: call button 36″ from floor Signage: use of symbols and Braille
		Promote independence	Environmental hardware: between 1 1/2 and 4 1/2 ft from floor for wheelchairs Public bathrooms: wide stalls/high toilet seats/low sinks with 5 ft depth clearance for wheelchairs/low towel dispensers Private bathrooms: roll-in shower stall; tub clearance 5 ft long and 4 ft out from tub; low sink with 5 ft depth clearance for wheelchairs Water fountains: 36″ high Telephones: 48″-mounting height; enclosure is adapted or 36″ wide Adapted kitchens: lower counter height and overhead cabinets; cut out in countertop to accommodate wheelchairs; front controls on stove
		Promote safety	Proper work height to prevent repetitive motion injuries Adequate space for using proper body alignment and good body mechanics Grab bars in the tub and near the toilet; tub seats; hand-held shower attachment Removal of small area rugs; put rubber mats in tub or shower Railings on ramps; non-skid surface on ramp Curb cuts located so individual is not discharged into parking lanes Smoke alarms; intercom systems Buzzers to denote arrival of elevator at floor
		Promote energy conservation, work simplification, and joint protection	Avoid stressful positions: high stools; tub seats; raised toilet seat Use loose grip: adapted handles on doorknobs/cabinets/faucets/drawers Reorganize storage: rarely used items stored at ceiling and floor level; lower clothes bar; slide out shelves; lazy Susan; easy flow of work Energy-saving appliances: self-defrosting refrigerator; microwave oven; self-cleaning oven; dishwasher; electric mixer; can opener; Utility cart for moving several small objects or one large object

Very few devices are available for the client with poor internal stability, like the patient with ataxia or athetoid-type spasticity. In fact, uncoordinated movements make most adaptive devices dangerous. Some rationales are diagnosis-specific, such as avoiding ulnar deviation for arthritic patients.

Adaptive devices are probably the most commonly used rehabilitation method, but they have demonstrated varied success. Geiger found that 54% of dressing devices were not used by patients with orthopaedic conditions after they went home (4). Half of the patients in the survey said they no longer needed the device. Even patients with long-term disabilities, such as stroke patients, reported a 25% disuse rate for dressing aids (5). Yet therapists said they thought only about 16% of adaptive devices were discarded after discharge (6). There is a discrepancy between therapists' and patients' perception of how helpful adaptive devices are at home.

Adaptive devices have three advantages. First, some adaptive devices have good face validity. Even cognitively impaired patients can usually understand their usefulness just by looking at them. Second, they have a strong placebo effect. They are a concrete, immediate solution, like taking a pill. Some patients respond positively to these technological gadgets. Third, many adaptive devices are inexpensive enough for patients on a fixed income if the devices are not covered by insurance.

Adaptive devices have two disadvantages. Some patients feel these devices stigmatize them as "handicapped." They would rather have a spouse cut up their meat in a restaurant than draw attention to themselves by pulling a rocker knife out of their purse or pocket. Adaptive devices also require intact perceptual skills. Patients who can't tell which side of a regular knife to place against the meat won't do any better with a rocker knife. Adaptive devices may provide a failure experience for patients with severe perceptual deficits, making them even more frustrated.

UPPER EXTREMITY ORTHOTICS

Orthotics are devices that patients can wear (e.g., a splint) or take with them throughout the day (e.g., a mobile arm support). Orthotics can do more than enhance independence. They can immobilize a painful or unstable joint, prevent deformities, and restore physical skills (7). Trombly divides upper extremity (UE) orthotics into proximal and distal. Proximal UE orthotics that enhance independence include overhead suspension slings, friction feeders, and mobile arm supports (MAS) that attach to wheelchairs. Distal UE orthotics that enhance independence include flexor hinge splints and universal cuffs.

The rationale for using proximal and distal upper extremity orthotics is to compensate for weak UE strength. They are most helpful with light tasks such as feeding, grooming, writing, and typing. They are not realistic for doing heavy tasks such as scrubbing floors or lifting heavy objects.

Orthotics have the same advantages and disadvantages as adaptive devices. They have the additional disadvantage of being bulky and uncosmetic. Since UE orthotics are often used in combination with adaptive devices, these two methods are combined in the rehabilitation postulates (see Tables 12.1 and 12.2).

ENVIRONMENTAL MODIFICATIONS

Environmental modifications include any equipment that changes the environment for everyone who shares space with the patient. A raised toilet seat affects everyone who uses that toilet.

Evaluation for architectural barriers is usually organized by rooms. For example, the bedroom is evaluated separately from the kitchen. This promotes the "catalog-ordering approach" for environmental modifications.

However, you should be guided by the prerequisite skills your patient lacks (see Table 12.2). Is he/she unable to access public facilities? Does he/she lack independence because of joint pain or fatigue? Does the patient need prompts to avoid hazards? Is he/she unsafe due to poor balance?

Perinchief identified four rationales that justify the need for environmental modifications (8). Two rationales, to provide access and to promote independence, are closely tied to wheelchair use. That is why most of the measurements listed under these two rationales in Table 12.2 are determined by the size of a standard wheelchair. For example, a standard wheelchair requires a MINIMUM opening of 32 inches to accommodate the 27-inch width of the chair, the 2-inch wide door that is blocking the hinge side of the opening, and 3 inches divided between the patient's two hands on the wheels. If you've added up these numbers, you can see that this is a very tight squeeze, especially when turning corners, so 36-inch openings are PREFERRED. Similarly, countertop and sink heights are determined by the lap height of someone sitting in a wheelchair that is 2 feet 3 inches. The only exception to this wheelchair "rule of thumb" is the height of raised toilet seats in public bathrooms. These seats are 17 to 19 inches high to accommodate patients with hip conditions who cannot squat down low enough for regular-height toilets.

A third rationale for using environmental modifications is to promote safety. This goal has traditionally included equipment that provides greater stability, such as grab bars and tub seats. However, repetitive motion injuries, such as carpal tunnel syndrome in computer users and low back injuries, have expanded the therapist's role in addressing safety issues. In one study, teaching good body mechanics was ineffective when environmental design did not support safe movement patterns (9). While workers who received training exhibited significantly improved body mechanics on a novel task, they still demonstrated poor body mechanics while on the job in a cafeteria line. These workers often had to assume awkward positions to lift and lower cooking supplies and equipment because of the awkward placement of storage shelves. Employers may have to modify their physical environment to make safety education effective.

The last rationale for using environmental modifications is to promote energy conservation, work simplification, and joint protection. For example, using a cart to transport supplies during cooking reduces physical stress on joints from heavy objects and reduces the number of trips taken, which therefore saves energy. Most texts restrict these types of environmental modifications to chapters on arthritis, cardiac conditions, or homemaking. However, these environmental modifications are helpful for people with many diagnoses. For example, a patient with spinal cord injury can benefit from reorganizing cabinets and closets so that the most commonly used items are at wheelchair height.

Environmental modifications are usually part of one giant list for a single diagnosis. For example, it is common to see a list of environmental modifications, adaptive devices, and adapted procedures that use joint protection principles. However, you should think of these methods as alternate approaches to the same problem. A patient may reject one method, so you may need to switch to other rehabilitation methods that protect joints. The overlap among rehabilitation methods allows the therapist to design an individualized mix of rehabilitation methods that are used to achieve a goal. That mix varies from patient to patient.

Environmental modifications are advantageous when some problems cannot be solved any other way. A wheelchair will not permit access to a given area or make someone independent if architectural barriers are present. Wheelchairs do not simplify work, protect joints, or promote safety. They usually complicate daily life. If a bathroom stall is too small to allow the door to close when you are in a wheelchair, who wants to use a public toilet? Environmental modifications can make the difference between regaining or losing a valued role.

Environmental modifications have three disadvantages. First, it usually costs more than adaptive devices. This is a problem because many insurance policies do not cover environmental modifications. Second, an environmental modification is not portable. If the deficit that causes dysfunction is temporary, the cost of environmental modification is not justified (8). Even for long-term disability, you need to ask how long your patient plans to live in a particular residence or work at a particular job. Third, environmental modifications make the patient dependent on the willingness of others. One mother did not want a wheelchair ramp built for the front door because she did not want her house to look different from the other houses in the neighborhood (8). Employers may not want to change the workplace for one employee.

WHEELCHAIR MODIFICATIONS

There are five rationales for prescribing specific wheelchair parts and models (see Tables 12.3 and 12.4). Three rationales for using wheelchair modifications are to facilitate transfers, to facilitate proper positioning, and to overcome architectural barriers. Every patient must be able to meet these three task demands. Otherwise, the wheelchair is useless. If a patient has sufficient motor skills left intact, he/she may need minimal modification of the wheelchair. Don't order parts that com-

pensate for these task demands unless the patient needs them.

Two additional rationales for using wheelchair modifications are to permit self-propulsion and transportation of objects. All patients do not have the cognitive skills to permit self-propulsion and transportation of objects while in the wheelchair, so prescribe these additional wheelchair modifications carefully.

One advantage of wheelchair modification is that the cost of a basic chair is usually covered by insurance. Expensive modifications may also be covered if their cost is justified. A second advantage is that long-distance locomotion may be more practical in a wheelchair than with ambulatory aids. How functional is walking at work when the employee is so tired that he/she can't continue to work after lunch?

Two disadvantages of wheelchair use are that many architectural barriers arise and the wheelchair itself creates social barriers. Many buildings do not have wheelchair ramps or electric-eye doors. Many rooms are too cluttered to provide a pathway for a wheelchair. The wheelchair also creates social barriers because the patient is no longer at eye level. The patient quickly loses status and is easily ignored when sitting in a wheelchair.

AMBULATORY DEVICES

There are six rationales for prescribing ambulatory devices (see Table 12.4). First, ambulatory aids reduce weightbearing on the lower extremities. Some patients need to temporarily eliminate weightbearing to protect damaged joints and fractured leg bones until they heal. Some patients, like paraplegics, can continue to walk if the weight on both legs is permanently reduced to a safe limit. Devices that achieve reduced weightbearing are crutches and canes that remove or reduce the load on the legs.

A second rationale for using ambulatory aids is to provide a wider base of support. Some patients can continue to walk even though they are unstable if they are given a wider base of support. Patients with poor balance may be more stable if they use a walker or quad cane.

A third rationale for using lower extremity orthotics is to support unstable LE joints. Lower extremity orthotics, such as short and long leg braces, will support unstable hip, knee, and ankle joints. A fourth rationale is to completely substitute for a lost limb, such as an above-the-knee or below-the-knee prosthesis.

A fifth rationale is to protect the arm during locomotion. An arm sling supports a subluxed shoulder and keeps the arm from swinging out of control while walking. The wheelchair arm trough and lapboard support the arm and keep it from getting caught in the spokes

Table 12.3.
Wheelchair Modifications

Goal	Method	Rationale	Examples
1. Independence in ADLs will be maximized by using	C. WHEELCHAIR MODIFICATIONS, which	Facilitate wheelchair transfers (Tx)	Back: zipper-back (permits sliding transfer backwards out of chair) Armrest: removable (permits sliding transfer sideways over rim of wheel) Legrest: swing-away (W/C close to furniture but uses wider turning space) detachable (permits wheelchair to get CLOSEST to furniture) Seat: transfer board (for sliding transfer; for safer sitting pivot transfer) Brakes: extension handle (better leverage; easier reach for sound hand to reach across body if hemiplegic arm is flaccid)

		Facilitate proper positioning	Back: reclining back (better trunk stability); reclines for low blood pressure head extension (for poor head control)
			Arm rest: adjustable height (to ensure proper arm and trunk support)
			   arm troughs/lapboards (UE positioning)
			   offset (increases inside width between uprights for wider hips)
			Overhead sling (UE positioning for hand use in gravity-eliminated plane)
			Legrest: elevating (for edema or problems with blood pressure);
			   calf pad (prevents leg from sliding off footrest)
			Footrest: heelstrap (prevents foot from sliding off footrest)
			Seat: narrow adult (sides are closer for better lateral stability)
			   lateral supports (for better lateral stability)
			   seatbelt (keeps hips back so pelvis and trunk can rest against backrest and trunk is erect)
			   hard seat (inhibits LE spasticity; promotes neutral pelvic tilt and symmetrical weightbearing)
			   ROHO seat cushion (for pressure relief)
			   Jay seat cushion (for pressure relief and lateral support)
			   numerous abductor devices (inhibits leg scissoring and extension which cause patient to slide out of wheelchair)

		Overcome architectural barriers	Seat: narrow adult (for narrow doorways; navigating congested rooms);
			   narrowing device (for narrow doorways)
			Legrest: detachable (considerably reduced turning space for W/C)
			Armrest: wrap around (2″ less in overall width)
			   desk arms; detachable armrests (to get closer to table)
			   lapboards (for when W/C won't fit under sink, table, etc.)

	C. WHEELCHAIR MODIFICATIONS, which	Permit self-propulsion of W/C	Seat: narrow adult (requires less UE abduction, which is tiring)
			   low hemi-seat (so propelling foot easily reaches floor)
			Wheels: 8″ diameter (more stable on rocks, curbs, etc.)
			   5″ diameter (tighter turns)
			Rims: spoke extensions (quad can push with palm or webspace);
			   double rims (hemiplegic can push chair with one hand)
			   flat rim (lighter weight)
			Electric W/C

		Permit transportation of objects	Pouches attached to W/C with Velcro straps Wheelchair laptray Crutch holders attached to wheelchair Loop over back of wheelchair (for hooking elbow while reaching for objects)

Table 12.4.
Ambulatory Aids

Goal	Method	Rationale	Examples
1. Independence in ADL will be maximized by using	D. AMBULATORY AIDS, which	Reduce weight bearing on LEs	Standard crutches; forearm (Loftstrand) crutches; platform crutches Standard cane; curved-top cane
		Widen base of support to increase stability	Standard walker; rolling walker; stair-climbing walker Quad cane
		Increase joint stability of LE	Short leg brace; long leg brace Plastic ankle-foot orthosis (AFO)
		Substitute for lost limb	Above-the-knee prosthesis Below-the-knee prosthesis
		Protect UE	Arm sling while walking W/C arm trough or lapboard
		Permit transportation of objects	Walker pouch Backpack while crutch-walking

of the wheelchair. Without these UE orthotics, some patients are not safe during locomotion.

The last rationale for using ambulatory aids is to permit transportation of needed objects. The ambulatory patient needs to carry objects like books, a purse, or a long-handled reacher. This may be possible by using a backpack while crutch-walking or a hanging pouch when using a walker.

Ambulatory aids permit a person to overcome architectural and social barriers. While removable leg-rests and desk arms enable a person to get the wheelchair closer to a toilet or desk, the chair can still be too wide to get into the toilet stall or office. The ambulatory patient can overcome these architectural barriers by walking the short distance required. The height achieved when standing also produces a more positive social response than sitting in a wheelchair. Equal height means equal status. When people look down at someone in a wheelchair, it negatively affects their expectations and attitudes toward the person in the chair.

Ambulatory aids also have several disadvantages. They require prolonged high-energy expenditure from UE muscles that are not designed for endurance. They require judgment. Crutch tips and the legs of walkers get caught on furniture unless motor planning is adjusted for the extra space needed to maneuver. Walking up and down stairs must be done in a specific sequence when ambulatory aids are used. Ambulatory aids also sacrifice the function of one or both hands. While trying to get something out of the refrigerator, the patient may have to use one hand to lean on the crutches, cane, or walker to keep from falling. When patients walk with ambulatory aids, they can't carry something in their hands. Finally, ambulatory aids

reduce walking speed, which some people find very frustrating.

ADAPTED PROCEDURES

There are five rationales for using adapted procedures (see Tables 12.5 and 12.6). One rationale for using adapted procedures is to substitute for lost motion. Table 12.5 lists the trick motions that patients with a spinal cord injury use. This is only one example of substitution. A hemiplegic patient can learn to dress the affected side first and push his/her wheelchair with the sound leg and arm. The UE amputee can learn to move his/her stump and shoulder to operate the prosthesis. For example, he/she can open the terminal device by flexing the shoulder. Patients are the best source of innovative ways to substitute for loss of AROM.

One rationale for using adapted procedures applies only to brain-damaged patients. When a patient has ataxia, there are three proprioceptive neuromuscular facilitation (PNF) techniques that help control the ataxia. "Chop" and "lift" are two-handed movement patterns that lock the arms together for greater stability (10). These bilateral patterns and their application to functional activities are shown in Trombly's textbook (11). "Surface contact" consists of sliding the ataxic hand along a stable surface for greater stability (12). To keep from knocking over a glass while picking it up, the patient can slide his/her hand along the table instead of reaching for the glass with his/her hand in the air. "Move and stop" consists of breaking a large movement into several small arcs by using external sources of support (12). For example, the patient can get a medicine bottle off the top shelf of the bathroom cabinet by resting

Table 12.5.
Adapted Procedures

Goal	Method	Rationale	Examples

1. Independence in ADL will be maximized by using	E. ADAPTED PROCEDURES, which	Substitute for lost AROM. The motions on the right are taught to SCI patients.
		
		Other examples: a hemiplegic patient propeling a W/C with the sound arm and leg; an UE amputee using shoulder flexion to open terminal device
			1. *Head movements* (C1–C4): use mouth stick or chin controls
			2. *Light shoulder motions* (C5 = partial deltoids and scapular muscles) e.g., ext rotation/abduction replaces supination to eat with M.A.S.
			3. *Hook with elbow* (C5 = biceps) e.g., hook elbow around W/C upright to lower self to reach floor
			4. *Extrinsic tightness* (C5 = selective tightening for hook-grasp)
			   e.g., fingers hook on edge of transfer board to slide it around
			   e.g., wedge typing tool between tight fingers
			5. *Elbow-walk* (C6 = more shoulder) roll onto side and push up onto elbow; depress scapula to shift off elbow to inch it forward to sit up
			6. *Lock elbow* (C6 = pectoralis major, which adducts shoulder) sit supported: fling arm behind body using shoulder extension and external rotation to lock elbow in extension with powerful adduction
			7. *Wrist extension* (C6 = ECRL & B)
			   e.g., pick up and hold light objects using tenodesis action
			   e.g., hang on extended wrist that is hooked behind W/C upright
			8. *Elbow extension* (C7 = triceps and rest of shoulder girdle)
			   e.g., trunk-balancing with extended arms held out to sides

		Provide stability during ataxic movements	1. *"Chop and lift"* (two-handed PNF patterns)
			   e.g., use reverse of "chop" to wash face and "lift" to reach for glass in cupboard (Trombly, Chapter 24D)
			2. *"Surface contact"* (PNF technique)
			   e.g., slide hand along tabletop to get glass
			3. *"Move and stop"* e.g., rest on every shelf of cabinet to lower hand

		Inhibit spasticity	1. *Use "distal key points of control"* (NDT technique)
			   e.g., clasp hands and reach forward to initiate chair transfer
			   e.g., put sound leg under spastic leg during bed mobility
			2. *Use "proximal key points of control"* (NDT technique)
			   e.g., lean forward to dangle spastic arm to use weight of arm to protract scapula and extend elbow while putting on a shirt
			   e.g., cross spastic leg over sound leg to relax extensor spasticity
			3. *Use placing, lowering, and weightbearing* (NDT technique)
			   e.g., lower spastic arm to table; hold arm there to hold down paper

		Conserve energy	1. Respect pain (i.e., don't work through the pain—stop when pain occurs; in the long run, you will be able to do what you want longer)
			2. *Rest frequently*
			   e.g., take mini-rests during activities
			   e.g., plan regular rest periods throughout the day
			3. *Prioritize activities* (don't tire self by taking shower when you want to play with children after breakfast)
			   e.g., do the most important activities first
			   e.g., don't worry about low-priority tasks once you're tired
			4. *Avoid isometrics*
			   e.g., rest elbow on table while eating instead of holding it up in air
			   e.g., stand up, roll in bed, etc. without holding your breath
			5. *Avoid stressful positions*
			   e.g., standing requires more energy than sitting (sit to shave, cook, etc.)
			   e.g., reaching over head is stressful (stand on stool)
			   e.g., prolonged squatting or bending at waist
			   e.g., crossing your legs (raises your blood pressure)

Table 12.5.
Adapted Procedures (continued)

Goal	Method	Rationale	Examples
			6. *Avoid exercise/hot showers after a meal* (this directs blood to both the peripheral and deep organs, which strains the heart) Use best work height/energy-saving equipment (see environmental modifications)
		Simplify work	1. *Organize storage* to eliminate wasted trips and stressful reaching e.g., keep frequently used clothing at W/C height e.g., put infrequently used baking equipment up high in cupboards 2. *Plan ahead* to eliminate wasted trips e.g., gather all clothing and jewelry before dressing e.g., gather all cooking supplies ahead of time 3. *Use an easy flow of work* (assembly-line style) e.g., lay out soap/towels/clothing in order they are needed e.g., lay out salad greens/cutting board/salad bowl/dressing in order needed 4. Eliminate steps and jobs e.g., use permanent press clothes; let dishes drip dry e.g., hook bra in front and then turn it around; leave tie knotted e.g., use premeasured bags of soap and bleach

the hand on the top shelf after grasping the bottle and then stopping to rest the hand on the middle shelf and then the bottom shelf. People without disabilities use this procedure to walk down the aisle of a moving train by stopping to control the sway of their body as the train lurches from side to side.

Another rationale for using adapted procedures applies only to patients with brain damage. These patients can benefit by learning to use reflex inhibiting patterns (RIPs) during ADLs to inhibit spasticity (13). For example, "distal key points of control" require the patient to learn to clasp hands together and lead with both arms extended in front of the body to stand up (see Fig. 8.2). Clasping hands together brings both scapulae forward into protraction, which inhibits the flexion synergy of the arm that would otherwise pull the patient back into the chair. Extending both arms in front of the body shifts the patient's center of gravity forward over the feet and helps to arch the low back so that anterior pelvic tilt occurs. Posterior pelvic tilt makes a patient very dysfunctional. It throws the patient's center of gravity backward and facilitates the extensor synergy in the LE, which thrusts the patient even farther back in the chair.

Patients can be taught to use "proximal key points of control" to inhibit spasticity (see Fig. 8.3). For example, the patient can learn to dangle the hemiplegic arm between his/her legs while putting the arm in the sleeve of a shirt or coat. The weight of the hemiplegic arm drags the scapula forward into protraction, which inhibits the flexion synergy and facilitates elbow extension, allowing the arm to slide easily into the open sleeve.

Brain-damaged patients can also learn to use normal movements to inhibit spasticity. "Placing" the hemiplegic arm in space and then lowering it using eccentric control until it is weightbearing on a surface inhibits spasticity. Even if the hemiplegic arm has to be assisted by the sound arm, muscle tone will be more normal than if the hemiplegic arm is flung into place using pathological synergies.

The last two rationales for using adapted procedures are to conserve energy and to simplify work (see Table 12.6). These procedures help any patient who has a permanent loss of physical skills. A patient who has fewer muscles to do the same work as healthy individuals no longer has the luxury of resting some muscles while working others. The high energy expenditure of the remaining muscles can make a patient dysfunctional if energy conservation and work simplification are not used.

The advantage of adapted procedures is that they are relatively inexpensive and are less visible to others. The cost is determined by the time the therapist spends training the patient, which may be less expensive than some wheelchair and many environmental modifications. Adapted procedures are also less visible than adapted devices and other equipment. Most people do not really scrutinize how another person gets into a car or slices meat. The "invisibility" of adapted procedures makes some people feel less self-conscious.

Table 12.6.
Safety Education

Goal	Method	Rationale	Examples
1. Independence in ADLs will be maximized by using	F. SAFETY EDUCATION, which	Ensures good body mechanics	Patient will consistently demonstrate the following principles 1. Keep objects/people close to body (social distance not acceptable!) 2. Keeps wide base of support: feet wide apart with no obstacles in way 3. Slides objects/people rather than lifting if possible 4. Lifts with legs not back by bending knees to squat and then stand up 5. Uses good pacing: lifts smoothly; doesn't jerk 6. Pivots whole body en bloc by moving feet instead of twisting torso
		Ensures safe transfers	Patient will consistently demonstrate the following principles: 1. Gets W/C as close as possible; removes W/C parts if necessary 2. Equalizes heights as much as possible 3. Locks W/C brakes 4. Moves hips forward to get close to edge of chair/bed 5. Places feet flat on floor and directly under knees before standing 6. Identifies safe landing site for fall before standing up 7. Moves smoothly; doesn't thrust self out of chair
		Ensures safety for somatosensory loss	Patient will consistently demonstrate the following principles: 1. Inspects skin daily 2. Differentiates between a pressure mark and pressure area 3. Relieves pressure at regular intervals 4. Wears protective splints and orthotics 5. Uses appropriate positioning 6. Moves desensate body part carefully using visual feedback
		Ensures cardiac precautions	Patient will consistently demonstrate the following cardiac precautions: 1. Rest if heart rate goes up more than 20 bpm from resting pulse 2. Rest if heart rate goes above 120 bpm or below 60 bpm 3. Rest if systolic BP goes above 150 or below 90 (normally SBP = 120) 4. Rest if diastolic BP goes above 90 or below 50 (normally DBP = 80) NOTE: CONSULT PHYSICIAN FOR EXCEPTIONS TO THESE GUIDELINES
		Ensures that hip precautions are followed	Patient will consistently demonstrate hip precautions: 1. *Avoids hip adduction* (e.g., don't cross legs to roll in bed) 2. *Avoids hip internal rotation* (e.g., don't line up foot with shoe by twisting leg into internal rotation) 3. Avoids hip flexion past 90° (e.g., stand up from chair by leaning back and sliding hips to edge of seat, then extend knee of operated leg, and push off from armrests)
		Other diagnosis-specific precautions	e.g., Stump protection e.g., Visual field deficit

Adapted procedures also have disadvantages. They may provoke resentment because the new procedure requires a change of habit. It is amazing to see how much emotional investment people have in minor habits like squeezing the toothpaste tube a certain way. Refusal to learn to do things a new way will make adapted procedures useless for some patients. Some patients feel that their privacy has been invaded when a therapist asks them how they make a bed or bathe their children. Some patients also take this type of analysis of their personal habits as a form of criticism. They may not understand why we need to know how they organize

		Table 12.6. **Safety Education (continued)**	
Goal	Method	Rationale	Examples

		Ensures joint protection
		
		(see also adapted devices and environmental modifications that ensure joint protection)
			Patient will consistently demonstrate the following principles:
			
			1. *Uses work simplification, energy conservation, good body mechanics*
			2. *Doesn't use fingers: Use strongest joint instead*
			   e.g., stands up from armchair by pushing with palms, not knuckles
			   e.g., stabilize mixing bowl in crook of elbow
			   e.g., carry purse on forearm instead of hand
			3. *Use a loose grip* (if fingers must be used)
			   e.g., place two hands under heavy object to carry it
			   e.g., press moisture out of sponges instead of wringing them dry
			4. *Avoids ulnar deviation*
			   e.g., hold knife like ice pick and use pulling action to cut
			   e.g., open jar with open palms and shoulder motion, not wrist motion
			   e.g., turn doorknob with two hands
			5. *Avoids lateral pressure on the fingers*
			   e.g., dial rotary phone with a pencil held like a dagger
			6. *Avoids static positions* (RA patient can stiffen in 20 minutes during flareup)
			   e.g., change regularly from sitting to standing and back
			7. *Avoids static flexion* (neutral position = most joint stability)
			   e.g., sleep flat in supine instead of fetal position on side
			   e.g., rest extended arms on table; don't lean flexed arms on armrests

their dresser drawers, unless we explain the concept of adapted procedures to them. Adapted procedures also lack external prompts to remind the patient to perform a task a new way. For this reason, adapted procedures may not be useful for patients with cognitive deficits.

SAFETY EDUCATION

Safety education is really a subcategory of adapted procedures. However, safety is so crucial for discharge planning that therapists have generated several procedures just to address safety issues. For this reason, it has been identified as a separate rehabilitation method.

Two rationales for using safety education apply to every patient. They are safety procedures that ensure good body mechanics and safe transfers (see Table 12.6). The remaining rationales for safety education are diagnosis-specific, such as joint protection for arthritis (see Table 12.6).

The advantage of safety education is that it may allow the patient to be discharged to a less restrictive environment and maintain valued roles and interests. Unfortunately, patients who are still relatively healthy do not always see the need for safety education. Until they are hurt or can see an imminent loss of function or need

for institutional care, some patients are unwilling to follow safety precautions.

One disadvantage of safety education is that it requires the vigilant application of abstract concepts. Cognitively impaired patients may not be able to visualize their prosthetic hip popping out of the socket or understand the purpose of moving their center of gravity closer to the object they are lifting. Even if these patients can memorize safety principles by practicing specific tasks, you may not be able to rely on them to generalize safety principles to new situations.

Even cognitively intact patients may find it difficult to implement safety education. Safety precautions can be hard to implement because it is difficult to view one's own body while performing a task. For example, patients must look down at their body parts and mentally visualize what their hip looks like from the side in order to evaluate whether they are flexing the hip more than 90°. Safety precautions also require mental vigilance. For example, extra mental effort is required to monitor how long one has been sitting in a static position or how many times one has fleetingly used ulnar deviation during a single task.

The second disadvantage of safety education is that it often requires a change of habit. It is difficult to remember not to grip a heavy pot by the handle when

Rehabilitation Postulates Regarding Intervention

Independence in ADLs, work, and leisure will be maximized by using:

A. *Adaptive devices and orthotics*, which
   1. Compensate for lack of full reach
   2. Compensate for lack of UE strength
   3. Compensate for lack of a hand to stabilize objects
   4. Compensate for lack of full hand closure
   5. Compensate for lack of power grip or pinch
   6. Compensate for lack of supination
   7. Eliminate spills
   8. Eliminate cuts
   9. Compensate for lack of internal stability (ataxia)
   10. Ensure joint protection
   11. Ensure hip precautions are followed
   12. Compensate for lack of vision

B. *Environmental modifications*, which
   1. Provide access to housing and public and private facilities
   2. Promote independence in a given environment
   3. Promote energy conservation and work simplification
   4. Promote safety and reduces hazards in a given environment
   5. Promote joint protection

C. *Wheelchair modifications*, which
   1. Facilitate wheelchair transfers
   2. Facilitate proper positioning
   3. Overcome architectural barriers
   4. Permit self-propulsion
   5. Permit transportation of needed objects

D. *Ambulatory devices*, which
   1. Reduce weightbearing on the LE
   2. Widen the base of support
   3. Increase joint stability of LE
   4. Substitute for lost limbs
   5. Protect UEs
   6. Permit transportation of needed objects

E. *Adapted procedures*, which
   1. Substitute for lost AROM
   2. Provide stability during ataxic movements (PNF)
   3. Inhibit spasticity (NDT)
   4. Conserve energy
   5. Simplify work

F. *Safety education*, which
   1. Ensures good body mechanics
   2. Ensures safe transfers
   3. Ensures safety during somatosensory loss
   4. Ensures that cardiac precautions are followed
   5. Ensures joint protection
   6. Ensures that hip precautions are followed

the handle is there to prompt us to use old habits. When a patient is already independent doing a task his/her way, it can be difficult to convince him/her that a preventative measure is worth the aggravation.

POSTULATES REGARDING INTERVENTION

Postulates regarding intervention in the rehabilitation frame of reference link functional outcomes and rehabilitation methods in a structured format: a *short-term func-tional outcome* will be achieved using *rehabilitation methods* that have *rationales* to guide selection of *specific rehabilitation equipment and procedures*. See Figure 12.1 for an example of solutions for one functional task. A single patient may not need all of these compensatory strategies, but you need to have a wide range of approaches to accommodate different needs and personalities.

Think carefully when writing the rationales in the center column. Third-party payers don't automatically know why a patient needs a piece of equipment or why an occupational therapist needs to train the patient to use adapted procedures. Insurance companies will not reimburse a policyholder for equipment and training without a clear and reasonable rationale.

Devices and procedures must be named and explained in the Specific Modality Column. Sometimes the name of an adaptive device makes its purpose self-evident (e.g., button-hook). However, the purpose of most equipment and adapted procedures is not obvious. Describe how it will be used (e.g., hook elbow on back of W/C upright while reaching down for clothes in dryer).

SUMMARY

This chapter attempts to teach you to consider compensatory strategies in a systematic way that it not restricted to diagnosis-specific choices. To help you remember all the rehabilitation methods and rationales, use Memory Aid 12.1. There is some redundancy in this table because every method is not successful with every patient. Each method has its own advantages and disadvantages that need to be matched to the patient.

STUDY QUESTIONS

1. What are the advantages and disadvantages of adaptive devices and UE orthotics?
2. The majority of adaptive devices compensate for what?
3. UE orthotics are most helpful with what type of tasks?
4. What factor determines most measurements for environmental modifications?
5. How has the occupational therapist's use of environmental modifications to promote safety been expanded?
6. Compare and contrast the advantages and disadvantages of environmental modifications, wheelchair modifications, and ambulatory aids.
7. What are the five rationales that should guide a therapist's thinking when ordering wheelchair equipment?
8. Who is your best resource for learning substitute motions?
9. What adapted procedures are used only for brain-damaged patients?

Figure 12.1.
Example of Rehabilitation Postulates Regarding Intervention

Dysfunction/Cause/Goals	Method/Rationale	Application/Explanation
Dysfunction: unable to brush hair	*Adaptive devices*, which compensate for weak tenodesis grip	1. Brush handle in universal holder 2. Adapted lever for hairspray can
Cause: complete deenervation of hands/ triceps/trunk/BLEs; partial deenervation and disuse atrophy of BUEs; somatosensory loss of fingers and ulnar side of BUEs due to C6 SCI	*Environmental modification*, which facilitate independence	1. Light switch about 4 ft high 2. Lower mirror to 4 ft at bottom 3. Bathroom door at least 36″ wide 4. Lever handles on faucets 5. Sink cut out; 29″ high for knees
Short-Term Functional Outcome: able to brush hair with moderate physical assistance	*Environmental modifications*, which ensure safety	1. No throw rugs (W/C propulsion) 2. Wrap exposed pipes under sink to prevent leg burns
Long-Term Functional Outcome: able to independently brush hair with adapted procedures and equipment	*Wheelchair modifications*, which overcome architectural barriers	1. Narrow adult W/C to get through door and maneuver between sink/tub 2. Detachable legrests and deskarms to get closer to sink
	Wheelchair modifications, which ensure proper positioning	1. Cushion for pressure relief 2. Narrow adult W/C with seatbelt for trunk support
	Adapted procedures, which substitute for trunk control and power grip	1. Intrinsic tightness to grasp hairspray can more tightly 2. Tenodesis action to grasp brush 3. Hook elbow to lean forward
	Adapted procedures, which simplify work	1. Organize storage: put all grooming supplies in one place 2. Plan ahead: get all supplies out before starting
	Safety education, which compensates for loss of sensation	1. Have patient use thumb to feel how hot water is to wet hair

10. Why is safety education separated from adapted procedures in this text?
11. What advantages and disadvantages do adapted procedures and safety education share?

References

1. Malik MH. Activities of daily living and homemaking. In: Hopkins HL, Smith HD, eds. Willard and Spackman's occupational therapy. 7th ed. Philadelphia: JB Lippincott, 1988:259.
2. Pedretti LW. Activities of daily living. In: Pedretti LW, Zoltan B, eds. Occupational therapy practice skills for physical dysfunction. St. Louis: CV Mosby, 1990:230.
3. Trombly CA, Quintana LA. Activities of daily living. In: Trombly CA, ed. Occupational therapy for physical dysfunction. 3rd ed. Baltimore: Williams & Wilkins, 1989:436.
4. Geiger CM. The utilization of assistive devices by patients post discharge from an acute rehabilitation setting. Unpublished master's thesis. Temple University, 1989.
5. Bynum H, Rogers J. The use and effectiveness of assistive devices possessed by patients seen in home care. Occup Ther J Res;1987;7:181.
6. Gitlin L, Levine R, Geiger C. Evaluation of extended equipment use by disabled elderly. Paper presented at the American Occupational Therapy Association Annual Meeting, Baltimore, 1989.
7. Trombly CA. Orthoses: purposes and types. In: Trombly CA, ed. Occupational therapy for physical dysfunction. 3rd ed. Baltimore: Williams & Wilkins, 1989:329.
8. Perinchief J. Environmental modification. Lecture presented at Temple University, 1990.
9. Carlton RS. The effects of body mechanics instruction on work performance. Am J Occup Ther 1987;41:16.
10. Voss DE, Ionta MK, Myers BJ. Proprioceptive neuromuscular facilitation. 3rd ed. New York: Harper & Row, 1985.
11. Myers BJ. Proprioceptive neuromuscular facilitation (PNF) approach. In: Trombly CA, ed. Occupational therapy for physical dysfunction. 3rd ed. Baltimore: Williams & Wilkins, 1989:141.
12. Becker P, Myers BJ, Mukoyama S. Two week workshop on proprioceptive neuromuscular facilitation. Rehabilitation Institute of Chicago, 1985.
13. Bobath B. Adult hemiplegia: evaluation and treatment. 2nd ed. London: William Heinemann Medical Books Limited, 1978.

Rehabilitation Case Simulation: Arthritis

CREATING NARRATIVE HYPOTHESES AND AN EVALUATION PLAN

Mrs. C. is a 54-year-old woman with an 5-year history of rheumatoid arthritis. She is taking nonsteroidal anti-inflammatory medication. She was recently admitted with an acute flare-up and referred to OT for resting hand splints.

She lives with her husband and two children in a two-story house. Her daughter attends high school and her son attends a local college. Her husband works with the highway department. She graduated from college with a degree in medical records and was working as a medical secretary.

Student's Narrative Hypotheses

Use this space to write your narrative hypotheses. Restrict yourself to ± 7 hypotheses by chunking related concerns. Review a chapter on rheumatoid arthritis BEFORE doing this assignment!! Use Memory Aid 2.2 to guide you.

Suggested Narrative Hypotheses

Based on the diagnosis and date of onset, I would expect:

1. Possible damage to the heart, lungs, or kidneys; fever; fatigue;
2. Joint inflammation and pain with possible joint instability and deformity, especially the MP and PIP joints of the hand;
3. Reduced ROM, strength, and coordination of involved joints, especially in the of the hand;
4. Possible loss of independence in self-care, leisure, and work skills;
5. Architectural barriers at home;
6. Stress reactions and hindered sexuality;
7. Possible lack of understanding about rheumatoid arthritis disease process.

Student's Evaluation Plan

Use this space to design an evaluation package. Identify the domains of concern you would test. Name the test you would use and justify why you would choose these tests. Remember, in-depth testing is not indicated all the time.

Concern	*Name of Tests*	*What the Data Will Be Used for*

Suggested Evaluation Plan

Based on the narrative hypotheses, I recommend initial evaluation of:

Concern	Name of Tests	What the Data Will Be Used for
Systemic disease	Read medical chart; test tolerance for a 10-minute activity bedside	Need to know whether precautions should be taken during evaluation and early treatment
Joint damage and pain, esp., MP and PIPs	Check for deformities in resting and moving hand; test for intrinsic tightness; subjective report of pain and stiffness	Deformities will affect splint design; must identify potential for further joint damage before choosing functional activities; need to know if pain will interfere with Rx
ROM	Active ROM of BUEs; observe LEs during ADLs	Need baseline to test effectiveness of joint protection training to preserve ROM
Strength	Active ROM of BUEs; observe grasp and LEs during AM self-care	Must choose early Rx activities that will not cause further joint damage due to excessive resistance
Coordination	Write name; button; cut meat; dial phone; handle mail and coins	Need to know how much coordination affects daily activities without using stressful coordination tests
ADLs	AM care; self-feeding; toileting	Need to maintain ROM/strength without overstressing joints during acute flare-up; full eval later
Architectural barriers	Informal conversation	Need to plan discharge goals as early as possible
Psychosocial issues	C.O.T.E. and informal conversation	I don't want to upset the patient with an in-depth interview until I get to know her better
Knowledge of disease	Informal conversation	Lack of understanding after 5 years will reduce compliance with adapted methods and rehabilitation potential

EVALUATION RESULTS

See Figure 13.1 for her AROM test results. She cannot oppose her thumb to the last two digits of either hand. Ulnar drift occurs during active MP flexion, but it disappears at rest. There is no intrinsic tightness and there are no permanent deformities. There is boggy swelling around both shoulders, wrists, and knees as well as around the MP and PIP joints of both hands. The skin around all of these joints looks red and feels warm. She complained of joint pain during the evaluation, but reported no paresthesias. She gets up an hour earlier to fix breakfast because of morning stiffness. She is currently ambulatory, but is worried about the effect of the pain in her knees on her future ambulation. She fatigued after 10 minutes of evaluation and was given a rest.

She is right-hand dominant. She has a gross grasp for light objects with a diameter of up to 3 inches. Handling coins, signing her name, and managing fastenings,

JOINT RANGE MEASUREMENTS

Patient's name _____ Chart no._____

Date of birth _____ Age _____ Sex _____

Diagnosis _____ Date of onset _____

Disability _____

3	LEFT 2	1	SPINE		1	RIGHT 2	3
			Cervical spine				
			Flexion	0-45			
			Extension	0-45			
			Lateral flexion	0-45			
			Rotation	0-60			
			Thoracic and lumbar spine				
			Flexion	0-80			
			Extension	0-30			
			Lateral flexion	0-40			
			Rotation	0-45			
			SHOULDER				
	0-90°		Flexion	0 to 170		0-90°	
			Extension	0 to 60			
	0-90°		Abduction	0 to 170		0-90°	
	0-5°		Horizontal abduction	0-40		0-5°	
	0-90°		Horizontal adduction	0-130		0-90°	
			Internal rotation	0 to 70			
			External rotation	0 to 90			
			ELBOW AND FOREARM				
	0-135°		Flexion	0 to 135-150		0-135°	
	0-80°		Supination	0 to 80- 90		0-80°	
	0-90°		Pronation	0 to 80- 90		0-90°	
			WRIST				
	0-50°		Flexion	0 to 80		0-50°	
	0-40°		Extension	0 to 70		0-40°	
			Ulnar deviation	0 to 30			
			Radial deviation	0 to 20			
			THUMB				
			MP flexion	0 to 50			
			IP flexion	0 to 80- 90			
			Abduction	0 to 50			
			FINGERS				
	0-30 to 40°		MP flexion	0 to 90		0-30 to 40°	
	0-30 to 40°		MP hyperextension	0 to 15- 45		0-30 to 40°	
			PIP flexion	0 to 110			
			DIP flexion	0 to 80			
			Abduction	0 to 25			
			HIP				
			Flexion	0 to 120			
			Extension	0 to 30			
			Abduction	0 to 40			
			Adduction	0 to 35			
			Internal rotation	0 to 45			
			External rotation	0 to 45			
			KNEE				
			Flexion	0 to 135			
			ANKLE AND FOOT				
			Plantar flexion	0 to 50			
			Dorsiflexion	0 to 15			
			Inversion	0 to 35			
			Eversion	0 to 20			

Figure 13.1.

A. ENGAGEMENT
  0 -Needs no encouragement to begin task
  ①-Encourage once to begin activity
  2 -Encourage two or three times to engage in activity
  3 -Engages in activity only after much encouragement
  4 -Does not engage in activity

B. CONCENTRATION
  ⓪-No difficulty concentrating during full session
  1 -Off task less than one-fourth time
  2 -Off task half the time
  3 -Off task three-fourths time
  4 -Loses concentration in less than 1 minute

C. RESPONSIBILITY
  ⓪-Takes responsibility for own actions
  1 -Denies responsibility for 1 or 2 actions
  2 -Denies responsibility for several actions
  3 -Denies responsibility for most actions
  4 -Denial of responsibility; messes up project and blames therapist or others

D. FOLLOW DIRECTIONS
  ⓪-Carries out directions without problems
  ①-Occasional trouble with more than three step directions
  2 -Carries out simple directions; has trouble with two-step directions
  3--Can carry out only very simple one step directions (demonstrated, written, or oral)
  4 -Unable to carry out any directions

E. ACTIVITY NEATNESS
  ⓪-Activity done neatly
  1 -Occasionally ignores fine detail
  2 -Often ignores fine detail; materials are scattered
  3 -Ignores fine detail; work habits disturbing to those around
  4 -Unaware of fine detail; so sloppy that therapist has to intervene

F. PROBLEM SOLVING
  ⓪-Solves problems without assistance
  1 -Solves problems after assistance given once
  2 -Can solve only after repeated instructions
  3 -Recognizes a problem but cannot solve it
  4 -Unable to recognize or solve a problem

G. SOCIABILITY
  ⓪-Socializes with staff and patients
  1 -Socializes with staff and occasionally with other patients or vice-versa
  2 -Socializes only with staff or with patients
  3 -Socializes only if approached
  4 -Does not join others in activities

H. COMPLEXITY AND ORGANIZATION OF TASK
  0 -Organizes and performs all tasks given
  ①-Occasional trouble organizing complex tasks he should be able to do
  2 -Organizes simple but not complex tasks
  3 -Can do only very simple activities with organization imposed by therapist
  4 -Unable to organize or carry out task when materials/directions available

I. INITIAL LEARNING
  ⓪-Learns new activity quickly and easily
  1 -Occasionally has difficulty learning a complex activity
  2 -Frequent difficulty learning complex activity but can learn simple one
  3 -Unable to learn complex activities; occasional difficulty learning
  4 -Unable to learn a new activity

K. INTEREST IN ACCOMPLISHMENT
  0 -Interested in finishing activities
  ①-Occasional lack of interest or pleasure in finishing a long-term activity
  2 -Interest or pleasure in accomplishment of short-term activity; lack of interest in a long-term activity
  3 -Only occasional interest in finishing
  4 -No interest or pleasure in finishing

L. DECISION MAKING
  ⓪-Makes own decisions
  1 -Makes decisions but occasionally seeks therapist approval
  2 -Makes decisions but often seeks therapist approval
  3 -Makes decision when given two choices
  4 -Refuses to or cannot make any decisions

M. FRUSTRATION TOLERANCE
  0 -Handles all tasks without becoming overly frustrated
  1 -Occasionally becomes frustrated with complex tasks; can handle simple ones
  ②-Often becomes frustrated with complex tasks; can handle simple ones
  3 -Often becomes frustrated with any task but attempts to continue
  4 -Becomes so frustrated with simple tasks that refuses or is unable to function

N. EXPRESSION
  ⓪-Expression consistent with situation and setting
  1 -Occasionally inappropriate
  2 -Inappropriate several times during session
  3 -Expression inconsistent with situation
  4 -Extremes of expression: bizarre, uncontrolled or no expression

Figure 13.2. Excerpts from COTE: Mrs. C.

such as buttons, are all very awkward due to the exclusive use of a lateral pinch and pain.

She reports that despite pain, she can do all her self-care except for fastening her bra. She reports no longer being able to do all her own housework, but she still drives herself to do her shopping. There are 12 steps with a railing to the second story. There is a powder room on the first floor, but laundry facilities are in the basement. She had to quit her full-time job due to decreased sitting tolerance and joint pain. She was working at home about 10 hours per week typing medical reports for a local hospital before this current flare-up.

She says she became depressed after the changes in her employment and the inability to do all her housework. She describes herself as a perfectionist, and she gets angry when her family members don't do the housework exactly as she'd like it done. See Figure 13.2 for psychosocial observations from the C.O.T.E. She likes to read and swim. Her goal is to "get rid of my pain and be able to move better."

INTERPRETING THE TEST RESULTS

On the two blank pages, list each hypothesis, *but* leave a generous space under each hypothesis to list the evaluation results that you believe are relevant to each hypothesis. In front of each cue, write one of the following symbols. A plus means a cue confirms and a minus means a cue disconfirms a hypothesis. A ± means a cue partially confirms and partially disconfirms a hypothesis. A question mark means the cue's relevance is unclear. Remember, these symbols are feedback to you about the accuracy of your hypotheses! They do not indicate the patient's assets and deficits! At the bottom of each list, conclude that each hypothesis was confirmed as written -OR- write a revised hypothesis. Cues that are completely unrelated to your hypotheses should be preceded by a capital N for New and added to the end of the list.

Student's Cue Interpretation List

1.

Student's Cue Interpretation List cont.

Student's Problem List

The cue interpretation list and hypothesis evaluation represents an inner dialogue that is too lengthy to put in a medical chart. A facility will want you to write a Problem List that consists of general deficits and dysfunction. At the bottom of this page, convert your confirmed hypotheses into a Problem List. By definition, a Problem List does not include assets and function, so delete them. Feel free to change the numbers and descriptions from the ones used in your hypotheses. Remember, working memory is limited to ± 7 pieces of information, so eliminate unconfirmed hypotheses, and chunk related problems. Don't forget to add new problems not anticipated by your hypotheses!

1.

2.

3.

4.

5.

6.

7.

8.

Suggested Cue Interpretation List

1. *Possible damage to heart/lungs/kidneys; fever; fatigue*
   - − Medical chart negative
   - − No fever noted in evaluation results
   - + Had to quit full-time job due to decreased sitting tolerance
   - ± Unable to do all her housework independently
   - + Fatigued after 10 minutes of evaluation

   Revision: significant fatigue is present

2. *Joint inflammation and pain; joint instability and deformity, esp. MP/PIPs*
   - + Boggy swelling of both wrists, shoulder, knees and MP/PIP of last two digits of both hands
   - + Skin feels warm and looks red around these joints
   - + Complained of joint pain
   - + Reported morning stiffness
   - + Ulnar drift during active MP flexion

   −   No permanent deformities

   −   No intrinsic tightness (which often leads to swan-neck deformity)

Revision: joint inflammation, edema, pain, and stiffness with instability and potential for joint deformity of MPs

3. *Reduced ROM, strength, and coordination, esp of hand*

   +   Limited AROM of both shoulders, wrists, and fingers

   +   Unable to oppose thumb to last two digits of either hand

   +   Gross grasp only for light objects with diameter up to 3″

   +   Handling coin/signing name/fastenings awkward due to pain/lateral pinch

   ±   Currently ambulatory

Hypothesis confirmed as written

4. *Possible loss of independence in self-care/leisure/work*

   ±   Currently independent in self-care except for fastening bra

   +   Handling coins/signing name/fastenings awkward due to pain and exclusive use of lateral pinch

   ±   Reports being unable to do all her housework

   ?   Enjoys reading and swimming

   +   Had to quit full-time job due to decreased sitting tolerance

   +   Currently unable to work at home for about 10 hours per week

   −   Able to drive car to do shopping

Revision: Partial dependence in dressing and housework; impact on leisure unknown; dependent in work

5. *Architectural barriers at home*

   +   Two-story house with bedrooms on second floor (12 steps with railing)

   +   Laundry facilities in the basement

   −   Powder room on first floor

Hypothesis confirmed as written

6. *Stress reactions and hindered sexuality*

   +   Worried about effect of knee pain on future ambulation

   +   Became depressed after changes in employment and housework

   +   Gets angry when family doesn't do housework "as she'd like it done"

   +   Needs encouragement to begin activity

   +   Occasional difficulty organizing activities that she should be able to do

   +   Often becomes frustrated with complex tasks but can handle simple tasks

Revision: stress reactions present; impact on sexuality unknown

7. *Possible lack of understanding about R.A.*

   ±   Goal is to "get rid of my pain and be able to move better"

   ±   Describes self as a perfectionist

   ±   Occasional lack of interest in new activity

   ±   Occasional lack of interest/pleasure in finishing long-term activity

Hypothesis needs to be further investigated

N = No paresthesias reported

Suggested Problem List

1. Significant fatigue
2. Joint inflammation, edema, pain, stiffness with MP joint instability and potential for joint deformity

3. AROM limited bilaterally in shoulders, wrists, and fingers
4. Impaired hand coordination and lack of mature prehension
5. Partial dependence in dressing and housework; dependent in work
6. Architectural barriers at home with pain in knees
7. Stress reactions present; possible lack of understanding about R.A.

Reflection on the Problem List

Note that some numbers have changed from the hypothesis list to the Problem List. This is customary since test results often redefine the therapist's focus. Feel free to chunk the problems differently. Chunking is a personal strategy that helps an individual remember the main treatment issues.

1. Significant fatigue.   The hypothesis about fever and damage to the heart, lungs, and kidneys is a good example of having to read between the lines of a medical report. If any of her vital organs showed dysfunction, it would have been clearly stated in the medical record. If the patient had appeared flushed or felt hot, the therapist would have indicated this in his/her notes. Assets are frequently omitted in medical writing. Assistance for housework was given a ± score since more than just fatigue may account for this loss.

2. Joint inflammation, edema, pain & stiffness; MP joint instability and potential deformity.   The probability of deformity without intervention is very high, so it is reasonable and necessary to include deformity in both the hypothesis and the Problem List, even though current test results show no current deformity (see two −'s listed with Hypothesis #2). A great deal of therapy time will be spent addressing potential deformity. Failure to mention this potential now creates internal consistency between the initial report and subsequent notes that will repeatedly discuss preventing future deformities.

3. Impaired AROM bilaterally in shoulder, wrist, and fingers.   The need to do an initial evaluation does not override the therapist's obligation to do no harm. Resistance is contraindicated at this time, so UE strength on the Manual Muscle Testing and grip strength on a dynamometer were not tested.

4. Impaired hand coordination and lack of mature prehension.   Coordination was listed as a separate problem on the Problem List because it is at a very low level right now. This creates immediate concerns for early ADL treatment. Coordination did not have to be extensively tested since clinical observation during ADLs confirmed that the patient was too low-functioning to perform stressful, timed tests of fine motor coordination requiring tip pinch, such as pegboard evaluations. This is a good example of the decision tree in action.

5. Partial dependence in dressing and housework; dependent in work.   Leisure activities were dropped from the Problem List. An in-depth interview about leisure interests could be upsetting during this acute stage. The grieving process is renewed every time a patient with arthritis experiences an exacerbation. After the therapist has established rapport, leisure interests may be more safely breached. Other therapists might disagree with this conservative approach to occupation in acute care. On the other hand, it is important to list self-care and work dysfunction in the initial Problem List because a.m. care will be an early treatment focus, and her work status already affects her current emotional state.

6. Architectural barriers at home with pain in knees.   These two concerns are chunked together in the Problem List because they are intimately related to each other and to discharge planning. Yet, it would also be appropriate to chunk knee pain with joint inflammation concerns.

7. Stress reactions and possible lack of understanding about R.A.   Notice that the hypothesis about sexuality was dropped from the Problem List. It is unlikely to have information about this intimate topic this early in the treatment process. Information about this sensitive topic may never be written in the chart. Possible lack of understanding about R.A. was chunked with stress reactions on the Problem List because they both have psychosocial components. Her comment about getting rid of her pain suggests an incomplete acceptance of rheumatoid arthritis after 5 years. The goal in R.A. is to control pain so that it does not interfere with functional activities.

However, note the repeated use of the ± sign under Hypothesis #7. This indicates that, while these data suggest a lack of understanding of the arthritis disease process and the need for significant life-style changes, taken alone, they are not conclusive. Occasional lack of interest in activities may reflect her current depression more than a lack of understanding of her disease. Additional information will be obtained when the therapist observes the patient's response to joint protection training.

Notice the omission of "no paresthesias reported" on the Problem List. A Problem List does not include assets by definition.

Student's List of Deficits Not Addressed by Rehabilitation

One narrative hypothesis raised concerns about her non-human environment. Use this space to identify additional two MOHO assets or deficits. Name each MOHO concern. Then give an example of a question that needs to be explored in future dialogue with this patient for each MOHO concern. Use Memory Aid 14.1 to guide you.

1.

2.

One psychosocial problem already identified is depression. Use this space to identify two additional psychosocial assets or deficits that are ignored by the MOHO frame of reference. Name each psychosocial concern. Then write a reasonable question regarding each concern that needs to answered in the future. Use Memory Aid 14.1 to guide you.

1.

2.

Use this space to identify two biomechanical deficits that are not addressed by the rehabilitation frame of reference. Name the specific biomechanical concern, and give a specific example from the evaluation results that proves your point.

1.

2.

Suggested List of Deficits Not Addressed by Rehabilitation

MOHO assets and deficits.   Note the use of question marks to indicate reasonable questions about issues not specifically stated in the results

Locus of control: How much internal control does she feel?

Expectations of success: What does she mean by being "able to move better"?

Meaning of activities: What do her medical records and housework skills really mean to her? (e.g., competence, pleasure, helping others?)

Interests: How recently has she participated in reading and swimming?

Family permeability:

Is her family open to the changes in housework that have taken place?

Have they discussed using outside resources?

Psychosocial assets and deficits ignored by MOHO.   Note the use of question marks to indicate reasonable questions about issues not stated in the results

Hospital-induced stressors

Is she experiencing stress due to pain and sleep deprivation?

Is she experiencing stress due to medical jargon and procedures?

Is she experiencing stress due to the inability to relieve stress with recreation, sex, exercise, and socializing with her family?

Sexuality:

Does her fatigue, shoulder pain, and knee pain interfere with sexual activity?

Does inability to do all her housework impair her feminine self-concept?

Biomechanical deficits not addressed by the rehabilitation frame of reference.

1. Joint instability of MPs
2. Very low-level endurance: e.g., tires after 10 minutes of evaluation
3. Joint edema/stiffness of MPs, IPs, wrists, shoulders, and knees
4. Limited AROM of shoulder, wrist, and fingers: e.g., wrist extension = 40°
5. Unable to test maximum strength since resistance is contraindicated now

GENERATING TREATMENT GOALS

Use the next page to write a rehabilitation goal spreadsheet. Divide your concerns into short- and long-term goals by thinking about what is safe, functional significance, goals that are possible in 1 week, and goals that must be treated directly. Prioritize within short-term and long-term goals by asking if one goal is a prerequisite for another goal. All goals must be measurable. Be sure to include compensatory devices and procedures if a full recovery is not possible.

Student's Goal Spreadsheet

Current Dysfunction.

To help you write appropriate functional goals, BRIEFLY list Mrs. C.'s current dysfunction.

Short-term Rehabilitation Goals (in 1 week during acute stage):

Long-term Rehabilitation Goals (after as much therapy as patient needs):

Suggested Rehabilitation Goal Spreadsheet

Current Dysfunction

1. Patient doesn't know how to perform a.m. care without injuring her joints; Potential for joint deformity during a.m. care

Short-term Rehabilitation Goals (in 1 week twice a day during acute stage):

1. Able to wash face and hands, brush teeth and hair, and toilet with intermittent supervision to implement joint protection procedures[a] and use adaptive devices and environmental modifications

Long-term Rehabilitation Goals (after as much therapy as patient needs):

1. Independent use of joint protection procedures[a], adaptive devices, and environmental modifications during self-care;
2. Independent use of joint protection procedures[a], adaptive devices, protective splints, and environmental modification during light housekeeping;
3. Independent use of joint protection procedures[a], protective splints, and environmental modification while typing 10 hours per week at home

Reflection on the Goal Spreadsheet

The list of current dysfunction documents her lack of training, which can cause joint damage. While it is true that she is currently dependent in bra-fastening and work and is partially dependent in housework, these tasks are too dangerous to use right now. In this stage of acute flare-up, fatigue and joint instability restrict the therapist's choices. The therapist must focus on patient education with very light, very brief tasks. Since documentation is supposed to help the clinician by focusing on upcoming treatment, there is no point in talking about bra-fastenings now. You would just have to explain in upcoming progress notes why it wasn't addressed. The two versions of a.m. dysfunction listed for Mrs. C. show two of several writing styles.

Notice that changing her level of independence is NOT the current focus of treatment because she is already independent in toileting and a.m. care. The current focus of treatment is to teach her new methods for doing self-care activities without harming her joints. Patient education is a service goal that states what the therapist will do. In order to be reimbursed, you must write outcome goals that state what skills the patient exhibits after treatment. Therefore, supervision is included in her short-term goals to document how much assistance is needed to support the patient's learning.

The initial statement about supervision also creates a baseline which permits you to document how well the patient acquires new knowledge. In this case, long-term goals state that she will demonstrate this new knowledge without prompting (i.e., independently). NOTE: standby supervision is NOT part of documenting the learning curve for this patient since standby supervision was designed for brain-damaged individuals who will always need supervision.

[a]Joint protection procedures also include energy conservation and work simplification.

DESIGNING A TREATMENT ACTIVITY

Use Figure 13.3 to design *ONE* rehabilitation treatment activity for one of your short-term rehabilitation goals. To show that you are fully prepared for the clinic, you must list every joint protection, every energy conservation, every work simplification, every adaptive device, and every environmental modification method that is possible for the activity that you've chosen. This leads to some redundancy, but you must be able to offer alternatives when your patient is unhappy with a particular solution. Being overprepared is a must when patients have emotional responses to such personal advice as how to organize their bedrooms or wipe themselves.

Remember, rationales are reviewed by third-party payers, so think carefully when writing them in the center column. Third-party reviewers don't automatically know WHY a patient needs what you have ordered.

Devices and procedures must be named *AND* explained. Sometimes the name of an adaptive device makes its purpose self-explanatory (e.g., button hook). However, the purpose of most equipment and adapted procedures is not obvious. Name the equipment or procedure AND describe how it will be used (e.g., hook elbow on back of wheelchair upright while reaching down for clothes in dryer).

Dysfunction/Cause/FO's	Method/Rationale	Specific Modality: Name, Description, Precautions

Figure 13.3a.   Student's Rehabilitation Activity

Dysfunction/Cause/FO's	Method/Rationale	Specific Modality: Name, Description, Precautions

Figure 13.3, continued   Student's Rehabilitation Activity

Dysfunction/Cause/FO's	Method/Rationale	Specific Modality: Name, Description, Precautions
Dysfunction: potential for joint deformity during a.m. care	*Adapted procedures* which simplify work	*Plan ahead:* gather wash cloth, towel, soap, toothbrush, toothpaste, and hairbrush to take to hospital bathroom in one trip in a small bag
Stage Specific Causes: 1. Pain and fatigue 2. Swelling which stretches ligaments, tendons, and joint capsules	*Adapted procedures* which conserve energy	*Respect pain:* stop activity and breathe deeply a few times if pain occurs (a longer activity might have to be stopped altogether) *Prioritize:* do important things first (e.g., toileting)
3. Joint hypermobility which erodes joint tissues and can result in cartilage necrosis	*Environmental modification* which promotes energy conservation, work simplification, and joint protection	*Avoid stressful positions:* sit down on a chair instead of standing to brush teeth and comb hair *Avoid tight grip:* use palms to operate lever handles on faucet at sink
Short-Term Functional Outcome: able to wash face and hands, brush teeth and hair, and toilet with intermittent supervision to use joint protection procedures, adaptive devices, and environmental modification	*Adapted devices* which ensure joint protection	*Avoid tight grip:* use built-up handles on toothbrush and hairbrush
Long-term Functional Outcome: independently use joint protection procedures, adaptive devices, and environmental modification during all self-care activities	*Safety education* which ensures joint protection	*Avoid ulnar deviation:* Turn bathroom doorknob by turning self sideways to door and using palm and wrist flexion/extension *Avoid a tight grip:* 1. Squeeze toothpaste against sink using palm 2. Let washcloth drip while hanging over spigot; when done with other activities, wrap it inside towel and press flat with palm on sink instead of wringing it *Use the strongest joint:* 1. Close drawer to night stand with buttock 2. Carry a.m. supplies to bathroom in bag with handle in crook of elbow instead of hand 3. Stand up from toilet by pushing with palms on toilet seat instead of using knuckles

Figure 13.4. Suggested Rehabilitation Activity.

SECTION V

DEFICITS NOT ADDRESSED

CHAPTER / 14

Psychosocial Issues

Historically, occupational therapy curricula, textbooks, and job opportunities have been divided into physical vs. psychiatric dysfunction. Therefore, it is not surprising that some experienced therapists working in physical disability settings feel uncomfortable about psychosocial issues in their practice (1, 2).

One source of the discomfort has been the criticism that psychosocial issues are not as concrete or measurable as physical concerns. Therapists worry about not being able to document the effectiveness of their psychosocial intervention. This has led some therapists working in physical disability settings to believe that psychosocial treatment is not reimbursable. Reimbursement is a real problem because few physically disabled patients have a psychosocial diagnosis and referral for treatment of psychosocial issues.

Some therapists have also reported feeling uncomfortable about getting too close to their patients. They may believe that emotional involvement with a patient will make them less objective or therapeutic. There is a fine line between feeling empathy and pity for what is happening to a patient. It is easy to cross this line without knowing it. This may be why therapists talk about keeping a professional distance in the therapist-patient relationship.

Many therapists working in these settings value a close therapist-patient relationship, but continue to feel ambivalent about reporting psychosocial concerns. They believe that expressing a personal interest in the patient is essential for establishing rapport, but they are still reluctant to talk about it with investigators or to include this data in medical records (1, 2). This lack of openness about and documentation of psychosocial issues led Fleming to call this part of treatment the "underground practice" (1).

Of course, new patients in physical disability settings can also have a psychiatric diagnosis (3). A premorbid condition may have even caused the traumatic physical injury. It is not uncommon to see alcoholics on a burn

ward because they fell asleep while smoking a cigarette in bed. Substance abuse may have caused an automobile accident. Personality disorders such as a generalized anxiety disorder, antisocial personalities, passive-aggressive personalities, and borderline personalities may also be present. Finally, even severe psychiatric conditions like bipolar disorders, chronic depression, and schizophrenia may be a part of the patient's history. These premorbid psychiatric conditions can have a severe impact on functional outcomes, which is why they are included in Memory Aid 14.1. For more information on these conditions, consult psychiatric textbooks. This vast topic is beyond the scope of this book.

There are three types of psychosocial issues that have been discussed in the physical disabilities literature. They are the model of human occupation (MOHO), sexuality, and stress reactions. This chapter explores these psychosocial issues. You should be able to identify these concerns in the mini-case study at the end of this chapter.

MODEL OF HUMAN OCCUPATION

Hierarchy

Kielhofner put psychosocial issues into a hierarchy that includes volition, habituation, and performance subsystems (4). Volition is the highest level in the hierarchy. **Volition** implies that individuals can make conscious choices about their behavior. Behavior is determined by more than just basic drives that build up pressure. Behavior can be influenced by personal causation, values, and interests. **Personal causation** is defined as the image of the self as a competent or incompetent person. **Values** are defined as the importance we place on activities that sustain our commitment to action. **Interests** are defined as the pleasure we associate with activities that create a preference for action. As therapists, we need to be aware of these kinds of motivation in our patients if our plans are to succeed. Patients are

---

Memory Aid 14.1.
Psychosocial Issues

I. Model of Human Occupation	II. Premorbid Conditions	IV. Stress Reactions

A. *Volition*
  1. *Personal Causation*
    a. Locus of control
    b. Expectations of success
    c. Efficacy of skill
  2. *Values*
    a. Life goals are life-long values
    b. Personal standards
    c. Meaning of activities
  3. *Interests*
    a. Pattern
    b. Potency
	1. Personality disorders
	2. Substance abuse/alcoholism
	3. Chronic depression
	4. Other psychiatric conditions
		A. Can have a positive or negative influence
		  1. Depression
		  2. Denial
		  3. Intellectualization
		  4. Anger
		  5. Dependency
		B. Usually have a negative effect
		  1. Repression
		  2. Projection
		  3. Self-abasement
		  4. Regression
		  5. Rationalization
		  6. Somatization

I. Model of Human Occupation	III. Sexuality Issues	V. HOSPITAL-INDUCED STRESSORS

B. *Habituation*
  1. *Roles*
    a. Types
    b. Conflict or balance
  2. *Habits* that support roles
    a. Degree of organization
    b. Social appropriateness
    c. Flexibility
	A. *Definition of Sexual Identity*
	  1. Physical appearance
	  2. Feminine and masculine personality traits
	  3. Emotional intimacy
	  4. Physical intimacy
	B. *Level of Therapist Involvement*
	  P: gives permission to be a sexual being by referring patient to appropriate resources
	  LI: gives limited information
	  SS: gives specific suggestions
	  IT: intensive therapy
		A. Stress due to the inability to communicate

		B. Stress due to fear of death/pain/ mutilation
		C. Stress due to medical jargon/ procedures that result in a feeling of helplessness
		D. Stress due to inability to relieve tension using familiar strategies like sex/food/ play/friends/work/exercise
		E. Stress due to sensory deprivation and separation from a familiar environment

I. Model of Human Occupation	Other Psychosocial Issues	V. HOSPITAL-INDUCED STRESSORS

C. *Environment*
  1. *Cultural influence* on
    a. Attitudes towards patients
    b. Expectations of workplace
    c. Expectations of community
  2. *Social groups*
    a. Expectations of family
    b. Permeability of family
  3. *Objects*
    a. Availability
    b. Complexity
    c. Symbolic meaning
	Some psychosocial issues fall between the cracks. Examples include frustration tolerance, cooperative attitude, and ability to socialize with staff and other patients.	F. Stress due to sleep deprivation caused by disruptive medical routines and pain

---

more likely to adopt new roles, habits, and skills if these new behaviors relate to their current interests, values, and sense of personal control.

Habituation is the middle level in the hierarchy. It is called **habituation** because it guides the performance of habitual patterns of behavior. Our values, interests, and belief about causation lead us to select certain roles and habits. **Roles** are defined as the images people have of themselves as holding certain positions in specific social groups and the expectations that accompany these positions. What values and interests influenced your choice of occupational therapy as a role? **Habits** are defined as the automatic routines that develop when an individual repeats certain actions. Habits operate largely below the level of consciousness. Try to recall the exact series of steps you go through to get

in and start your car. Habits are very important because many of them support our roles, like the habit of getting to work on time. Patients are often challenged by new habits, such as joint protection and modified bowel and bladder care. The concept of habits asks not whether the patient has the necessary skills to carry out a task, but whether he/she is willing to consistently use necessary routines.

Performance is the lowest level in the hierarchy. The roles and habits we choose lead us to develop specific prerequisite and functional skills. The majority of this text focuses on these skills, but MOHO puts them in the proper perspective—at the bottom of the hierarchy. It isn't enough to know that a bone has healed or a muscle is stronger. Our discharge plans also depend on what the patient intends to do with that newly healed arm. In fact, the MOHO hierarchy emphasizes a unity of body and mind that is lacking in the medical model.

Environment

The environment is a holistic MOHO concept that is based on the idea of an open system where individuals constantly interact with their surroundings. No attempt to understand a person's behavior is complete without understanding the expectations of the environment, called "environmental press." Environment is divided into culture, social groups, and objects (4).

Culture is defined as the beliefs, perceptions, values, norms, and customs that are shared by a group and passed from one generation to the next by formal and informal education. Cultural expectations define what types of jobs have status, whether work and play should be balanced in a person's life, and how a valued member of society should look and act. Cultures use informal and formal methods of transmitting these expectations. Informal learning is a powerful mechanism for teaching attitudes towards the physically challenged. Because this group does not visibly meet the expectations of society, they often have to overcome negative attitudes toward the handicapped in themselves and in others.

The spread factor is a common negative attitude that leads people to believe that physically challenged people are also mentally incapacitated and assume that they are more restricted than they really are (5). Other negative reactions include avoidance, nonacceptance, and enforced segregation (5). As a result of these negative attitudes, physically challenged people are often relegated to minority group status (5).

One patient talked about how these negative cultural attitudes toward the handicapped affected her: "As I wheeled to my room past a group of patients gathered in the second-floor lobby, I felt I had been abandoned in a netherworld populated by freaks: slack-jawed people staring wide-eyed into nothingness or contorted like corkscrews; people lying prone on wheeled stretchers or wearing strange helmets that made them look like hockey goalies" (6, p. 25). Attitudes toward the handicapped can negatively affect participation in a rehabilitation program and reintegration into the community.

Cultural expectations may produce a conflict between therapist and patient. In some communities, housewives have a lot of status, while in others, working women are more valued. In some communities, sustaining personal relationships is the most important sign of your worth as a human being, while in others, having a productive job is the most important way to judge how you have spent your life. The therapist may not share these or other cultural expectations. Trying to convince a patient in a few short weeks to ignore the cultural expectations of his/her own community is usually not effective. Discharge plans have to be made with the patient's cultural milieu in mind.

Social groups also influence patients. **Social groups** are collective units of individuals that create opportunities for people to assume certain roles. One of the most important groups a patient belongs to is his/her family. Each family has a dominant purpose that creates a press for time, commitment, and role definition. Some families are **permeable**, which means they are open to outside influences and able to change. Other families are **impermeable**. They have rigid hierarchies and cannot accept change in the dominance order. The therapist's and patient's plans for the future cannot be made without awareness of these family dynamics.

Discharge plans need to take into account that family members have a right to their own life. For example, we have empathy for children who feel that their handicapped sibling is getting all the attention in the family. We worry about mothers who fixate on their handicapped child to the exclusion of their other children and their marriage. We should also worry about caregivers of adult patients who try to change their whole life so it revolves around the disabled adult in the family.

Consent of family members is important in all settings. In pediatric settings, consent takes the form of legal documents that have to be signed by the parents. In adult settings, consent takes the form of informal negotiations. Talk to the family member *before* you plan treatment goals that rely on family members. Don't assume the social worker or psychologist will ask everything you need to know. These other team members don't know the details of your discharge plan. Don't assume that everything your patient tells you about the family is a shared perception. Remember the Newlywed Game? That's the TV show where couples lose the game because they recall the life they live together differently.

Finally, the environment affects people's lives through objects—from houses to toothbrushes. **Objects** vary according to their availability, complexity, and symbolic meaning. Therapists are painfully aware of the availability of objects when patients can't afford a major modification of their home or expensive adaptive devices. We also need to remember that many of the objects we recommend to our patients also have a range of complexity and symbolic meaning. To one patient, a rocker knife may be easy to manipulate and may represent independence. To other patients, a rocker knife may be confusing to use and may draw unwanted attention to them.

One patient shared her reaction to her wheelchair. "The patients were required to use wheelchairs even if they were ambulatory. The chair, in my mind, quickly became a symbol of dependency, almost a badge of shame. I remember that the first time I passed a good-looking 'upright'—a staff member walking by—I looked away, as if, by not looking, I would be invisible to him" (6, p. 25). When we think about changing the objects in our patients' lives, we need to remember that objects have psychosocial attributes as well as physical ones.

The assessment of environmental issues begins with reading the patient's social history in the medical chart. The social history identifies the patient's family and significant social contacts. It identifies financial concerns such as whether money is available for respite care. It may identify environmental barriers at home and at work. More subtle environmental concerns such as cultural values, family permeability, and the patient's response to adaptive equipment have to be assessed informally as patient and family training sessions unfold.

Concepts

The MOHO concepts make sense in terms of the discharge decisions that have to be made. For example, the team needs to know what types of roles the patient hopes to resume. Common sense also tells us that discharge plans will be adversely affected if the patient does not feel in control of his/her life and does not expect to succeed. Team members also need to know if the patient is socially appropriate and flexible when selecting appropriate discharge settings. Read Chapters 2 and 4 of *The Model of Human Occupation* (3) to become proficient with the MOHO concepts listed in Memory Aid 14.1.

Assumptions

The model of human occupation assumes that emotional stability is present. If this skill is absent, evaluation can be a problem. For example, an emotionally distraught patient may react negatively when asked about her daily routines at home soon after she is told that she will never walk again or that she has terminal cancer. It would also be pointless from a MOHO perspective to ask a patient with delusions about being Napoleon to describe his roles.

MOHO also assumes that cognitive skills are present. Cognitively impaired patients can make data collection difficult. They may not understand subtle concepts such as values and expectations of success. Functionally illiterate patients will have difficulty filling out the complex checklists and questionnaires that require six different answers to each question. For this reason, MOHO is most helpful with emotionally stable, cognitively intact patients.

Evaluation Tools

The Interest Checklist, Role Checklist, Time Inventory, Life Goals Inventory, and other evaluation tools used in Kielhofner's case studies are not fully standardized (4). Kielhofner responded by developing a manual for the Occupational Performance History Interview (OPHI). This interview tool asks patients about their perceptions of their ability and responsibility; interests, values, and goals; life roles; organization of daily living routines; and environmental influences (7).

Test-retest reliability for the OPHI varied from .55 to .68 for questions about the past and from .31 to .49 for the present. Responses were obviously more reliable for the past. When 21 patients who did not appear to give honest answers were eliminated from the sample of 153 subjects, the reliability coefficients increased to a mean of .75 for the past and a mean of .54 for the present. These correlations for test-retest reliability are acceptable for research purposes (see Appendix).

Inter-rater reliability coefficients ranged from .38 to .55 for the past and from −.08 to .46 for the present. These coefficients are low even by research standards. Kielhofner believes that the use of audiotapes instead of videotapes and the lack of a formal training program to teach raters how to use the manual may have produced these results.

An alternative tool that gathers some MOHO data is the Comprehensive Occupational Therapy Evaluation (8). This scale ranks a variety of behaviors observed during a one-hour therapy session on a scale of 0 to 4. Excerpts from the COTE are shown in Table 14.1. Inter-rater reliability ranged from .36 to .84. The centers that contributed the case simulations for this book do not use the OPHI, so portions of the COTE, based on several days of observation, and social history were used instead.

SEXUALITY

Sexuality is discussed in physical dysfunction texts (9). Most of the discussion focuses on how physical dysfunction affects sexual performance. I would like to talk about sexuality as a psychosocial issue because so many students are uncomfortable about discussing the role of sexual partner.

Definition

When students were asked "what makes you feel like a woman or a man," sexual intercourse was only one of the many responses (11). The list below is not exhaustive, but it gives you an idea of the wide variety of responses.

Table 14.1.

Comprehensive Occupational Therapy Evaluation Scale Definitions

Part I. General Behavior	

A. APPEARANCE

The following six factors are involved: (1) clean skin, (2) clean hair, (3) hair combed, (4) clean clothes, (5) clothes ironed, and (6) clothes suitable for the occasion.
0—No problems in any area.
1—Problems in 1 area.
2—Problems in 2 areas.
3—Problems in 3 or 4 areas.
4—Problems in 5 or 6 areas.

B. NONPRODUCTIVE BEHAVIOR

(Rocking, playing with hands, repetitive statements, appears to be talking to self, preoccupied with own thoughts, etc.)
0—No nonproductive behavior during session.
1—Nonproductive behavior occasionally during session.
2—Nonproductive behavior for half of session.
3—Nonproductive behavior for three-fourths of session.
4—Nonproductive behavior for the entire session.

C. ACTIVITY LEVEL (a or b)
(a) 0—No hypoactivity.
1—Occasional hypoactivity.
2—Hypoactivity attracts the attention of other patients and therapists but participates.
3—Hypoactivity level such that can participate but with great difficulty.
4—So hypoactivity that patient cannot participate in activity.

(b) 0—No hyperactivity.
1—Occasional spurts of hyperactivity.
2—Hyperactivity attracts the attention of other patients and therapists but participates.
3—Hyperactivity level such that can participate but with great difficulty.
4—So hyperactive that patient cannot participate in activity.

D. EXPRESSION

0—Expression consistent with situation and setting.
1—Communicates with expression, occasionally inappropriate.
2—Shows inappropriate expression several times during session.
3—Shows expression but inconsistent with situation.
4—Extremes of expression—bizarre, uncontrolled or no expression.

E. RESPONSIBILITY

0—Takes responsibility for own actions.
1—Denies responsibility for one or two actions.
2—Denies responsibility for several actions.
3—Denies responsibility for most actions.
4—Denial of all responsibility—messes up project and blames therapist or others.

F. PUNCTUALITY

0—On time.
1—5–10 minutes late.
2—10–20 minutes late.
3—20–30 minutes late.
4—30 minutes or more late.

G. REALITY ORIENTATION

0—Complete awareness of person, place, time, and situation.
1—General awareness but inconsistency in one area.
2—Awareness of 2 areas.
3—Awareness of 1 area.
4—Lack of awareness of person, place, time, and situation (who, where, what, and why).

Part II. Interpersonal	

A. INDEPENDENCE

0—Independent functioning.
1—Only 1 or 2 dependent actions.
2—Half independent and half dependent actions.
3—Only 1 or 2 independent actions.
4—No independent actions.

B. COOPERATION

0—Cooperates with program.
1—Follows most directions, opposes less than one-half.
2—Follows half, opposes half.
3—Opposes three-fourths of directions.
4—Opposes all directions and suggestions.

C. SELF-ASSERTION (a or b)
(a) 0—Assertive when necessary.
1—Compliant less than half of the session.
2—Compliant half of the session.
3—Compliant three-fourths of the session.
4—Total passive and compliant.

(b) 0—Assertive when necessary.
1—Dominant less than half of the session.
2—Dominant half of the session.
3—Dominant three-fourths of the session.
4—Totally dominates the session.

D. SOCIABILITY

0—Socializes with staff and patients.
1—Socializes with staff and occasionally with other patients or vice-versa.
2—Socializes only with staff or with patients.
3—Socializes only if approached.
4—Does not join others in activities, unable to carry on casual conversation even if approached.

E. ATTENTION-GETTING BEHAVIOR

0—No unreasonable attention-getting behavior.
1—Less than one-half time spent in attention-getting behavior.
2—Half-time spent in attention-getting behavior.
3—Three-fourths of time sent in attention-getting behavior.
4—Verbally or nonverbally demands constant attention.

F. NEGATIVE RESPONSE FROM OTHERS

0—Evokes no negative responses.
1—Evokes 1 negative response.
2—Evokes 2 negative responses.
3—Evokes 3 or more negative responses during session.
4—Evokes numerous negative responses from others, and therapist must take some action.

	Feel Like a Man	Feel Like a Woman
Physical appearance	Hairy chest Handsome Wearing work boots	Smooth legs Pretty Wearing high heels
Personality traits	Decisive Responsible	Sensitive Nurturing

Emotional intimacy	Fun to be with
	Can't get too close
	  to women friends
		Good at
		  relationships
		Allowed to touch
		  the people I care
		  about

Physical intimacy	Able to participate in sexual intercourse Able to have children in the future	

Hospitalization interferes with all these aspects of sexuality. It is difficult to look attractive while you are in the hospital. The role of dependent patient doesn't utilize all of our feminine and masculine personality traits. The hospital separates us from our loved ones, and it impedes our social and physical intimacy when our loved ones visit.

Illness threatens a person's femininity or masculinity in many ways (11). Patients worry that their partner won't want to be seen with them because of their appearance, will be afraid to touch them for fear of hurting them, will be reluctant to talk to them about personal problems or negative feelings for fear of upsetting them, will be unable to accept the fact that they can't have children, or won't be able to rely on them to take care of the family. Single patients worry about going out alone, having no one to talk to, and being unable to find a life-long partner.

Therapists' Role

You will very likely deal with sexual issues as a therapist. We are often the first person a patient talks to about sex because of our prolonged contact with them and our empathy. Since our initial response can have a big impact on whether the patient pursues his/her concerns, here are some counseling tips you need to keep in mind (9).

One, don't overemphasize the genital aspect of sex. When the word "sex" first comes up, think of the bigger picture, discussed earlier. Two, don't overreact to sexual language. Street language may be the only words a patient knows to identify body parts. Anatomical terminology is a part of our professional subculture. Three, don't overreact to sexual behavior. Erections during self-care activities can have a reflexogenic origin as well as a psychogenic origin. Four, don't be seductive or use locker room humor. Patients get confused when we try to reassure them that they are still a sexual being by responding sexually to them. If a patient acts seductively

or gets upset during physical contact, stop and explain your intentions. You can prevent misunderstandings by apologizing for inadvertent physical contact, by explaining why physical contact is necessary, and by keeping the genital and breast areas covered whenever possible. Five, don't impose your own values on the patient. Your beliefs about sex outside of marriage and acceptable sexual practices are not on trial, so don't judge your patient's beliefs. If you cannot suspend judgment, refer your patient to someone else. Finally, don't do sexual counseling if you don't feel comfortable with it. Tell the patient about your discomfort with the subject matter and refer him/her to another resource instead of making the patient feel that his/her questions are inappropriate.

The PLISSIT model for counseling will help you find the level of counseling that is most comfortable for you (9). The "P" stands for permission. This first level of counseling gives the patient permission to be a sexual being. Being old or sick doesn't turn patients into sexless entities. If patients are people, and all people have a sexual nature, then our patients must have sexual concerns (11). You can give permission by referring the patient to an appropriate resource.

The "LI" stands for limited information. This second level of counseling gives the patient some information about sexual dysfunction. You can give your patients handouts about diagnosis-related sexual dysfunction or a list of resource organizations. You may help them improve their physical appearance and help them plan opportunities for privacy, such as home visits. Make sure you have accurate information before you engage in this second level of counseling (9).

The "SS" stands for specific suggestions. This is the third level of counseling. Chapter 6 on adapted methods and Chapter 7 on devices in *Choices: A Guide to Sexual Counseling with Physically Disabled Adults* are two excellent resources (9).

The "IT" stands for intensive therapy. This fourth level is not possible in an open-therapy department. This type of counseling requires a private environment and sufficient time to discuss intensely personal problems. It is usually done by psychologists, social workers, or marriage counselors.

The level in the PLISSIT model you choose depends on your comfort level, your academic training, and on each physician's preference for handling sexual counseling. Some physicians feel they should be the only member of the team to talk to patients about sexual dysfunction. Other physicians prefer a team approach. Don't presume that you are free to do sexual counseling without clearing it with the doctor first.

STRESS REACTIONS

Positive and Negative Effects

Stress reactions have been called coping mechanisms (4), adaptive mechanisms (8), and stress responses (12) in physical disability textbooks. Stress reactions are reasonable responses of emotionally intact individuals to stressful conditions. They are different from defense mechanisms, which are seen as chronic, neurotic responses to stress. The stress reactions listed in Memory Aid 14.1 are familiar concepts used by health professionals in physical disability settings.

Some stress reactions can have either a negative or a positive influence. Depression means a patient has acknowledged that a disability exists, which is good, but severe depression can emotionally paralyze a patient. Denial is good when it enables a patient to carry on in the face of crushing tragedy. Therapists talk to patients about taking one day at a time without worrying about everything that has to be resolved in the future. Prolonged denial, however, can lead to noncompliance because the patient may not think he/she needs therapy. Intellectualization is good when it channels intellectual energy into solving problems, but it also permits strong emotions, like anger, to go unresolved. Anger is helpful when it encourages a patient to pursue rehabilitation goals, but it can disrupt treatment when anger turns into hostility toward self and others. Dependency enables the patient to accept the advice and assistance of health professionals. It can become a problem if the patient tries to avoid responsibility or completely rejects dependency and refuses to accept help that is truly needed. Fantasy is wonderful for creative problem solving and relieving tension, but can block recovery when the patient rejects reality.

One patient's story shows how stress reactions can have either a positive or a negative effect: "It takes a good deal of impatience—of dissatisfaction with the status quo—to fuel the internal mechanism for its fight back to health. We feared our progress was slowed by too much patience. It was anger and stubbornness that kept me alive in those crucial first weeks after the strangulation. However, once the immediate crisis passed, that unfocused anger became terribly draining" (5, p. 37).

Some stress reactions have only a negative impact. Repression goes beyond denial by completely suppressing painful thoughts so they can't even be discussed. Projection often produces a negative reaction from the secondary target, which undermines relationships. Self-abasement and rationalization may procure assistance, but they don't produce a positive self-image. Regression is an emotional retreat to infantile behaviors that make all rehabilitation difficult. Somatization is dangerous to physical well-being.

Hospital-Induced Stressors

Stress reactions appear first in acute care where survival is threatened. One of the most frightening stressors is the inability to communicate because of respiratory apparatus. Equipment that substitutes for the loss of a vibratory chamber, like the Olympic trach talk, can restore verbal communication (see Table 14.2). Alternative communication systems are available to replace verbal communication. Strategies such as lip-reading and writing with a nondominant hand can be difficult to implement, but they are preferable to no communication. The inability to communicate means the staff cannot assess how much the patient understands and has difficulty understanding the patient's requests. Not knowing what happened to them and suffering from thirst are a few of many consequences that patients experience when they can't communicate.

Fear of death and mutilation is also very threatening. Verbalization of these fears can permit catharsis, legitimize fears, and sensitize staff to fears that need to be addressed.

Yet, physical mutilation doesn't have to be massive to create emotional distress. Traumatic hand injuries can produce a profound sense of loss that results in the grieving process associated with death or terminal illness (13). Even partial loss of hand function can be devastating because the hand allows the individual to control the environment. Because most hand injuries are caused by accidents, patients often have the added burden of guilt. They may blame themselves and can end up with divorces and loss of employment if they cannot communicate and deal with their feelings.

More subtle stressors are also present in acute care. Intensive care units have many strange-looking devices and unusual procedures. Stress due to the lack of understanding of medical jargon and procedures can result in a feeling of powerlessness and lack of compliance. Patient education should begin as soon as possible. Even if the patient doesn't understand everything the first time around, the willingness to share information is comforting.

Intensive care units also create stress by interfering with the inability to relieve stress using familiar strategies like sex, exercise, work, eating, talking to friends and family, and recreation. The patient can be taught to use alternate stress management techniques like progressive relaxation. Make yourself familiar with the specific techniques discussed by Neistadt in *Willard and Spackman's Occupational Therapy* (12).

Stress due to sensory deprivation and separation from a familiar routine created by the intensive care unit can be relieved by sensory stimulation. However, random overstimulation is not helpful. Stimuli need to be organized into an orderly and familiar routine. Finally, stress due to a lack of sleep can undermine all treatment goals. Unfortunately, hospitals are noisy places that impose night-time procedures such as checks

Table 14.2.
Hospital-Induced Stressors

Goals	Method/Rationale	Activity Examples
Stress due to *lack of communication* will be reduced by using	*Equipment*, which substitutes for the loss of a vibratory chamber to restore speech	1. Olympic trach talk 2. Fenistrated trach 3. Artificial larynx
	Communication systems, which replace speech	1. Lip reading 2. Zygo communication board
Stress due to *fear of death and mutilation* will be reduced by using	*Verbalization*, which will sensitize staff to fears that patients have, enable staff to legitimize fears, and permit catharsis	1. Talking to the staff 2. Group discussions with other patients
Stress due to a *lack of understanding* of medical jargon and procedures that can result in a *feeling of powerlessness* will be reduced by using	*Patient education*, which will explain medical jargon and procedures and enable patient to take an active role in the decision-making process and accept responsibility for his/her own care	1. Spinal cord handbook 2. Family conferences 3. Informal discussions with the OT
Stress due to the *inability to relieve tension* using familiar strategies will be reduced by using	*Stress management techniques*, which can replace tension-relieving strategies such as sex, exercise, eating, and recreation	1. Visualization 2. Progressive relaxation 3. Meditation
Stress due to *sensory deprivation* and *separation from a familiar routine* will be reduced by using	*Sensory stimulation*, which will reintroduce an orderly and familiar routine	1. Self-feeding 2. Adapted remote control for TV
Stress due *sleep deprivation* will be reduced by using	*Negotiation* will staff to modify the hospital routine	1. Lower lights at night 2. Schedule naps

for vital signs. No one truly sleeps well until they go home, but negotiations with staff to modify normal hospital routines can reduce the severity of sleep deprivation. A few suggestions include lowering lights at night, scheduling naps, and permitting self-pacing during early morning routines when poor arousal affects performance most.

While patients are most likely to be exposed to these stressors in acute care settings, many of these stressors continue to be present in later stages of treatment. While the inability to communicate and fear of imminent death may recede, all inpatient programs stress patients by using unfamiliar medical procedures, imposing some sensory deprivation (especially on weekends), and interfering with sleep and normal routines for relieving stress.

MINI-CASE STUDY

None of the clinical sites that provided case studies for this book formally collect MOHO data. The following case study comes from *The Model of Human Occupation* (3).

Creating Narrative Hypotheses

Sally is a 37-year-old woman with rheumatoid arthritis. She was recently referred to occupational therapy, but is 5 years postonset. A variety of medications have failed to put her arthritis into remission. Her current complaints are pain and swelling in her wrists, fingers, knees, ankles, and feet. She was a high school teacher for 1 year, but quit work to become a full-time housewife to raise her two sons, who are now teenagers.

Based on her poor response to medication, I wonder whether Sally perceives her locus of control as internal or external (hypothesis #1). What values prompted her to quit work when her children were young (#2)? How has the arthritis changed her interests and daily routine (#3)? What roles does she hope to pursue now that her children are almost grown (#3)? How supportive is her family and what do they expect of her (#4)? How will Sally respond to adaptive procedures and devices prescribed for joint protection (#5)? Has the arthritis impaired her sexuality (#6)? Is she depressed or angry (#7)? Is she experiencing stress and sleep deprivation due to pain (#7)?

Designing an Evaluation Package

A comprehensive evaluation of MOHO issues was planned. It consisted of an Occupational History, an informal interview about her values, an Interest Checklist, a Role Checklist, and an Activity Questionnaire, which asked questions about her daily activities over a 2-day period. Other psychosocial issues, such as sexuality and stress reactions, are usually explored through informal discussions once treatment begins.

It is essential to chunk the MOHO data, or your thoughts will wander from giving up bowling to her belief that she does housework well only 1% of the time. Chunking the results by evaluation tool is not helpful because some tests collect data about several MOHO concepts. You end up with information about a single concept scattered throughout your report. Chunking the data by MOHO concepts is more helpful.

Naming the MOHO concepts in your report is important. Other frames of reference imply the concept that was evaluated when data are reported. For example, when you read 65° in a biomechanical report, you know it refers to range of motion. The significance of personal information about a patient may not be self-evident to other team members. I have italicized the MOHO concepts in the results section to reinforce the discipline of chunking MOHO data by concepts.

Test Results. Sally has a decreased sense of personal causation. Her *locus of control* appears to be external. During the Occupational History, she reported that arthritis forced her to give up two cherished roles. She had planned to return to teaching once her sons were grown, but she is now thinking only vaguely about substitute teaching. After arthritis set in, she had to stop volunteering at her church. She had been running an education program for senior citizens. Now Sally is anxious to learn joint protection techniques to reduce pain and joint deformity. Perhaps this will give her a greater sense of internal control over her life in the future. Her *efficacy of skill* is unclear. When asked to rank her own skill for daily activities on the Activity Questionnaire, she said she did well 1% of the time, average 79% of the time, and poorly only 19% of the time. Yet, the OT reported "difficulty" during some self-care and homemaking tasks due to pain, loss of grip strength, and fatigue. She has a low *expectation of success*. She now seems apprehensive and uncertain about her future.

The interview revealed Sally's *occupational goals*. She values fulfilling the expectations of others very highly and places much less emphasis on personal satisfaction and self-development. This impression was supported by the Occupational History. She apparently became a homemaker out of a sense of obligation to her children. When asked how much her daily activities meant to others on the Activity Questionnaire, she said 56% meant a lot to others, 35% to some, and 8% to very few people or no one. The *meaning of current activities* is negative. The Occupational History revealed that her homemaker role does not satisfy her or appear important to her self-esteem. Her sense of competence as a homemaker is unclear (see belief in skill). Unfortunately, she had to give up volunteer work, which was very satisfying and important to her.

Sally has severely limited current *interests*. Out of 11 past strong interests, she has maintained only singing and mending since the onset of her arthritis. Past interests had both a physical and social component (e.g., bowling). Swimming is her only new interest, which she perceives as therapy. However, she wants to develop a wide variety of new interests in the future. When asked how well she enjoyed her daily activities on the Activity Questionnaire, she said 51% some, 24% very little or not at all, and 24% a lot. She expressed a desire to get more enjoyment out of her daily activities.

Sally reports that her current *roles* are: caregiver, home maintainer, friend, family member, and religious participant. In the future, she would like to add the role of volunteer. She did not list worker as a future role. The only data collected on her *habits* showed that she spends only 1% of her day resting.

Interpreting the Test Results

Generating a Cue Identification List

1. *What is locus of control?*
   Feels external locus of control for health
2. *What are her values?*
   Devalues personal satisfaction and development
   Values fulfilling expectations of others
3. *What are her interest/roles?*
   Limited current interests
   Wants to develop new interests
   Caregiver/teacher roles are not satisfying
   Unable to perform valued volunteer work
   Uncertain about future roles
   Wants to get more enjoyment out of daily routine
4. *What is family support?*
   No data
5. *Will she accept joint protection?*
   Wants to learn joint protection
   Only rests 1% of day while at home
6. *Is sexuality affected?*
   No data
7. *Are stress reactions present?*
   No data
N. *Efficacy of skill*
   OT reports "difficulty" in some self-care/home-care tasks due to pain, loss of grip strength, and fatigue
   By self-report, 79% of daily activities are done with "average" skill, while only 19% of daily activities are done "poorly"

Evaluating the Narrative Hypotheses. Hypotheses about her locus of control, what values prompted her to quit work, and her current interests, roles, and daily routine (hypotheses #1–3) were only partially answered.

We still don't know much about her personal standards, temporal orientation, her perception of role balance, potency of current interests, pattern of future interests, her family's expectations and level of support, and her acceptance of joint protection principles (hypotheses #2–5).

We still don't know whether arthritis has interfered with her sexuality (hypothesis #6) or whether she is experiencing stress related to pain, the inability to relieve tension using familiar strategies, or sleep deprivation (hypothesis #7). This psychosocial information that is ignored by MOHO usually comes out during informal conversations with the therapist during treatment sessions.

These gaps in the MOHO database are not unusual. The MOHO frame of reference requires a patient to reveal very personal information. It is common to have gaps in the initial database until the patient feels more comfortable with the therapist. Some of this psychosocial information may never be revealed. Only the patient can determine where the dividing line is between the invasion of privacy and the therapist's need to know.

Here is an example of how sharing personal feelings evolves gradually. It was unclear how much Sally valued teaching (hypothesis #3) from the initial evaluation. She did not list worker as a future role. In subsequent discussions during treatment sessions, Sally said that teaching had never been a strong career choice. She got into teaching because of family pressure and a lack of clear career choice. She now expresses a strong interest in health care and is exploring the career of medical technology.

New information about the efficacy of her skills is confusing. The OT describes her as having "difficulty" doing some ADLs, while she says she performs daily activities with average ability 79% of the time. More precise information about ADL skills is needed.

Deficits Not Addressed by the Biomechanical Frame of Reference. Rheumatoid arthritis is commonly treated with the biomechanical frame of reference. However, this approach ignores a significant number of pyschosocial issues that will affect functional outcomes. If Sally believes that control over her life is external, does not believe in her own skills, and expects to fail, therapy is not likely to succeed in changing her life. These are significant deficits if they continue. Another potential deficit is her family's expectations. If they are not supportive of her, Sally could have a very difficult time changing her life.

Her life-long goal of satisfying others is a noble value. However, she does not find her homemaker and teacher roles very satisfying. She is currently exploring medical technology as a new role. Perhaps this choice will balance the goals of self-development and satisfying the needs of others.

Sally's interests are currently severely curtailed. Interests represent the joy we feel in life, and Sally cannot

live without joy indefinitely. Fortunately, she realizes this, so her current dissatisfaction with life may change. New interests that are compatible with her arthritis must be found.

Her habit of resting only 1% of the day will definitely have to change. An important aspect of joint protection is scheduling regular rest breaks, even if a task is not completed. If she does not change her habit of minimal rest, her arthritis will continue to produce joint damage. Her flexibility when exposed to joint protection procedures and adaptive devices must be determined as these techniques are introduced in therapy.

SUMMARY

Psychosocial issues have been called the "underground practice" of therapists working in adult physical disability settings. Three approaches to talking about these issues have been accepted in these settings. They are the model of human occupation, sexual dysfunction, and stress reactions. Even these three approaches do not cover all psychosocial issues. Therapists frequently comment on a patient's frustration tolerance, cooperative attitude, or ability to socialize with staff and other patients (see Memory Aid 14.1).

There is no way to synthesize these three approaches. Therapists often use two or more simultaneously. Which approach you use may be a function of how well it is accepted by other team members. Any of these three approaches provides legitimate concepts for conveying psychosocial information in the subjective section of a progress note. Look for these issues in the database for every case simulation.

You are more likely to get reimbursement for remediation of psychosocial skills in physical disability settings if you link them to functional outcomes (14). For example, you could state that decreasing depression will decrease the number of refusals to perform independent self-dressing. If you show that functional changes occurred, it should be difficult for third-party payers to deny coverage.

STUDY QUESTIONS

1. Why are psychosocial issues an "underground practice" in physical disabilities?
2. How do personal causation, values, interests, roles, habits, culture, social groups, and objects affect treatment goals?
3. What is the MOHO hierarchy?
4. Name four general characteristics that define sexuality.
5. What does PLISSIT stand for?
6. What are the positive effects of stress reactions?
7. What stressors are especially prevalent in acute care?

References

1. Fleming MH. The therapist with the three track mind. Paper presented at the annual meeting of the American Occupational Therapy Association, Baltimore, 1989.
2. Rogers JC, Masagatani G. Clinical reasoning of occupational therapists during the initial assessment of physically disabled patients. Occupational Therapy and Journal of Research 1982;9:195.
3. Versluys HP. Psychosocial accommodation to physical disability. In: Trombly CA, ed. Occupational therapy for physical dysfunction. 3rd ed. Baltimore: Williams & Wilkins, 1989.
4. Kielhofner G. The model of human occupation. Baltimore: Williams & Wilkins, 1985.
5. Pedretti LW. Psychosocial aspects of physical dysfunction. In: Pedretti LW, Zoltan B, eds. Occupational therapy practice skills in physical dysfunction. 3rd ed. St. Louis: CV Mosby, 1990.
6. Gruson K. The long road. New York Times, June 25, 1985.
7. Kielhofner G, Henry AD. Development and investigation of the occupational performance history interview. Am J Occup Ther 1988;42:489.
8. Brayman SJ, et al. Comprehensive occupational therapy evaluation scale. Am J Occup Ther 1976;30:94.
9. Neistadt ME, Freda M. Choices: a guide to sexual counseling with physically disabled adults. Malabar, FL: Krieger Publishing.
10. Dahl MR. Human sexuality. In: Hopkins HL, Smith HD, eds. Willard and Spackman's occupational therapy. 7th ed. Philadelphia: JB Lippincott, 1988:354.
11. Dahl MR. Sexual dysfunction. Lecture presented at Temple University School of Occupational Therapy, 1989.
12. Neistadt ME. Stress management. In: Hopkins HL, Smith HD, eds. Willard and Spackman's occupational therapy. 7th ed. Philadelphia: JB Lippincott, 1988:321.
13. Brown EJ. Specialized OTs take pride in "handiwork." Advance for Occupational Therapists 1989;5:1.
14. Dahl M. Money and reimbursement of occupational therapy practice. Pennsylvania Occupational Therapy Association workshop, Philadelphia, 1990.

CHAPTER 15

Perceptual-Cognitive Issues

This chapter is designed to help you identify perceptual-cognitive deficits that are left unaddressed by the physically oriented frames of reference. Included is a taxonomy, which organizes the perceptual-cognitive concepts that are relevant to physical disabilities. This chapter also provides an overview of treatment and evaluation to make you aware of the current state of the art in this area.

Historical Perspectives

Occupational therapy's understanding of perceptual-cognitive issues was strongly influenced by Jean Ayres' theory of sensory integration and perceptual-motor theories by Frostig and Kephart, and others. These theorists worked with learning disabled children who had normal intelligence. This enabled these theorists to assume that cognition was intact and to focus on sensory and perceptual deficits. Therefore, when clinicians applied their theories to brain-damaged patients who had a combination of sensory, perceptual, and cognitive deficits, there was a blind spot. Cognitive skills, like memory and problem solving, were being ignored.

Incorrect conclusions about the performance of brain-damaged patients on perceptual tests are possible when perceptual skills are tested in isolation. For example, a patient may fail the form perception subtest of the Santa Clara Perceptual Motor Evaluation because he/she is distractible or has impaired memory for instructions.

The taxonomy used here corrects this blind spot by combining perceptual and cognitive skills into one continuum (see Memory Aid 15.1). It is an expansion of the continuum suggested by Abreu and Toglia, who in turn based their continuum on Luria's three brain blocks (1). Brain block #1, which involves damage to the brainstem, is listed in column I of Memory Aid 15.1. The brainstem regulates arousal. Brain block #2, which involves damage to the temporal, parietal, and occipital lobes, is listed in column II. These cortical areas analyze raw sensory input, organize it into recognizable entities, and store

the information. Brain block #3, which involves damage of the frontal lobe, is listed in column III. The frontal lobe plans, monitors, and corrects actions.

Current Treatment Approaches

This chapter reflects the current lack of continuity in treatment. It is a confusing time, which requires the ability to tolerate ambiguity and a willingness to experiment. Only time will show which approaches will survive our scrutiny. Currently accepted treatment approaches are listed below.

The Rancho Los Amigos Scale describes cognition and behavior following head injury or coma (2). These descriptions follow a hierarchical sequence that outlines stages of recovery. There are no standardized tasks to determine the patient's level of function. The team tries to pick the description that best fits each patient. The **Manzi and Weaver approach** used the Rancho scale to generate suggestions for intervention (3).

The **Allen approach** describes cognitive function at each of six levels (4). Level 1 patients are interested in automatic reactions, like swallowing food, that briefly get the patient's attention. Level 2 patients are interested in postural reactions that feel good, like riding a bicycle. Level 3 patients are interested in repetitive manual actions that enable them to perseverate on familiar manipulation of objects, like peeling potatoes. Level 4 patients are interested in goal-directed actions that enable them to replicate a sample project or demonstrated activity. Level 5 patients are interested in exploratory actions that enable them to use overt trial and error to explore new ideas. Level 6 patients are able to perform planned actions that require discovering new means through mental imagery.

Allen's activity analysis enables the student to identify the type of activities and amount of assistance used at these six levels (4). Her ordinal scale was initially developed on psychiatric patients, but is now being used to address cognitive issues in brain-injured patients. The

Memory Aid 15.1.
Perceptual-Cognitive Issues

I. Arousal/Attention/Confounding Variables	II. Visual Perception/Praxis/Memory	III. Higher Cognitive Processes
A. *Arousal/Orientation* 　1. No response to stimuli 　2. Generalized response 　3. Localized response 　　(Rancho levels I–III)	A. *Simple Visual Perception* 　1. Matches objects 　2. Matches shapes 　3. Matches color 　4. Matches line orientation	A. *Abstract thought* 　1. Classification 　2. Sequencing 　3. Conservation 　4. Abstract reasoning
B. *Attention* 　1. Agitated; fleeting attention only to large motions; needs physical prompts; uses only automatically used tools 　2. Inappropriate; attends to repetitive manual actions; needs visual prompts; learns simple ADLs; difficulty switching attention; uses only habitually used tools	B. *Complex Visual Perception* 　1. Recognizes what objects are used for 　2. Visual figure-ground discrimination 　3. Form constancy 　4. Spatial relations 　5. Topographical orientation	B. *Executive Functions @* 　1. Metacognition 　　a. Awareness of skill 　　b. Self-monitoring, like error detection, self-questioning 　2. Processing strategies 　　a. Nonsituational, like goal formation, prioritizing, initiating, time management 　　b. Situational, like verbal rehearsal, chunking, visual imagery, scanning 　3. Generalizing learning 　　a. Recognize relevance of previous experiences 　　b. Transfer: near to very far
C. *Rule Out CNS Impairment* 　1. Visual field deficits 　2. Visual neglect 　3. Unilateral neglect 　4. Aphasia % 　5. Auditory figure-ground discrimination	C. *Praxis** 　1. Body Scheme # 　2. Dressing apraxia 　3. Ideational praxis 　4. Ideomotor praxis 　　(imitates gestures/postures) 　5. Constructional apraxia	
D. *Ocular-Motor Control* 　1. Quick localization 　2. Convergence 　3. Visual acuity 　4. Ocular persistence 　5. Visual pursuits 　6. Saccades for reading	D. *Memory* 　1. Attend to immediate memory 　2. Encoding % (can't remember what you don't understand) 　3. Storage and retrieval for: short-term, long-term, prospective, declarative and procedural memory	*WHAT'S BEEN DE-EMPHASIZED?* # Proprioceptive, tactile, vestibular basis for praxis * Oral apraxia, dysarthria % Language @ Volition and habituation

Allen descriptions correspond to the Rancho levels when the number two is added to the Allen level (e.g., Allen level 4 = Rancho level VI). Her concrete suggestions are especially helpful to students who are treating a low-functioning patient who is dangerous to him/herself and others for the first time.

The **functional approach** assumes that recovery of perceptual and cognitive skills is not possible (5). This approach uses both adaptation and compensation. **Adaptation** ensures that the environment will be appropriately modified to substitute for lost function. **Compensation** teaches the patient to use adapted procedures, which substitute for the lost function and to use the modified environment. Teaching takes the form of drills for specific functional tasks in specific contexts. For example, a patient would be taught by rote to do a wheelchair transfer to the bathtub in exactly the same layout as his/her bathroom at home.

The **remedial approach** assumes that a perceptual or cognitive deficit can be reversed. There are no common suggestions for treatment because each regime is deficit-specific. Zoltan et al. call the remedial approach the **transfer of training approach** (5). This approach the assumes that specific skills, such as form constancy, can

be remediated by paper and pencil tasks and then transferred with no additional training to real-life situations.

The **information-processing approach** assumes that the brain functions as a whole rather than as separate specific skills (1). Information processing is defined as the ability to handle increasing amounts of information by using a variety of mental strategies that control the flow of input. Emphasis is placed not on the ability to perform specific skills, but on general cognitive strategies that can be used in many different situations. The therapist controls the amount of information that has to be processed at any one time by: (*a*) grading activity and (*b*) teaching cognitive strategies. The therapist grades activity by regulating the rate of response time provided, amount of stimuli present, the duration of the activity, type of sensory modality used, and complexity of the task. The patient develops cognitive strategies including planning ahead, controlling the speed of work, checking the work, and generating alternatives.

AROUSAL AND ORIENTATION

Numerous animal studies have confirmed that arousal is a function of the reticular formation. None of these research studies has suggested how to manipulate the reticular formation in brain-damaged patients. The only practical approach to remediating severe deficits in arousal is based on the Ranchos Los Amigos Scale. Manzi and Weaver don't cite a theoretical base for their treatment suggestions (3).

A patient at Rancho level I exhibits no observable response to sensory stimuli. The goal is to increase arousal enough to get a **generalized response** (3). This includes indiscriminate moaning, blinking, and mass movements after every stimulus (see Table 15.1). Treatment modalities are noxious stimuli such as loud noises and unpleasant odors.

A patient at Rancho level II exhibits a generalized response to stimuli. The goal is to increase arousal to achieve **localized responses** that have a logical connection to the kind of stimulus that is given (3). For example, a moving light should stimulate ocular tracking. Treatment modalities are familiar activities such as manipulating familiar objects, looking at photographs of familiar people, performing weight shifts within a posture such as rolling over in bed, listening to familiar music, and eating familiar food. All the sensory modalities should be used, BUT it is best to use only one modality at a time in a quiet, stark environment. You may need to wait from 1 to 2 *minutes* between administration of stimuli to see if you get a localized response because the reticular formation is still not functioning normally.

A patient at Rancho level III exhibits delayed and inconsistent localized responses. The goals are to increase the speed and consistency of localized responses and to improve orientation to time and place (3). Familiar stimuli are still used, but can now be combined. For example, you might have a patient look at familiar photographs while moving slightly side to side with Bobath handling techniques. Gross motor activities are believed to have a particularly strong organizing effect because proprioceptive and vestibular input quickly get the attention of the reticular formation. The speed and consistency of appropriate responses are also facilitated with simple purposeful activities like self-feeding with full physical assistance.

Purposeful activities also help to orient the level III patient (3). Suggestions for facilitating orientation to time and place include: (*a*) giving cues rather than information (tell the patient, "This is the first day of the week") ; and (*b*) concentrating on concrete times and places (e.g., time for lunch; layout of hospital room) before asking for more abstract orientation (e.g., current events).

At Rancho levels I through III, you need to be aware of signs of sensory overload (3). These include flushing, perspiration, prolonged increase in respiratory rate, and agitation. Eye-closing and a sudden decrease in attention can also signify a need to withdraw from overstimulation. Carefully document negative reactions as well as the increase in number of desired responses.

ATTENTION

The next step on the continuum is attention. Once arousal is sufficiently high, the brain can begin to focus more selectively. There are a number of theoretical models of attention (6). One model states that attention can be divided into automatic attention (e.g., driving a car while talking) and conscious attention (e.g., scanning a telephone book to find the Smiths). Another theory suggests that some sensory input can be suppressed at a peripheral gate so that higher centers do not need to attend to these stimuli. For example, one researcher found that the cochlear nucleus, which controls auditory input, showed decreased electrical activity when a cat was watching a mouse in a jar. This peripheral filter theory was studied repeatedly with conflicting results

TABLE 15.1.
Generalized to Localized Responses

Generalized Responses	Stimulus	Localized Responses
1. Responds inappropriately, e.g., always blinking, grimacing, or groaning regardless of type of stimulus.	Visual	Moving light → head moves in direction of light; eyes track light
	Auditory	Speech → looks at the speaker; tries to follow verbal commands
2. General responses to all types of stimuli like skin flushing, mass movements, agitation, or increased respiration.	Tactile	Various textures → pushes stimulus away; moves extremity away
	Kinesthetic	Move the patient → looks at body as it is moved; tries to reposition self; assists desired motion
	Gustatory	Food presented → swallows; moves lips; turns head toward food

(6). There is no comprehensive model of attention that predicts and explains all of the attentional deficits seen in the clinic. Nor do any of the theoretical models suggest how to treat brain-damaged patients.

Manzi and Weaver described treatment for low-functioning patients based on Rancho levels (3). A patient at Rancho level IV is confused and agitated. Responses to stimuli are frequently bizarre. Movement is nonpurposeful and part of an agitated state. Verbalization is often incoherent and inappropriate. Attention span is limited to 5 to 10 minutes. These behaviors can be frightening unless you understand their cause. This type of patient has a fully aroused reticular formation that is unable to regulate attention to outside events and internal confusion.

The goal with the Rancho level IV patient is to increase attention while decreasing agitation (3). Manzi and Weaver believe that gross motor activities that target a specific movement like ankle dorsiflexion may be too frustrating at this cognitive level. Physical goals must be secondary to cognitive goals during this stage of recovery. Overlearned movements like eating and ambulation may be used to calm the patient rather than to improve the quality of oral control or gait. They also recommend the use of inhibition techniques devised by Rood to calm the patient, like slow rocking. Treat the patient in a stark environment: feed the patient with just a dish and a spoon on the table. Use physical assistance in addition to verbal cues or demonstration. Provide frequent breaks and use environmental changes, like turning off the lights or leaving momentarily, to break up the agitation before it gets out of control.

Allen (4) provides additional suggestions for dealing with a Rancho level IV patient/Allen level 2 (see Table 15.2). A patient at this level attends only to "postural reactions," which are body-centered movements that "feel good" but have no real purpose. For example, these patients like to move to music and repetitively catch balls. The completion of a purposeful activity is irrelevant to the patient. Memories are disorganized, so the therapist can't use past preferences to guide selection of activities. The therapist is instructed to:

1. Focus on imitation of movements;
2. Use a stark environment with materials out of reach;
3. Provide no choices;
4. Limit activities to 5 to 15 minutes;
5. Restrict verbal commands to a noun plus a verb (e.g., "raise arms") in combination with a *physical* prompt;
6. Be ready to prevent damage to objects and people such as throwing a ball at a window; and
7. Use a few "automatically used tools."

Automatically used tools are defined as tools that require only brief attention to initiate the action followed by repetitive movements. Examples include a spoon and a glass.

All patients do not have such a disabling loss of attention (3). A Rancho level V patient is confused and inappropriate, but is able to focus his/her attention if prompted. This patient can respond to simple verbal commands fairly consistently. He can perform familiar ADLs with constant supervision. Complex tasks and lack of supervision results in inappropriate behavior. The goal is to increase attention and orientation while decreasing confusion. Manzi and Weaver suggest teaching functional activities one step at a time instead of trying to teach the whole activity at once: put on clothing one piece at a time. Limit demands on attention to what can be completed in one session. Limit environmental stimuli. For example, the patient will be less distracted if you hand clothes to him/her one piece at a time. Use one-step verbal commands with visual/tactile cuing. Practice orientation to person, place, and time at every session.

Allen (4) provides additional suggestions for the Rancho level V patient/Allen level 3 patient. This type of patient is interested in manual actions that enable the patient to perseverate on manipulation of familiar objects. This patient likes activities with one or two repetitive steps like bead-stringing and tile trivets with NO pattern to follow. Choices about materials are meaningless since completion of a project is irrelevant to a level 3 patient. It would be typical to see such a patient put a few beads each on several separate pieces of string (see Fig. 15.1). The patient ignores even clearly visible errors, like forgetting to leave space between tiles for the grout, unless the error physically interrupts the motor sequence, like running out of room for tiles on the trivet form. Current activities may trigger fragments of previous experiences, but the patient may perseverate on these memories even if they are not appropriate for the current task (see Fig. 15.2).

The therapist is instructed to:

1. Focus on repetitive manipulation of objects;
2. Hand supplies to the patient for only one step at a time;
3. Permit no choices about projects on materials;
4. Expect the patient to be on task only 30 out of 60 minutes;
5. Restrict verbal commands to three to four word phrases (e.g., "give me the shirt") in combination with *visual* demonstrations; and
6. Choose a few "habitually used tools."

Habitually used tools require prolonged attention to a changing task to monitor effective use. Examples include a pencil and hairbrush.

TABLE 15.2.
Guidelines for Attention Training

Rancho IV: Confused-Agitated

1. Limit movement activities to ones that calm patient
2. Take frequent breaks
3. Interrupt agitation with environmental/task changes
4. Use stark environment
5. Use physical prompt in addition to verbal/visual cues
6. Use Rood inhibition techniques

Rancho V: Confused-Inappropriate

1. Increase attention and decrease inappropriate behavior
2. Limit attention to one session
3. Limit environmental stimulation
4. Use one-step commands with visual/tactile cues
5. Teach functional activities like feeding and dressing
6. Orient patient to person, place, and time every treatment session

Allen 2: Postural Actions

1. Attends only to gross motor actions because they "feel good"
2. Attends maximum of 5–15 minutes
3. Completion of task is irrelevant
4. Use stark environment
5. Name body part and verb and pair them with physical prompt
6. Learn from others = imitate motion
7. Recall familiar tasks = incoherent
8. Tools use = "automatically used" tools can be used (e.g., spoon, glass)
9. Error detection = OT must prevent damage to objects and people
10. Choices given = none

Allen 3: Manual Actions

1. Attends only to repetitive manual actions (e.g., peeling potatoes)
2. Attends 30 out of 60 minutes
3. Completion of task = irrelevant
4. Stark environment: hand supplies to patient for only one step at a time
5. Use single command of three to four words paired with visual cuing
6. Familiar tasks trigger recall of memory fragments; perseverates
7. Learns from others = brief regard
8. Tool use = "habitually used" tools (e.g., pencil, comb) can be used but does better using hands
9. Ignores clearly visible errors unless they interrupt movement
10. Choices given = none

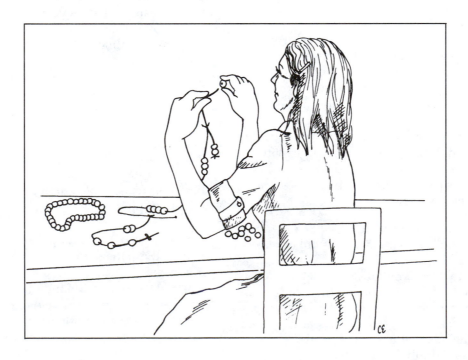

Figure 15.1. Allen Level 3: a repetitive action with a disregard for a goal.

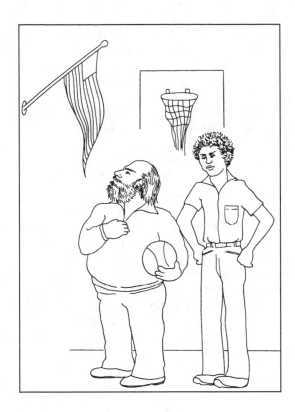

Figure 15.2. Allen Level 3: a chance awareness of a familiar object may elicit a familiar action.

Researchers have just begun to investigate the efficacy of attention training. For example, Sohlberg and Mateer used a system of 19 audiotapes and 13 visual stimulus sheets with visual distraction overlays to remediate attention in four patients with closed head injuries who were 1½ to 6½ years post-injury (7). All four patients had an attention deficit on the Paced Auditory Serial Addition Test (PASAT). Two subjects who had a mild to moderate attention deficit on the PASAT improved to within normal limits. Two subjects who had a severe attention deficit on the PASAT improved to a mild impairment. All four subjects maintained their gains for 8 months after treatment was stopped.

RULING OUT CENTRAL NERVOUS SYSTEM DEFICITS

A number of central nervous system (CNS) deficits can mimic inattention and perceptual deficits. Inappropriate interpretation of test results will occur unless you rule out these CNS deficits.

Visual field deficits are the result of damage to the visual pathways in the brain. Damage to different locations results in six types of visual field deficits. These deficits are described in Chapter 2 of Zoltan et al. (5). **Homonymous hemianopsia,** which is the most common

type, causes the patient to be blind to all visual stimuli on one side. It is very dangerous because patients forget that objects are present on that side. For example, one stroke patient was able to see the furniture in the hallway when the objects were on his intact side, but as soon as he turned around to walk in the opposite direction, he forgot that they were there and repeatedly walked into them. A student wearing hemianopsia glasses left one side of the wheelchair locked for an entire 3-hour lab. She couldn't figure out why the wheelchair was so hard to push until she took the glasses off. The most common treatment is the functional approach, which places as many objects on the uninvolved side as possible. Clinicians are also reporting that prism glasses prescribed by optometrists enable some patients to compensate for their visual field deficits.

Visual neglect is the inability to attend to visual stimuli on one side when there are competing visual stimuli on the other side. If no competing stimuli are present, the patient attends to visual input on the involved side. Treatment for visual neglect includes four strategies: anchoring, controlling density, pacing, and giving feedback. Make sure you are familiar with these strategies described in Chapter 2 of Zoltan et al. (5).

Unilateral neglect is the inability to attend to one side of the body. Neglect can be so severe that patients deny that the hemiplegic arm and leg belong to them or are completely unaware that the affected arm or leg are moving. This deficit can occur by itself or be compounded by loss of proprioceptive and tactile sensation, visual field deficits, or visual neglect. The transfer of training approach uses sensory stimulation of the affected side to regain awareness of it. This enables the patient with unilateral neglect to use the motor return on the affected side. The functional approach focuses on teaching: (*a*) compensatory strategies, like always looking at the affected side before moving it; and (*b*) adaptation of the environment, like placing the telephone on the unaffected side.

Aphasia is the inability to express oneself verbally (Broca's aphasia), to understand the spoken word (Wernicke's aphasia), or a combination of both (global aphasia). Aphasia is associated with left hemisphere damage. Treatment recommendations are usually made by the team's speech pathologist. A few common sense rules include: (*a*) don't shout, (*b*) allow enough time for a response, (*c*) assume patients can understand what you say when you talk about them, and (*d*) use visual demonstration.

Auditory figure-ground discrimination is the inability to distinguish foreground sounds from background noise. You use this skill at a party where loud conversations are taking place around you while you are trying to listen to the person in front of you. Elderly people often loose this skill, which makes it difficult for them to hear in noisy situations, like a clinic. Poor auditory figure-ground discrimination can mimic poor attention and confusion.

OCULAR-MOTOR DEFICITS

Before assessing visual perception, it is essential to rule out ocular-motor deficits that can cause poor visual processing. Ocular-motor skills are controlled by structures that are physically far apart in the brain. Damage in one location will not affect all ocular-motor skills. Therefore, you cannot sample one ocular skill, like convergence, and assume it is representative of all the other ocular-motor skills. Different ocular-motor deficits also have different effects on higher-level skills.

Quick localization is the ability to detect and locate objects in space. It is controlled by the superior colliculus (8). When the superior colliculus was bilaterally ablated in hamsters, they were able to discriminate between pebbles and sunflower seeds, as seen by persistent reaching towards the seeds (9). However, they were never able to identify the exact location of the seeds in order to pick them up. The effect of poor localization on higher visual skills needs to be studied in humans.

Convergence is the ability to turn both eyes inward to form a single image. It is controlled by nuclei in the Medial Longitudinal Fasciculus (8). Without proper convergence, patients have double vision and lack accurate depth perception, making visual tests difficult.

Visual acuity (accommodation) is the ability to bring objects into sharp focus using the intraocular eye muscles. These muscles are controlled by nuclei in the MLF (8). Visual acuity is needed by every patient who takes a paper and pencil test. Screening is essential to rule out cataracts, diabetic retinopathy, glaucoma, eye injury, and other deficits that affect visual acuity. If visual acuity remains uncorrected with glasses, all visual perception test results are suspect.

Next there is the issue of **ocular persistence** (5). This skill is also called visual attention and the visual fixation reflex. The occipital lobes tell the oculomotor nuclei to keep both eyes focused on an object for several seconds (10). Without this skill, it is difficult to gather sufficient information to perform higher-level discrimination. Perceptual and cognitive tests that rely on visual stimulus items could be adversely affected by poor ocular persistence, especially tests that briefly present a stimulus and then remove it.

Visual pursuits are the ability to smoothly track a moving object. This ability is controlled by areas 17, 18, and 19 in the occipital lobe (10). Whether visual pursuits are needed for good visual processing is unclear. Patients with nystagmus at rest have demonstrated the ability to read.

Finally, **saccades** are rapid, lateral step-like eye movements that change visual fixation points (10). Saccades enable us to automatically scan the environment (visual association area #18) and to read (motor association area #8).

Treatment of ocular-motor dysfunction was pioneered by pediatric optometrists. The efficacy of ocular-motor training is still contested. Zoltan et al. recommends the four strategies of anchoring, pacing, density, and feedback that are also used for visual neglect (5).

SIMPLE VISUAL PERCEPTION

Visual perception used to be treated as a single entity. Today it is divided into simple and complex processing skills. Toglia defined simple visual processing as the ability to recognize objects, color, and shapes without naming them and to make gross discrimination about size, position, and direction with little effort (11). Bernspång referred to simple visual processing as low-order perception (12). Low-order perception includes the ability to point to body parts and identify form, color, and shape. Bernspång found that only 10% of 109 hemiplegic patients had low-order perception deficits. Warrington and Taylor found that basic discrimination of single attributes such as length, contour, and brightness remain intact in many brain-damaged patients (13).

Simple visual perception is rarely impaired because massive damage to several redundant sites in the brain is required (14). The ability to match colors is mediated by areas V1, V2, and V4 in the visual cortex. However, color is also mediated by the lateral geniculate body, which has a high concentration of blood vessels, so it is often spared even when areas V1, V2, and V4 are damaged. Simple line orientation and shape recognition are mediated by area V1. This part of the primary visual cortex is relatively safe from outside blows because it is well tucked on the medial sides of the two occipital lobes that face each other. Simple line orientation and shape recognition are also mediated by areas V2–V4 in the visual cortex. Even when one patient had damage to areas V2–V4 from a stroke, he was able to use his spared V1 area to copy a picture of a church, although he could not name what he was drawing (14).

Many simple perceptual tests involve matching colors, lines in different spatial orientations, common objects, and simple geometric shapes such as circles and squares. Treatment has consisted of "teaching the test". Adult patients are drilled in matching tasks originally designed for preschoolers. Perhaps the low incidence of impaired simple visual perception has not created the need for more sophisticated remediation.

COMPLEX VISUAL PERCEPTION

Complex visual perception requires concentrated effort and skill to make subtle visual distinctions (11).

Bernspång referred to these complex skills as high-order perception. They include spatial relations, visual figure-ground, and object constancy (12). Factor analysis of test scores for brain-damaged patients showed that complex visual perception deficits clustered together (15). If a patient did poorly with spatial perception, he/she also did poorly with overlapping figures and object constancy.

Studies of brain metabolism during PET scans support the idea that simple visual discrimination tasks require just the primary visual cortex, while complex tasks recruit additional areas of the brain (16). Complex tasks activate the visual association areas in the occipital lobe and inferior temporal lobe where synthesis of visual impressions and formation of visual memories occur. Complex tasks also activate prefrontal areas where task organization, sampling strategies, and decision making occur.

Excellent definitions of complex visual perception skills are available in Zoltan's chapter on Spatial Relations Syndrome (5). It is especially important to learn the definitions for object identification (gnosia), visual figure-ground discrimination, object and form constancy, spatial relations, and topographical orientation. Object and form constancy skills are often misunderstood. This complex skill is different from matching identical objects and geometric shapes. Object and form constancy is a primitive form of categorization that enables you to recognize a particular shape or object regardless of its size, orientation in space, or background material.

The transfer of training approach, which remediates complex visual deficits, is discussed at length in Zoltan et al.'s text (5). For example, poor spatial relations may be remediated by copying pegboard or parquetry block designs. Preliminary efficacy studies show that visual spatial training for stroke patients can produce a significantly greater improvement than traditional ADL training alone for hygiene, dressing, bathing, and toileting, but not for feeding (17).

The functional approach also offers suggestions for complex visual perception. For example, visual figure-ground deficits can be compensated for by removing the visual clutter in the environment. This includes removing objects from the nightstand and organizing drawers and leaving space between the articles.

The information-processing approach generated treatment recommendations for improving complex object recognition (11). A 66-year-old business executive had no difficulty recognizing objects when they were presented one at a time or when he was told what object to look for and where to look for it. However, when the task was unstructured and he was asked to tell the therapist what objects were on his desk, he omitted and misidentified objects.

The therapist facilitated information processing by grading the activity of object recognition (11). The therapist gradually increased the difficulty level of: (a) the environment, starting with a familiar context like his desk; (b) familiarity of the objects; (c) directions given, from specific to general requests; (d) number of objects presented at one time; (e) spatial arrangement, such as linear vs. scattered and overlapping; and (f) response rate allowed per object. The patient was encouraged to develop cognitive strategies such as: scanning consistently from left to right; visual imagery of the object before searching for it; organizing his desk so that important items were always kept in specific locations; and self-monitoring such as looking again to double-check for errors.

PRAXIS

Apraxia is defined as the inability to perform complex movements on command even though habitual movements, like drinking from a glass, and simple movements, like repeatedly making a fist, can be performed spontaneously (16). Many authors break apraxia down into constructional, ideational, ideomotor, and dressing apraxia, but these different types of praxis are controversial. Some authors believe that ideational and ideomotor apraxia are different kinds of apraxia caused by damage to different brain centers, while others claim that they represent different levels of severity (16). Even constructional apraxia is not truly well defined. There is a wide variety of constructional tasks, such as copying block designs and drawing shapes, but there is a low correlation among these tests (16). These "constructional tests" are not measuring the same thing.

Researchers found that both left and right adult hemiplegics could have one or all of these "types" of apraxia simultaneously (18, 19). These researchers concluded that the relationship of one type of apraxia to another is uncertain and that the labels have not been useful. However, the literature still discusses all these types of apraxia, and clinicians continue to test them separately even though treatment has not developed sufficiently to provide a separate approach for each type of apraxia.

Praxis is not even well differentiated from complex visual perception. Both of these skills are controlled by the parietal and occipital lobes. Factor-analytic studies do not support the separation of these two skills. Katz found that an ideational praxis test (use of objects) clustered with complex visual perception tasks, such as object constancy and overlapping figures, in 96 adult patients with closed-head injury and stroke (15). Bernspång found that tests of constructional apraxia, such as copying geometric shapes, clustered with tests of complex visual perception, such as object constancy, in a study of 109 adult stroke patients (12).

The only treatment specific to apraxia is the **sensory integrative approach** of Jean Ayres (20). This approach assumes that organization of sensory input is necessary for producing purposeful, goal-directed responses to environmental challenges (20). Ayres emphasized the importance of somatosensation such as tactile, proprioceptive, and vestibular input as a foundation for visual and auditory processing. Ayres postulated that most somatosensory processing takes place at subcortical levels. The brainstem integrates somatosensory input in the thalamus and vestibular nuclei. The cerebellum also processes somatosensory information. When this subcortical integration is intact, the cortical areas are free to perform more abstract functions.

MEMORY

There are several theoretical models of memory. A well-accepted model divides memory into immediate, short-term, and long-term memory (21). **Immediate memories** are fleeting images that last for milliseconds. For example, when you ask someone to repeat what he just said, you may suddenly realize that you can retrieve what he said before he can repeat it. **Short-term memory** is the ability to remember information for several minutes. It is the ability to recall a small amount of information after a short period of time with total accuracy. For example, normal adults can remember a digit span of five to nine numbers. A typical short-term memory test is the ability to remember a therapist's name at the end of a conversation. Short-term memory is also called working memory because this is where knowledge is briefly stored while information is being manipulated. **Long-term memory** is your personal history and the facts you learned in the past.

Another theoretical model divides memory into declarative and procedural memory (21). **Declarative memory** is the ability to remember facts and specific events. Retrieval includes time-tagging, which is the ability to remember when something happened. **Procedural memory** is the ability to perform learned skills that the patient may not remember learning. For example, a world-famous musician does not remember getting his degree in music or conducting a world class symphony, but he can still read music, play the piano, and conduct a quartet (22). Sohlberg and Mateer call this "learning without awareness" (23). The problem with theoretical models is that no single theory predicts and explains all the combinations of memory loss seen in the clinic.

In the clinic, memory drills were used because of their good face validity (see Appendix). However, drills produced no significant gains in recall in brain-damaged adults (24). Therefore, memory training was believed to be ineffective.

The failure of recall drills produced a paradigm shift in memory training (24). Memory is now believed to require information processing, which includes: (a) attention, (b) encoding, (c) storage, and (d) retrieval (21). When people learn something, they must attend to it and try to give it meaning (encoding). Making the material meaningful can be achieved by looking for an organizing theme or relating it to previous experiences. How can you memorize something that was said in French if you don't understand French to begin with? Drills for recall assumed that attention and encoding were present in brain-damaged patients.

Sohlberg and Mateer (25) developed a three-prong approach to memory training that uses the information-processing approach. The three-prong approach includes:

1. Attention training;
2. Prospective memory training, which includes encoding; and
3. Retrieval using external memory aids.

This approach produced dramatic changes is three patients with closed head injury who were 15 to 36 months post-injury. Initially, only two of the three patients could remember to perform a task 30 seconds later. At the end of training, all three could remember to perform a task 15 minutes later (the 15-minute limit was dictated by practical time constraints on the staff). All three patients also showed improvement on the Randt Memory Test.

Another paradigm shift in memory training is the new focus on training for **prospective memory** (24). This is the ability to remember to do something in the future. Adult brain-injured patients have complained the most about this type of memory loss. This may be due to the severe consequences they experience for forgetting to show up for a therapy appointment or for work.

Sohlberg and Geyer divide prospective memory training into two stages (25). A "Single Task Paradigm" requires a patient to remember to do something in the immediate future with no distractions. The patient does nothing until the time for the event arrives. A "Multiple Task Paradigm" requires a patient to perform a distractor task until the time for the event arrives. Both stages are graded by: (a) the duration of the time delay, starting with as little as 15 seconds; and (b) the complexity of both the distractor and target tasks to be carried out (see Fig. 15.3). For example, a patient may be asked to remember to do Theraputty exercises after working on a puzzle for 3 minutes, with the Theraputty and clock clearly in view (25).

The treatment for retrieval has focused heavily on the use of external memory aids (24). **External memory aids** include memory notebooks, marking a calendar,

GOOD SAMARITAN HOSPITAL
CENTER FOR COGNITIVE REHABILITATION

Prospective Memory With Distraction*

*Distraction means another task was assigned simultaneously

Date	Duration of Time	Type of Task Remembered	Distractor Task	Correct Task Initiated	Task Initiated at Target Time	Comments

Figure 15.3.

using a timer on the oven, and making a list. **Internal memory aids** include pairing words or faces with visual images, verbal rehearsal of steps in a task, and memorizing the first letter in a chain of words (mnemonics). Internal aids are not used as often because they require abstract skills that brain-damaged patients may lack. External aids are more concrete and adaptable to a wide variety of real-life situations. Normal college students also report a much higher frequency of use for external memory aids than internal aids (26), so why not teach what normal people use?

It is still not easy to introduce external memory aids to brain-damaged adults. Sohlberg and Mateer divide the training for a memory notebook into three phases (24). The first phase is **Acquisition,** where the patient learns the name and purpose of each section of the memory notebook. Sections can include a memory log of what happened every hour, a calendar with scheduled events, a list of things to do, a transportation section on places and how to get there, autobiographical data, and a section of names and descriptions of familiar people (see Fig. 15.4). Patients learn what these sections are for by first watching the staff make entries for them. The second phase is **Application,** which involves learning when and where to use the memory notebook in role-playing situations. The third phase is **Adaptation,** which involves using the memory notebook in a variety of functional settings such as a sheltered workshop. Initially, staff accompany the patient to ensure adaptation to novel situations. Later, the patient uses the notebook independently in functional settings.

The use of a memory notebook can have profound functional consequences. For example, F.S. lived at home with 24-hour supervision before training with his memory notebook. After training, he was able to live alone with 1 hour of supervision in the early evening and work in a sheltered workshop (24).

Preliminary research shows that patients with memory loss perform best when procedural training closely resembles what the environment requires. Even small modifications, such as changing the type case, can reduce gains in procedural recall (21). Four patients with closed head injury who learned to use a computer to type simple sentences like "Elizabeth is here" were unable to independently type simple math equations like $8 + 2 = 10$ (27).

Finally, Sohlberg and Geyer emphasize the need for repetition in memory training (25). We may be bored, but the patient needs the repetition. For example, it took F.S. 17 program days to correctly identify all four sections of his memory notebook with 100% accuracy for 5 consecutive days (24). They also stress the importance of data collection for designing an individualized program. For example, it is important to document both the type of task to be remembered and the duration of time waited in each prospective memory training session. Patients can show progress in one area but not the other. Upgrading should be done only when the data show the patient's readiness.

EXECUTIVE FUNCTIONS

The concept of executive functions came out of clinical observation of patients with frontal lobe damage (28). This damage had little effect on highly structured cognitive tests such as intelligence tests. Yet, these patients exhibited a willingness to do nothing for extended periods of time and to do anything they were told. At first, this behavior was called "chronic social dependency." These patients also lacked self-regulation, such as a lack of concern about their appearance and childish or crude behavior. Occupational therapists have been aware of executive functions for a long time because of their activity orientation. Purposeful activity confronts the patient with an unstructured task in a highly distracting environment, which makes executive function deficits more obvious.

Memory Aid 15.1 shows that cognitive skills were traditionally identified as classification, sequencing, conservation, and abstract reasoning (15). The ability to classify a grocery list and sequence a laundry task are important cognitive skills for function in the community. These types of cognitive skills are still routinely tested. More recently, the concept of cognition has been broadened to include executive functions. Executive functions can be divided into three categories: metacognition, processing strategies, and the ability to generalize.

Metacognition is the ability to think about one's own thought processes. Metacognition is divided into the awareness of cognitive deficits and self-monitoring (29). Lack of awareness of cognitive deficits is one of the major stumbling blocks to cognitive rehabilitation in brain-injured patients. Brain-damaged individuals also lack self-monitoring strategies. These strategies include self-questioning, self-evaluation, self-estimation, and role reversal (29). Self-questioning is an internal dialogue carried on during an activity. Self-evaluation is the ability to accurately assess one's own performance after a task is completed. Self-estimation is the ability to predict the task difficulty, time, and amount of assistance needed, and degree of personal success before a task begins. Role reversal is the ability to identify and explain the errors made by someone else, usually the therapist.

Processing strategies include situational and nonsituational strategies that we use to solve problems (29). **Situational strategies** work best in specific situations. For example, visual scanning works best when stimuli

Examples: Date:																			
1. What is the memory log for?																			
2. When do you write in the memory log?																			
3. Where do you write your schedule?																			
4. Where do you write down errands?																			
5. What do you do when you complete an errand?																			
6. How many times should you write in the evening?																			
7. Where do you find information about appointments?																			
8. Where do you find information about your accident?																			
9. How often do you write on the weekends?																			
10. Where do you write down information about a new attendant?																			
Total % correct																			

Figure 15.4. Good Samaritan Hospital Center for Cognitive Rehabilitation Prospective Memory Notebook: Sample Form

are organized horizontally, and verbal rehearsal works best when there are few items to remember. Other examples of situational strategies include chunking and visual imagery.

On the other hand, **nonsituational strategies** are used across a wide range of situations. Toglia said that nonsituational strategies include planning ahead, prioritizing, time-management, and self-monitoring (28). Lezak called them goal formation, initiation, effectively carrying out activities, switching, and error detection (28). Zoltan et al. called them initiation, planning and organizing, mental flexibility, and problem solving (5). Obviously, consensus about what to call these nonsituational strategies does not yet exist. Notice also that self-monitoring and error detection appear under both metacognition and processing strategies. This overlap is typical of the current discussion on executive functions.

The third executive function is the **ability to generalize**. This involves the ability to recognize the relevance of a current activity to previous experience and to transfer previously learned skills to a wide variety of tasks and situations that are increasingly different from the original (29). The ability to generalize can be graded from "near transfer," where the task and environment are almost identical to the original, to "very far transfer," where strategies are applied to a task and environment that are completely different (29).

Two treatment approaches for executive functions are currently in the occupational therapy literature. Allen's approach to executive function deficits uses activity analysis, which looks at what the environment can provide to structure cognitively impaired patients (4). Allen offers practical suggestions to help patients makes choices, organize materials, detect errors, complete tasks, and work with other people. Note that Allen levels 4 and 5 correspond to the Rancho levels VI and VII (see Table 15.3). Toglia recommends information processing from a multicontext approach that includes metacognition, situational and nonsituational strategies, and the ability to generalize from near to very far transfer (29).

TABLE 15.3.
Guidelines for Executive Function Training

Rancho VI: Confused-Appropriate

1. Shows goal-directed behavior
2. Attention span = 30 minutes
3. Shows carryover for relearned tasks (e.g., self-care)
4. Needs cuing
5. Follows simple directions
6. Vaguely recognizes some of staff
7. Increased awareness of own needs
8. Selective attention may be impaired
9. Maximum assistance needed for learning new tasks with little carryover

Allen 4: Goal-Centered Actions

1. Focuses on goal-centered actions
2. Attends 45 out of 60 minutes
3. Completes task in one to two sessions
4. Can get supplies if previously oriented to storage area
5. One-step commands in simple sentences with visual cuing
6. Can learn in a parallel group
7. Socially inappropriate in a group
8. Recognizes and corrects errors only if required action is clearly visible
9. Tool use = a few unfamiliar *hand* tools
10. Choices given = can change one striking feature such as color

Rancho VII: Automatic-Appropriate

1. Lacks realistic planning for future
2. Goes through daily routine automatically
3. Shows carryover of new learning
4. Requires at least minimum supervision to learn new tasks
5. Decreased awareness of others
6. Decreased judgment and problem solving
7. Requires supervision for safety purposes
8. Requires structure to initiate social/recreational activities

Allen 5: Exploratory Actions

1. Uses trial and error for problem solving
2. Attention = well oriented
3. Completion of task = can extend project over two to five sessions
4. Can get supplies from unfamiliar storage area with supervision
5. Can follow several verbal commands IF they are related (e.g., "get book and open it")
6. Can learn in an associative group
7. Rigid approach to social protocol
8. Recognizes clearly visible errors BUT makes them anyway because of impulsivity
9. Tool use = impulsivity and poor judgment make power tools unsafe
10. Choices given = can make several decisions about supplies and patterns

Research is needed to determine which approaches work best or whether combining approaches might be helpful.

WHAT'S BEEN DE-EMPHASIZED?

Unfortunately, even this complex taxonomy has several blind spots. First, the proprioceptive, vestibular, and tactile foundations of praxis are often ignored by neuropsychologists. Even Zoltan et al. discusses somatosensory deficits such as poor body scheme in a chapter separate from praxis. This omission can be corrected by using the sensory integrative frame of reference. Second, oral apraxia and dysarthria are usually divorced from the discussion of apraxia. These deficits are addressed separately in the pediatric literature. Third, the entire area of language is mentioned in passing in the form of aphasia in the CNS impairment section and as encoding in the memory section. Skills such as encoding are important because patients can't remember what they don't understand. These passing references oversimplify a vast and complex topic. Finally, deficits in executive function, like lack of initiation and error detection, are usually discussed outside the context of emotional, social, and cultural influences. However, what patients value and what their culture expects of them can influ-

ence whether a patient chooses to perform a task and how well he/she decides to execute it.

EVALUATION OVERVIEW

Screening

Screening is the first step in evaluation. Patients who should have obvious perceptual-cognitive deficits don't need to be screened, such as people with traumatic brain injury. However, these deficits can appear unexpectedly in patients with congestive heart failure, high blood pressure, diabetes, and many other diagnoses. Kiernan (30) described a patient who exhibited delusions and hallucinations 3 days before he became febrile and developed seizures due to viral encephalitis. A screening test called the Neurobehavioral Cognitive Status Examination (NCSE) provided early diagnosis of the neurological cause of this patient's psychotic symptoms.

The NCSE is a standardized test that can be administered at bedside in 10 to 20 minutes (30). It briefly samples attention, language, visual constructions, memory, calculations, and abstract reasoning. Inter-rater reliability data are not available, but construct validity is present, as seen by the test's ability to discriminate between subjects who are already known to be normal or abnor-

Table 15.4.
Comprehensive Occupational Therapy Evaluation Scale (COTE): Part III. Task Beahvior

A. ENGAGEMENT
  0—Needs no encouragement to being task.
  1—Encourage once to begin activity.
  2—Encourage 2 or 3 times to engage in activity.
  3—Engages in activity only after much encouragement.
  4—Does not engage in activity.

B. CONCENTRATION
  0—No difficulty concentrating during full session.
  1—Off task less than one-fourth time.
  2—Off task half the time.
  3—Off task three-fourths time.
  4—Loses concentration on task in less than 1 minute.

C. COORDINATION
  0—No problems with coordination.
  1—Occasionally has trouble with fine detail, manipulating tools or materials.
  2—Occasional trouble manipulating tools and materials but has frequent trouble with fine detail.
  3—Some difficulty in gross movement-unable to manipulate some tools and materials.
  4—Great difficulty in movement (gross motor); virtually unable to manipulate tools and materials (fine motor).

D. FOLLOW DIRECTIONS
  0—Carries out of directions without problems.
  1—Occasional trouble with more than 3 step directions.
  2—Carries out simple directions—has trouble with 2.
  3—Can carry out only very simple one step directions (demonstrated, written, or oral).
  4—Unable to carry out any directions.

*E. ACTIVITY NEATNESS
  0—Activity neatly done.
  1—Occasionally ignores fine detail.
  2—Often ignores fine detail and materials are scattered.
  3—Ignores fine detail and work habits disturbing to those around.
  4—Unaware of fine detail, so sloppy that therapist has to intervene.

*F. ATTENTION TO DETAIL
  0—Pays attention to detail apropriately.
  1—Occasionally too concise.
  2—More attention to several details than is required.
  3—So concise that project will take twice as long as expected.
  4—So concerned that project will never get finished.

G. PROBLEM SOLVING
  0—Solves problems without assistance.
  1—Solves problems after assistance given once.
  2—Can solve only after repeated instructions.
  3.—Recognizes a problem but cannot solve it.
  4.—Unable to recognize or solve a problem.

H. COMPLEXITY AND ORGANIZATION OF TASK
  0—Organizes and performs all tasks given.
  1—Occasionally has trouble with organization of complex activities that should be able to do.
  2—Can organize simple but not complex activities.
  3—Can do only very simple activities with organization imposed by therapists.
  4—Unable to organize or carry out an activity when all tools, materials, and directions are available.

I. INITIAL LEARNING
  0—Learns a new activity quickly and without difficulty.
  1—Occasionally has difficulty learning a complex activity.
  2—Has frequent difficulty learning a complex activity, but can learn a simple activity.
  3—Unable to learn complex activities; occasional difficulty learning simle activities.
  4—Unable to learn a new activity.

J. INTEREST IN ACTIVITIES
  0—Interested in a variety of activities.
  1—Occasionally not interested in new activity.
  2—Shows occasional interest in a part of an activity.
  3—Engages in activities but shows no interest.
  4—Does not participate.

K. INTEREST IN ACCOMPLISHMENT
  0—Interested in finishing activities.
  1—Occasional lack of interest or pleasure in finishing a long term activity.
  2—Interest or pleasure in accomplishment of a short term activity—lack of interest in a long term activity.
  3—Only occasional interest in finishing any activity.
  4—No interest or pleasure in finishing an activity.

L. DECISION MAKING
  0—Makes own decisions.
  1—Makes decisions but occasionally seeks therapist approval.
  2—Makes decisions but often seeks therapist approval.
  3—Makes decision when given only 2 choices.
  4—Cannot make any decisions or refuses to make a decision.

M. FRUSTRATION TOLERANCE
  0—Handles all tasks without becoming overly frustrated.
  1—Occasionally becomes frustrated with more complex tasks; can handle simple tasks.
  2—Often becomes frustrated with more complex tasks but is able to handle simple tasks.
  3—Often becomes frustrated with any tasks but attempts to continue.
  4—Becomes so frustrated with simple tasks that she refuses or is unable to function.

*Rate either Activity Neatness or Attention to Detail, *not both.*

mal (see Appendix). The NCSE has fewer false-negatives (deficits that go undetected) than other well-known screening tests such as the Mini-Mental State Examination. The NCSE is normed for ages 20 through 92. The NCSE cut-off scores take into account the normal decline of cognitive skills in the healthy aging population. This helps separate the effects of aging from the effects of

brain damage on test scores of geriatric patients. The NCSE results in a profile of strengths and weakness that enables you to choose specific deficit areas for further testing.

The Comprehensive Occupational Therapy Evaluation Scale (COTE) is also a quick way to screen for perceptual-cognitive deficits (31). See Table 15.4 for the

Task Behavior Scale. Be aware, however, that psychosocial deficits can produce some of these same behaviors. For example, depression can present as a need for encouragement to begin an activity and a lack of interest in new activities. Psychosocial issues must be ruled out when using the COTE as an indicator for perceptual-cognitive testing.

Comprehensive Testing

Comprehensive testing is the second stage of evaluation. For years, tests for adults could only be administered by psychologists or psychiatrists. Today, many tests can be administered by therapists. Abrue (32) recommends that therapists use a battery of standardized tests, like the Modified Stroop Test and the Cancellation Test. This battery requires 5 to 10 hours to administer. Its length is not practical in some settings and may duplicate testing done by other team members.

More recently, therapists have developed their own tests. The Santa Clara Perceptual Motor Evaluation was designed for therapists to evaluate visual perception and motor planning in adult patients (33). It ignores cognitive issues like attention, memory, and executive functions. However, the Santa Clara is the only test routinely used by occupational therapists that evaluates ocular-motor skills in adults. Inter-rater reliability coefficients range from .61, which is unacceptable in the clinic, to 1.0, which is ideal (see Appendix).

A practical comprehensive test that was standardized on adults has become available. It is called the Lowenstein Occupational Therapy Assessment (LOTCA). This battery samples attention and evaluates orientation, visual perception, visuomotor organization, and thinking operations (34). It does not test memory. It can be administered to patients with aphasia and does not require any writing. It takes 30 to 45 minutes to administer and results in a profile of strengths and weaknesses that enable the therapist to pinpoint specific areas for specialty testing. Inter-rater reliability coefficients range from .82 to .97, which is acceptable to excellent for the clinic (see Appendix). Construct validity was confirmed by the test's ability to differentiate between normal and abnormal subjects at the .0001 level of significance.

The final stage of testing is specialty testing. This complex topic is beyond the scope of this chapter. Table 15.5 is a partial list of the specialty tests on the market.

Functional Assessments

All of the comprehensive tests just described evaluate underlying deficits that cause dysfunction. They enable

TABLE 15.5.
Specialty Tests for Perceptual-Cognitive Skills

Arousal: Glascow Coma Scale

Attention
 Paced Auditory Serial Attention Test (PASAT)
 Digit Repetition Test
 Symbol Digit Modalities Test
 Modified Stroop Test
 Modified Trail-Making Test
 Cancellation Test

Orientation
 Galveston Orientation and Amnesia Test
 Benton Temporal Orientation Test

CNS Impairment
 Visual field deficits: Confrontation Test
 Visual neglect: Confrontation Test with simultaneous stimuli
 Unilateral neglect: Cancellation Test
  Draw a Man, clock, tree, and house

Ocular-Motor Deficits: subtest of the Santa Clara Perceptual Motor Evaluation

Complex Visual Perception
 Santa Clara Perceptual Motor Evaluation
 Motor-Free Visual Perception Test
 Subtests of the Lowenstein Occupational Therapy Cognitive Assessment (LOTCA)

Praxis
 Bender Visual Motor Gestalt Test
 Beery Butenica Test of Visual Motor Integration
 Subtests of Santa Clara Perceptual Motor Evaluation

Somatognosia
 Finger Identification
 Right-Left Discrimination
 Localization of Tactile Stimuli
 Kinesthetic Memory

Memory
 Rivermead Behavioral Memory Test
 Weschler Memory Scale
 Benton Visual Retention Test
 Randt Memory Test

Executive Functions
 Lezak's Tinkertoy Test

the therapist to design an individually prescribed remedial program. Yet, they cannot predict how the patient will function in the community. There are numerous functional assessments on the market, but they focus on the amount of physical assistance that is needed. This is a serious omission for students, who must then use intuition to predict how perceptual-cognitive deficits will affect functional outcomes and discharge recommendations. You will be asked if your patient can be left home alone or if he/she has to be institutionalized because of perceptual-cognitive deficits.

One method for assessing the impact of perceptual-cognitive deficits on functional outcomes is to use clinical observation during functional activities. The prob-

---

TABLE 15.6.
Sample of Routine Task Inventory

C. Bathing
  5. Bathes without assistance, using shampoo, deodorant, and other desirable toiletries.
  4. Bathes the front of the body.
      May not bathe the back of the body, or
      May not rinse shampoo from the back of the hair, or
      May not remember to use deodorant, or
      May not obtain a safe water temperature.
  3. Uses soap and washcloth in a repetitive action.
      May not bathe entire body unless given verbal or tactile direction, or
      May refuse to soap the entire body.
  2. Stands in the shower or sits in the bathtub.
      May not try to wash self, or
      May move body parts to assist the caregiver, or
      May resist the caregiver's help, or
      May refuse to enter the shower or bathtub.
  1. Does not try to wash self and is given a sponge bath by another person.
      May move body position on command.

D. Walking
  5. Goes about new grounds or city and finds way home.
  4. Walks in familiar surroundings without getting lost.
      May require an escort in unfamiliar surroundings, or
      May refuse to go to unfamiliar places.
  3. Initiates walking within a room to do a familiar activity.
      May get lost unless escorted from room to room, or
      May follow the lead of other people to the correct or incorrect location, or
      May pace or wander about and manipulate physical objects that happen to capture attention.
  2. Follows the lead or pointed direction of others.
      May not initiate movement to do a familiar activity such as going to the dinner table, or
      May pace or wander about aimlessly without regard for objects unless they obstruct his or her path, or
      May resist the guidance of others.
  1. Walks or transfers from bed to chair with physical guidance.
      May be bedridden, or
      May remain in a supportive chair, or
      May not notice objects that obstruct his or her path, or
      May require tactile assistance to bend knees.

---

lem with this method is that patients often have several deficits (35). Complex, multiple-domain tasks, like self-care, make it difficult to determine which deficits are present during a specific task. For example, it is difficult to determine whether dependence in dressing is due to an attention, perceptual, memory, or executive function problem or some combination of these problems.

Árnadóttir increased the reliability of identifying perceptual-cognitive deficits during functional activities.

The Árnadóttir Occupational Therapy Neurobehavioral Evaluation (A-ONE) provides a list of specific behaviors that the therapist chooses from to identify specific perceptual-cognitive deficits (17). For example, her Specific Symptom Subscale tells the therapist that poor spatial relations may be exhibited by the inability to find the correct armhole of a shirt or by overreaching for faucet handles. This descriptive approach reduces the need for individual judgment. Inter-rater agreement is at the .84 level, which is acceptable in the clinic (see Appendix).

The Routine Task Inventory (RTI) also uses a descriptive approach. The RTI describes cognitive errors that are made at six different levels on the Physical and Instrumental daily living scales (4). Descriptions of cognitive errors include forgetting to wash the back of the body, burning food, and having trouble finding infrequently used telephone numbers in an address book (see Table 15.6). The RTI was originally designed for use with psychiatric patients, but is currently being validated with adults with strokes and head injuries. Reliability for patient report was low. When the tasks were observed by a therapist, the RTI inter-rater reliability coefficient was .98 and the test-retest reliability coefficient was .91 (36).

The Expanded Routine Task Inventory (ERTI) is now available. The RTI describes cognitive errors that are made at six different levels on four scales (37). The **physical scale** includes grooming, dressing, bathing, walking, exercising, feeding, toileting, taking medication, and using adaptive equipment. The **community scale** includes housekeeping, preparing food, spending money, doing laundry, traveling, shopping, telephoning, and child care. The **communication scale** includes listening, talking, reading, and writing. The **work scale** includes following directions, performing simple to complex tasks, maintaining pace/schedule, getting along with co-workers, avoiding accidents, and supervising/planning work (see Table 15.7).

SUMMARY

The occupational therapist's understanding of attention, perception, and cognition must synthesize all these prerequisite skills into a cohesive treatment model. Even though this subject is still evolving, a taxonomy was presented that puts them together on a continuum based on Luria's three brain blocks.

Many theoretical models of attention, perception, and cognition are available, but they do not explain and predict many of the problems seen by clinicians. This chapter has provided an overview of clinical models of treatment, but the lack of continuity in today's knowledge base is evident. To help you compare the clinical

TABLE 15.7.

Expanded Routine Task Inventory: Work Scale

Maintaining Pace/Schedule

3. Unable to alter pace or follow a schedule.

4. Works at less than 75% of normal pace and inflexibly follows a set schedule:
> May not alter pace in response to prompting to hurry up or slow down, or
> May not recognize need to change pace, or
> Once a schedule is learned, may resist any changes, or
> May require a schedule established by others, or
> May need to follow schedule for several months before it is learned, or
> May require external allowances for reduced pace and productivity, or
> May become bored or frustrated and quit.

5. Works at a reduced or normal pace within an established schedule:
> May not anticipate need to adjust pace, or
> May need to be told when an adjustment in pace or schedule is required, or
> May have a high frequence of tardiness, or
> May not return from breaks on time.

6. Sets own pace and plans own schedule, considering relevant factors, other perspectives, priorities, and time constraints.

Planning Work/Supervising Others

3. Unable to plan work or supervise others.

4. Establishes personal goals and gives orders, but:
> May not establish personal goals relevant to the work situation, or
> May not distinguish between personal goals and job requirements of subordinates, or
> May give orders to authorities/co-workers who don't report to him/her, or
> May demand immediate and unquestioning compliance with orders that seem unreasonable to co-workers, or
> May avoid planning and supervising activities.

5. Plans inductively and negotiates with trial and error with subordinates, so:
> May not analyze, evaluate, or synthesize data objectively, or
> May not recognize significant details or may overvalue selected information based on personal prejudices, or
> May not be able to influence subordinates through negotiation, explanation, or persuasion, or
> May not be able to anticipate changes in work conditions, or
> May attack or ignore subordinates who offer evaluation or criticism.

6. Plans objectively via inductive and deductive reasoning and influences subordinates and is influenced by subordinates.

Table 15.8.

Summary of Clinical Treatment Approaches

Arousal

1. Generalized vs. localized responses (Manzi and Weaver)
2. Neurodevelopmental treatment to increase arousal (Bobath)
3. Facilitation techniques (Rood)

Attention

1. Attention training based on Rancho levels IV/V (Manzi and Weaver)
2. Inhibition techniques to reduce agitation (Rood)
3. Allen's activity analysis for gross motor-centered vs. manual action-centered patient (Allen levels 2 and 3)
4. Attention-training tapes/visual distraction overlays (Sohlberg and Mateer)

CNS Impairment

1. Visual field deficits: optometry consultation for lenses
2. Visual neglect: anchoring, density, pacing, feedback (Zoltan)
3. Unilateral neglect: transfer of training/functional approach (Zoltan)
4. Auditory: Speech Pathology consultation

Ocular-Motor Deficits: Optometry consultation for training programs

Simple Visual Perception: Treatment usually not needed

Complex Visual Perception

1. Transfer of training/functional approach (Zoltan)
2. Information processing approach (Toglia)

Praxis/Body Scheme: Sensory integration approach (Ayres)

Memory

1. Attention; see above
2. Encoding: make sure individual understands what he/she is trying to memorize (Sohlberg and Mateer)
3. Storage: Prospective memory training using single and multiple paradigms (Sohlberg and Mateer)
4. Retrieval: use of external memory aids (Sohlberg and Mateer)

Executive Functions

1. Information processing with a multicontext approach (Toglia)
   a. Metacognition: awareness of deficits and self-monitoring strategies
   b. Processing strategies: Situational and nonsituational
   c. Generalize learning to a wide variety of tasks and environments
2. Activity analysis for goal-centered vs. exploratory-centered patients (Allen levels 4 and 5)

---

models, review Table 15.8. This table oversimplifies the application of these approaches. For example, the information-processing approach is probably applicable to more concerns than those I have described, but there is not much in print about this new approach. The table shows that no one approach is effective at every stage on the continuum. Research may eventually show that multiple approaches may have to be used.

Assessment must cover both prerequisite skills, such as complex visual perception, and functional abilities. Therapists now have reliable perceptual and cognitive tests of reasonable length and reliability. Consultation with other team members is still needed to rule out CNS, ocular-motor, and language deficits that mimic poor attention and visual perception. Functional assessments are emerging to augment therapists' intuition for predicting how perceptual-cognitive deficits will affect performance after discharge.

STUDY QUESTIONS

1. What important skills were ignored by the early perceptual-motor theorists?
2. Identify the two methods used in the functional approach.
3. What is the difference between a generalized response to stimuli and localized response to stimuli?

4. What are the weaknesses of the theoretical attention models?

5. What is the difference between "automatically used tools" and "habitually used tools"? Give an example of each.

6. What is the difference between visual and unilateral neglect?

7. Why is it so important to rule out ocular-motor deficits before proceeding with perceptual and cognitive testing?

8. What is the difference between simple and complex visual perception?

9. What is the controversy surrounding apraxia?

10. What are the weaknesses of the theoretical models of memory?

11. What are declarative, procedural, and prospective memory?

12. What is the major paradigm shift in memory training today?

13. What is the "three-prong approach" to memory training?

14. What are the three phases for training a patient to use a memory notebook?

15. Executive functions can be divided into what three categories?

16. What is the difference between situational and non-situational processing strategies?

17. What four domains of concern are missing from the taxonomy used in this chapter?

18. When should you screen for perceptual-cognitive deficits?

19. Name two screening tests for perceptual-cognitive deficits.

20. Why are functional assessments of perceptual-cognitive skills necessary?

21. Name two functional tests of perceptual-cognitive skills.

References

1. Abreu BC, Toglia JP. Cognitive rehabilitation: a model for occupational therapy. Am J Occup Ther 1987;41:439.

2. Malkmus D, Booth BJ, Kodimer C. Rehabilitation of the head injured adult: comprehensive cognitive management. Professional Staff Association of Ranchos Los Amigos Hospital, Los Angeles, 1980.

3. Manzi DB, Weaver PA. Head injury: the acute care phase. Thorofare, NJ: Slack Incorporated, 1987.

4. Allen CK. Occupational therapy for psychiatric diseases. Boston: Little, Brown & Company, 1985.

5. Zoltan B, Siev E, Freishtat B. Perceptual and cognitive dysfunction in the adult stroke patient. Thorofare, NJ: Slack Incorporated, 1986.

6. Yingling C. Neuropsychology of attention. Paper presented at the Neuropsychology of Memory, Attention, and Judgment workshop. California Neuropsychology Services, Philadelphia, 1988.

7. Sohlberg MM, Mateer CA. Effectiveness of an attention-training program. J Clin Exp Neuropsychol 1987;9:117.

8. Carpenter MB. Human neuroanatomy, 7th ed. Baltimore: Williams & Wilkins, 1976.

9. Stockmeyer S. Foundations of motor control. Graduate course taught at Boston University, Boston, 1978.

10. Gilman S, Newman SW. Manter and Gantz's essentials of clinical neuroanatomy and neurophysiology. 7th ed. Philadelphia: F.A. Davis, 1987.

11. Toglia JP. Visual perception of objects: an approach to assessment and intervention. Am J Occup Ther 1989;43:587.

12. Bernspång B, Viitanen M, Eriksson S. Impairments of perceptual and motor functions: their influence on self-care ability 4 to 6 years after a stroke. Occupational Therapy and Journal of Research 1989;9:27.

13. Warrington E, Taylor M. Visual apperceptive agnosia: a clinico-anatomical study of three cases. Cortex 1988;24:13.

14. Zeki S. The visual image in mind and brain. Sci Am 1992;9:69.

15. Katz N, et al. Loewenstein Occupational Therapy Cognitive Assessment (LOTCA) Battery for brain-injured patients: reliability and validity. Am J Occup Ther 1989;43:184.

16. Árnadóttir G. The brain and behavior—assessing cortical dysfunction through activities of daily living. St. Louis: CV Mosby, 1990.

17. Carter LT, et al. Relationship of cognitive skill performance to activities of daily living in stroke patients. Am J Occup Ther 1988;42:449.

18. Geschwind N. Disconnection syndromes in animals and man. In: Boston Studies of the Philosophy of Science, vol. 16. Reidel, Boston, 1974:189.

19. Hécaen H. Human neuropsychology. New York: John Wiley & Sons, 1978:100.

20. Clark F: Ayres. Sensory integration. In: Clark PN, Allen AS, eds. Occupational therapy for children. St. Louis: CV Mosby, 1985:42.

21. Squire LR. Memory and brain. New York: Oxford University Press, 1987.

22. Hemingway J. The search for mind. Television series produced by WNET, New York, 1988.

23. Sohlberg MM, Mateer CA. Rehabilitation of memory deficits. Paper presented at the Neuropsychology of Memory, Attention, and Judgment workshop. California Neuropsychology Services, Philadelphia, 1988.

24. Sohlberg MM, Mateer CA. Training use of compensatory memory books: a three stage behavioral approach. J Clin Exp Neuropsychol 1989;11:871–891.

25. Sohlberg MM, Geyer S. Prospective memory: description and treatment tasks. Paper presented at the Neuropsychology of Memory, Attention, and Judgment workshop. California Neuropsychology Services, Philadelphia, 1988.

26. Harris J. Memory aides people use: two interview studies. Memory and Cognition 1980;8:31.

27. Glisky EL, Schacter DL, Tulving E. Computer learning by memory-impaired patients: acquisition and retention of complex knowledge. Neuropsychologia 1986;24:313.

28. Lezak MD. The problem of assessing executive functions. Int J Psycholphysio 1982;17:281.

29. Toglia JP. Generalization of treatment: a multicontext approach to cognitive perceptual impairment in adults with brain injury. Am J Occup Ther 1991;45:505.

30. Kiernan RJ, et al. The neurobehavioral cognitive status examination: a brief but differentiated approach to cognitive assessment. Ann Intern Med 1987;107:481.

31. Brayman SJ. Comprehensive occupational therapy evaluation scale. Am J Occup Ther 1976;30:94.

32. Abrue BC. Rehabilitation of perceptual-cognitive dysfunction. Workshop, 1987.

33. Perceptual motor evaluation for head injured and other neurologically impaired adults. Santa Clara Valley Medical Center, Occupational Therapy Department, 1987.

34. Loewenstein occupational therapy cognitive assessment. Pequannock, NJ: Maddax, Inc., 1990.

35. Toglia JP. Approaches to cognitive assessment of the brain-injured adult: traditional methods and dynamic investigation. Occupational Therapy and Practice 1989;1:38.

36. Heimann NE, Allen CA, Yerxa EJ. The routine task inventory: a tool for describing the functional behavior of the cognitively disabled. Occupational Therapy and Practice 1989;1:67.

37. Allen CA, Earhart CA. Cognitive disabilities: expanded activity analysis. Workbook introduced at the Institute on Cognitive Disabilities, AOTA National Conference, Phoenix, AZ, 1988.

CHAPTER / 16

Sensory-Motor Issues

This chapter addresses issues such as tactile defensiveness, debilitating pain, loss of somatosensory discrimination, and poor coordination, which are ignored by other frames of reference.

Jean Ayres addressed some of these issues in the sensory integrative (SI) frame of reference. Yet, an assumption of her frame of reference doesn't apply to all patients with physical disabilities. Ayres assumed that peripheral structures like the skin are intact, while the brain is damaged and unable to process sensory input, resulting in poorly executed movement (1).

Many physically disabled adults have the exact opposite problem. They have damaged peripheral structures that impair sensory input, but have an intact brain. For example, a physically disabled patient may have distorted somatosensory input due to a burn, peripheral nerve injury, pain, impaired circulation of the skin, arthritic joints, trophic changes of the skin, irritable scar tissue, stabilization devices, and severe edema. Even an intact brain can produce poorly coordinated movements when peripheral conditions impair sensory feedback. Since many medical conditions violate the SI assumption that brain damage is present, it is not appropriate to refer to incoordination due to peripheral sensory deficits as SI concerns. It is more appropriate to refer to them as sensory-motor issues.

The biomechanical frame of reference does not address sensory-motor issues. The fourth assumption of the biomechanical frame of reference states that the patient must have an intact brain and be able to perform smoothly coordinated movements (2). However, coordinated movement is dependent on accurate somatosensory feedback. The biomechanical frame of reference assumes that sensation is intact. It ignores the need for sensory reeducation, which involves retraining the brain to process new sensory input from recovering peripheral structures.

In addition, biomechanical treatment techniques do not necessarily promote good coordination. Exercises tend to be done in linear, anatomical planes with a constant rhythm while focusing on isolated motions, like flexing and extending your elbow with a free weight in your hand (3). Yet, normal movements are diagonal, which includes a rotary component, and are performed with irregular rhythm using large numbers of muscles acting together (4). Elbow motion while combing your hair requires far more coordination than repeatedly lifting a free weight. Hair-combing also requires the patient to deal with the frustration of not having his/her hair look just right. Stretching, strengthening, and endurance exercises do not remind the patient that movements must be performed in an complex, unpredictable environment that requires good coordination for ideal results.

Biomechanical treatment techniques can actually conflict with coordination goals (3). It is difficult to perform fine motor coordination when maximum resistance is being applied to strengthen a muscle. While 20 pounds on a patient's wrist will strengthen the wrist extensors, it also makes it difficult for the patient to feed him/herself neatly or keep an even stitch while knitting. It is also difficult to perform fine motor coordination when active stretch is done at the end of range. A patient may find it too frustrating to try to tie knots in a rug with his/her arms fully extended over the head.

Even the neurodevelopmental treatment (NDT) frame of reference does not focus directly on somatosensation and coordination (5). While the Bobaths talked about giving the sensation of what normal movement feels like, NDT techniques are not designed to reduce tactile defensiveness, reduce pain, or regain somatosensory discrimination, like stereognosis. Nor does NDT recommend coordination training for complex tasks such as gait and bilateral hand use. NDT assumes that good coordination will naturally follow if underlying deficits such as abnormal muscle tone are remediated. However, this assumption is often false, especially with patients who have perceptual-cognitive deficits. It isn't realistic to expect individuals who have perceptual-cognitive deficits to generalize skills learned during handling exercises to coordinated movement during a functional activity.

It is vital for you to understand the sensory-motor concerns listed in Memory Aid 16.1. Patients who have pain and abnormal sensation may not be able to tolerate routine treatment if they cannot tolerate being touched or moved. Until these sensory concerns are addressed, it may be impossible to use the NDT or biomechanical frames of reference. Coordination is an essential skill that affects return to the community. It isn't enough to be strong and have good endurance if you are clumsy. Coordination training is usually done after increased range and strength have been achieved. You should be able to identify sensory-motor concerns in the mini-case study at the end of this chapter.

SOMATOSENSATION

Somatic Hypersensitivity

Hypersensitivity to somatic input can take the form of tactile defensiveness. **Tactile defensiveness** is defined as a consistently present, irritable response to nonthreatening tactile stimuli like a therapist's hand (1). Adult patients report paresthesias such as burning or stabbing pain or the sensation of something crawling over their skin. These abnormal sensations are consistently present even when the patient can see that all you did was touch him/her once lightly. Tactually defensive patients may repeatedly refuse to allow the therapist to touch them. Avoidance can be subtle, such as repeatedly distracting the therapist with conversation in an attempt to interrupt touching procedures. Avoidance can also be very aggressive, such as hitting the therapist.

A good example of tactile defensiveness due to a peripheral condition is a gentleman who had a brachial plexus injury from a gunshot wound. He received physical therapy for his shoulder for 1 month before occupational therapy started. When the OT finally saw him, he had not washed his hand or let anyone touch it for an entire month. When he walked into OT, he said, "You're not going to touch my hand are you"?

Treatment for tactile defensiveness involves getting the patient to tolerate sensory stimulation that will inhibit the overactive spinothalamic system. Once this protective tactile system is normalized, the patient can begin to distinguish between truly harmful touch and safe touch.

Treatment for tactile defensiveness must be applied in three major stages (1). The first stage is firm, prolonged pressure over the hypersensitive skin. However, firm pressure must be applied in a mini-treatment sequence.

Initially, severely defensive patients may tolerate firm, prolonged pressure only when it is applied by inanimate objects such as sandbags, a mattress, or firmly tucked sheets. After this first mini-step, the patient may feel comfortable applying firm, prolonged manual pressure to him/herself. Lastly, the therapist applies firm, prolonged manual pressure over the patient's hypersensitive body parts. When you apply pressure with your hand, DON'T SLIDE it around to get a comfortable grip. This gives the sensation of something crawling over the skin. Instead, take your hand off the patient's skin and place it in the new position you want.

In the second stage, constant rubbing touch is used. When rubbing extremities with lots of hair, ask the patient if rubbing in the opposite direction from the hair growth is irritating. Textures should initially be nonthreatening, like the patient's hand, a piece of flannel cloth, or a soft, wide paintbrush. Later, you can grade up to more irritating textures, like rubbing the body with cotton balls and burlap or by moving the hand around in a bucket filled with sand, dried beans, or rice.

In the third stage, changing light touch is applied. An effective way to apply changing touch is self-directed interaction with objects such as dressing and bathing. These external sources of tactile input will inherently touch the patient in unexpected patterns.

It is essential to give the patient control over the tactile stimulation program. You will be more successful if you respect the patient's fear by letting the stimulation occur at the patient's own pace and stop when he/she wants it to stop. Patients who are tactually defensive have had touch repeatedly imposed on them during medical procedures. Letting the patient control the input helps to break the cycle of irrational fear and loss of control from imposed touch. Initially, the patient will not be able to tolerate all three stages of tactile input within a single treatment session. With nonthreatening treatment, the problem will subside, and the patient will be able to tolerate several kinds of tactile input.

Another form of somatic hypersensitivity is **vestibular hypersensitivity,** which is defined as an exaggerated fear of falling even when there is no danger of falling (1). Fear may stem from actual movement or from anticipation of movement. It is an exaggerated fear that does not respond to reason. It doesn't help to get out a ruler to prove to the patient that the step is only 5 inches high. Vestibular hypersensitivity is also called **postural or gravitational insecurity** (6). Adult patients may acquire it from decreased vestibular input due to prolonged bed rest, spasticity that evolves into rigid fixing, paralysis that makes the patient feel vulnerable, and medication or brain damage that affects the vestibular system.

Treatment for vestibular hypersensitivity must be applied in three stages (1). The first stage involves slow, linear movement. For adult patients who are larger and harder to support than children, this movement should occur in miniature ranges with maximal support from furniture. Examples of slow linear movement for adults include leaning slightly forward and backward while sitting, rolling the wheelchair slowly forward, or rising a few inches off of a chair and immediately sitting back down. These movements may need to be repeated several times at the beginning of every treatment session until hypersensitivity subsides.

The second stage of treatment for vestibular hypersensitivity involves irregular movements performed at functional speed. Interaction with objects and other people inherently produces irregular movements. Speed should be graded to whatever is functional for the activity that is being used. When a patient leans diagonally forward and backward to put on socks and shoes or walks around obstacles in a congested room, his/her head is moving in irregular patterns. This type of natural vestibular input makes more sense than having the patient perform irregular head movements in a nonsense sequence. The third stage of vestibular desensitization involves rotary movements in the form of spinning. This is used ONLY WITH CHILDREN! Even healthy adults do not readily tolerate this third stage of treatment.

Again, it is important to respect the patient's fear. If you back off as soon as the patient becomes frightened, he/she will trust you more and tolerate more movement in the long run.

Pain

Pain is such a little word for such a powerful and frequently occurring human experience. The success of an entire treatment program can depend on successful control of pain. Control is the key word because pain may never be completely relieved. You need to emphasize that your goal is to achieve tolerable discomfort that does not interfere with function. Telling patients that you will not hurt them and that they will be pain-free may be an impossible promise to keep. Promising no pain if it isn't possible will eventually destroy the patient's trust in you.

It is important to establish functional goals as early as possible when a patient has pain (7). Patients often misinterpret the persistence of pain as failure. They need to learn to see progress as a return of functional skills despite their pain. Patients need to develop a sense of mastery over pain instead of feeling controlled by it. By establishing functional goals early, we are teaching our patients to work around discomfort instead of giving up valued activities. Therapists also need to see if targeted functional goals are achieved to determine if the pain program is working.

To further assess treatment effectiveness, you may want to get a subjective pain baseline. Subjective data include having the patient rate the pain on a scale of 1 to 10 and then describe its characteristics. The patient may describe it as a burning or itching sensation, as cramping or throbbing, or as a dull ache or sharp pain. It may be constant or intermittent. Patients can also be asked to color in the parts of their body that hurt on an anatomical drawing.

When severe pain interferes with all treatment, objective data on pain are essential. Time that normally would be spent on ROM, strength, and other physical goals must be set aside for pain control. Objective pain data enable you to show immediate change and justify the need for treatment even when physical deficits have not improved or when progress is slower than expected.

One objective way to document pain is to mark **trigger points** on an anatomical drawing. These are small, extremely tender spots in muscles that are painful to the slightest pressure. They are scored as present or absent. The etiology of trigger points has not been determined. They may be pockets of accumulated lactic acid, calcium deposits, or an aberration of the autonomic nervous system (8).

Another common way to document pain objectively is to report which activities are impossible or difficult to perform because of the pain. The patient may move too slowly, have to stop too many times, or be able to work for such a short period of time that he/she is dysfunctional.

Maitland developed an objective method for documenting pain, called a pain baseline (9). This procedure takes too much time to administer to every patient, but it is useful when severe pain interferes with every initial evaluation procedure. When the patient with severe pain won't let you do anything, you can establish rapport and document how much pain limits movement by using Maitland's procedure.

First, you draw a chart for a specific joint motion. Maitland used rectangular boxes, but drawings of joint motions can also be used (see Fig. 16.1). It is not necessary to use a goniometer to measure exactly where in the range the patient reports discomfort or pain. There are too many factors that can alter the awareness of pain. Anxiety, fatigue, distractions, and antecedent events such as administration of hot packs or pain medication, can make awareness of pain vary. General estimates of where pain emerged such as "at mid-range," "around 45°", or "in the first one-third of the range" are sufficient.

After your chart is ready, you need to establish P1, which marks the end of the pain-free range. Ask the patient if pain is present at rest. If pain is present at rest, make a mark on the zero line. If pain is not present at

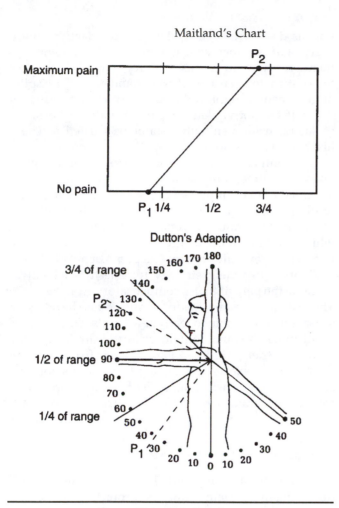

Figure 16.1. Pain Baselines.

rest, slowly move that joint at almost imperceptible speed and ask the patient to immediately report any discomfort. Tell the patient you will stop as soon as he/she reports any discomfort. This is a two-sided contract. You must stop to gain your patient's trust. The patient must report discomfort accurately to give you a reliable baseline. If the patient has trouble identifying exactly when discomfort first emerges, you can perform small oscillatory movements, starting in the pain-free range and gradually moving further into the range until discomfort is felt. Estimate where in the range discomfort is first felt and mark it as P1 on your chart. Your first treatment goal may be to move P1, which shows an increase in the degrees of pain-free range.

Next, tell the patient you will continue to slowly move the limb beyond P1, but will stop when his/her limit for discomfort is reached. The limit is just short of intolerable pain. This limit is determined by what the therapist is prepared to provoke (9). DO NOT continue past the patient's limit for discomfort. This is a pain baseline, not a test of full range of motion! Estimate where in the range the patient's limit for discomfort appears and

mark it as P2 on your chart. P2 is where range is limited by pain tolerance. Ideally, you would like to get rid of pain, but it may be more realistic to move P2. The patient will still experience discomfort, but it won't be intolerable pain and he/she may use more of the available range.

Pain control is possible because of the "gate theory" (10). This theory postulates that painful stimuli that pass through the substantia gelatinosa in the dorsal horn of the spinal cord can be blocked by competing stimuli. Only a limited amount of sensory information can pass through the gate. Thus, therapist-applied sensory input appears to cancel out the painful sensations. You close the sensory gate when you rub yourself after you've run into a piece of furniture.

Therapists talk about closing the sensory gate with a pain kit (11). Relief may initially be very brief. Outpatients are usually taught to use the pain kit at home for more extended relief. This kit includes applying prolonged ice to a painful body part, repeatedly applying fingertip vibration for 7 seconds over a trigger point (which is very tiring), using an electric vibrator over a trigger point or painful areas for 25 to 45 minutes, wearing a transcutaneous electrical nerve stimulation (TENS) unit over a painful area all day, learning biofeedback to reverse the temperature of a cold or hot body part, and using proprioceptive neuromuscular facilitation (PNF) diagonals in combination with rhythmic breathing.

Proprioceptive neuromuscular facilitation requires the patient to move the extremity in a diagonal pattern that combines flexion/extension components, abduction/adduction components, and rotation (4). For example, have the patient open his/her hand with the arm out to the side in about 45° of shoulder abduction. The elbow should be extended and the palm turned to face the wall behind the patient. Then ask the patient to "close your hand, turn it palm up, and bring it up and across your body." Then tell the patient to "open your hand, turn it palm down, and bring it back down to your side." Patients have reported a decrease in pain when doing these complex diagonal movements instead of simple, linear movements in anatomical planes such as simply opening and closing the fist (12). When PNF diagonals are combined with rhythmical breathing, the reduction of pain is even more dramatic. For example, the patient should time breathing so that he/she breathes in while closing the hand, and blows out while opening the hand.

Pain is often accompanied by edema, joint stiffness, and muscle weakness. While these symptoms are not as distressing to the patient as pain, they can be an early warning sign. For example, doctors found that muscle weakness, spasms, and difficulty initiating movement preceded the onset of reflex sympathetic dystrophy (RSD) by weeks or months (13). Reflex sympathetic dystrophy is a crippling condition that results in a painful frozen shoulder and a claw-hand that cannot tolerate being touched. It is essential to aggressively treat edema, stiffness, and weakness early. Once RSD sets in, aggressive handling exacerbates the problem. Any additional trauma can cause RSD to flare up (13).

When pain is severe or becomes chronic, patients become phobic (14). They begin to believe that if they develop a rigid posture and become sedentary, their pain will diminish. The treatment for a phobia is to relax the person and to reintroduce him/her to the feared activity. Relaxation techniques, such as progressive relaxation, are discussed in *Willard and Spackman's Occupational Therapy* (15). Relaxation tapes and low-pitched music with a tempo of 70 to 80 beats per minute are soothing (8). Yet, relaxation techniques are helpful only if they are followed by movement that the patient fears, so that desensitization occurs. Self-care or job-related activities are good ways to reintroduce feared movements. Purposeful tasks have the added benefit of distracting the patient. Patients have reported pain relief as long as the purposeful activity lasts (8).

Environmental modification should also be considered if chronic pain is present. Employers may need to modify work heights and require regular rest periods for workers who perform repetitive motions. For example, cafeteria workers with repeated low back injuries did not generalize a body mechanics lecture to the workplace because of environmental constraints (16). The fast work pace of the cafeteria line and awkward arrangement of storage cabinets made it difficult to use good body mechanics. Suggestions to modify the environment can generate resistance because they require money and a change of habits, but they may be essential to alleviate some types of chronic pain (14).

Finally, if a patient has intractable pain, more drastic steps can be taken. These include nerve blocks, dorsal rhizotomies, and narcotic pain relievers. These methods have side effects and may produce only transient relief from pain. The autonomic nervous system seems to be particularly adept at finding alternate pathways for carrying pain messages.

Anesthesia/Unilateral Neglect

Anesthesia is defined as the absence of somatosensation. When it is severe, it is called **unilateral neglect**. Unilateral neglect can be so severe that such patients adamantly deny that the extremity they see by their side belongs to them.

The therapist's main concern is to prevent structural damage to the involved extremity. Protective positioning (sandbags, seat cushions, wheelchair arm troughs) and protective orthoses (resting hand splints; arm slings) should be used from the moment either of these conditions is discovered. These devices are effective only if every staff member who works with the patient uses them properly and checks them regularly. It is possible for a patient to sleep all night on a hand in a resting splint or get a hand caught in the spokes of the wheelchair if the staff are not vigilant. A patient with anesthesia or unilateral neglect initially cannot be trusted to check his/her own positioning.

Environmental modification for unilateral neglect takes more time to implement because it requires team discussion. For example, everyone has to agree to consistently put important objects, like the telephone and nurse call button, on the unaffected side and to speak while standing on the unaffected side. Zoltan et al. discusses these modifications in Chapter 4 of her book (17).

Another treatment strategy for anesthesia involves teaching the patient to use compensatory strategies (17). The patient must be made aware of his/her lack of sensation and be able to learn new habits. For example, a patient with a spinal cord injury must learn to carefully watch his/her paralyzed legs to keep from banging them against objects or dragging them across abrasive surfaces when transferring. Patients with severe cognitive deficits cannot achieve this final strategy of preventing harm to the anesthetic extremity through vigilance.

Somatic Discrimination

Tactile sensation is divided into the protective and discriminative systems (18). The **protective tactile system** is called the protopathic or the spinothalamic system. This primitive system provides: (*a*) detection of light touch, deep pressure, and pain; and (*b*) differentiation of hot/cold and sharp/dull. The purpose of the protective system is to produce a ''fight or flight response'' in the presence of a threatening stimulus, such as a hot stove or a knife. The five types of protective sensation just listed are sent up through the spinothalamic tracks to terminate in the thalamus, which initiates quick, protective responses. Life-threatening stimuli reach the cortex later by indirect, slower pathways. The cortex is good at subtle discrimination, but it responds too slowly where safety is concerned.

The **discriminative tactile system** is called the epicritic or the medial lemniscal system. Tactile discrimination includes:

1. Two-point discrimination;
2. Localization of tactile stimuli (LTS);
3. Finger identification (FI);
4. Stereognosis or manual form perception; and
5. Graphesthesia.

The five types of discriminative sensation just listed are sent up the medial lemniscal track to terminate in the cortex, where sophisticated judgments can be made based on previous experience.

Somatosensation also includes the proprioceptive system. Proprioception is divided into the automatic and conscious systems (19). Proprioceptive input for both systems includes information about muscle length, muscle tension, the speed of movement, the direction of movement, the force of contractions, and joint position. However, these proprioceptive stimuli are sent to two different locations in the brain.

The conscious proprioceptive system sends proprioceptive input to the cortex. The person consciously attends to the proprioceptive input and watches his/her own movements while the therapist gives him/her feedback. This input is used when the person is trying to learn a new movement or relearn a lost movement. Conscious proprioception is called **kinesthesia** in the AOTA uniform terminology (20). Formal test procedures evaluate the conscious awareness of proprioceptive input with vision occluded and with no cognitive challenges other than concentrating on limb movement. Test procedures include asking the patient to tell you whether you are moving a particular joint up or down, duplicating the position you have placed one limb in by placing the other limb in the same position, or moving an index finger back to a specific point on the table after you have moved it away.

Unlike conscious kinesthesia, the automatic system sends input to the cerebellum, which frees the cortex for abstract thought. The automatic system, referred to as **proprioception,** is used during preplanned movements (19). The cerebellum compares the current proprioceptive input to previously learned sensory traces for an activity, like riding a bicycle. The cerebellum checks to see if the feedback matches the sensory trace. If no discrepancy is noted, the cerebellum continues to run the motor program.

Proprioception can be tested only while the patient is performing an automatic movement. When a patient was told to walk down the hallway, she was distracted by being asked to hold a folded newspaper under her arm. She dropped the paper after her first step. She was concentrating so hard on walking correctly that she lost track of the muscle tension needed to keep the paper under her arm.

Patients can demonstrate good kinesthesia during formal evaluations and still have poor automatic proprioception. One patient was able to identify when joints were being moved up and down when he was given sufficient time and was not distracted, but when he was engaged in a purposeful activity, his hemiplegic arm consistently floated up into the air. The patient never knew where his hemiplegic arm was until it was pointed out to him.

Proprioception and kinesthesia disappear only in the most severe cases and are the first somatosensory modalities to return. When protective tactile sensation and proprioception do not return quickly, the patient has a poor prognosis for further sensory and motor return (see #1 on Memory Aid 16.1).

Discriminative tactile sensation is used for early detection of slowly emerging compression conditions, such as carpal tunnel syndrome (see #2 in Memory Aid 16.1). Stereognosis and graphesthesia are often the first discriminative modalities to disappear and the last to return (21). They disappear even before muscle weakness can be detected. Only when compression becomes more severe do localization of tactile stimuli, finger identification and two-point discrimination disappear (21).

There is extensive information on how to evaluate tactile sensation and kinesthesia. Read Chapter 3 of Trombly's text (22). You must know: (*a*) the general suggestions for testing, (*b*) how to apply the stimuli properly, and (*c*) how to score the patient's responses. Patient responses are usually mapped on diagnosis-specific sensory charts such as spinal cord injury, hemiplegia, peripheral nerve injury, and hand injury test forms.

Information about sensory retraining is limited to treatment of patients with peripheral nerve injuries (PNI). Sensory retraining teaches the brain to interpret new sensory input (22). Wynn-Perry suggested that the speedy return of tactile discrimination in patients with PNI occurred in too short a time period to be explained by the regeneration rate of peripheral nerves. Peripheral nerves regenerate at a rate of only one inch per month (23). Once the regenerated peripheral nerve grows to the end of its myelin sheath, the brain quickly learns how to interpret the distal tactile input. Yet, retraining the brain in PNI can be a real challenge because the surgeon can line up the bundles of nerve fibers called fascicles, but not the 20,000+ fibers within each nerve (24). Mismatches of individual fibers with their original connections in the sensory-motor strip can produce bizarre sensory-motor experiences. Patients have reported feeling one finger move while actually moving a different finger.

The early phase of sensory retraining in PNI focuses on the recovery of protective sensation (22). Treatment begins with the detection of moving touch. For example, the patient tries to detect when the therapist is stroking the patient's body part with a cotton ball while vision is occluded. Once moving touch can be detected consistently, treatment progresses to detection of constant touch, such as being touched for several seconds with the eraser of a pencil.

Treatment for discriminative sensation in PNI begins only when detection of both constant and moving touch are intact at the fingertips (22). There is no treatment

---

Memory Aid 16.1.
Sensory Motor Concerns

I. Somatosensation	II. Coordination = Smoothness	III. Coordinate 2+ Structures
A. *Somatic Hypersensitivity* 　1. Tactile defensiveness 　　a. Firm/prolonged pressure 　　b. Constant rubbing touch 　　c. Changing light touch 　2. Vestibular hypersensitivity 　　a. Linear slow motions 　　b. Irregular/functional speed 　　c. CHILD ONLY: spinning	A. *Rule Out Cerebellar Dysfunction* 　1. Dysdiadochokinesis 　2. Dysmetria 　3. Dyssynergia 　4. Intention tremor 　5. Ataxic gait 　6. Dysarthria	A. *Basic Eye-Hand Coordination* 　1. Ocular-Manual Split 　2. Fleeting Eye-Hand Coordination 　3. Prolonged Eye-Hand Coordination
B. *Pain* 　1. Establish functional goals 　2. Close the "sensory gate" 　3. Reduce edema and stiffness 　4. Teach relaxation techniques 　5. Environmental modification 　6. Medication/surgery	B. *Screening for Smoothness* 　Screening procedures include writing, the Nine-Hole Pegtest, and fastenings on clothing like buttons and zippers.	B. *Coordination of the Two Eyes*[a] 　1. Convergence 　2. Ocular fixation 　3. Visual Pursuits 　4. Quick Localization 　5. Saccades
C. *Anesthesia/Unilateral Neglect* 　1. Protective positioning 　2. Protective orthotics 　3. Environmental modification 　4. Compensatory strategies	C. *Manual Dexterity* 　Standardized tests such as the Minnesota Rate of Manipulation Test use speed to assess smooth movement.	C. *Bilateral Limb Coordination* 　1. Reciprocal (e.g., walk/swim) 　2. Symmetrical (e.g., catch a ball, jump on 2 feet) 　3. Asymmetrical (e.g., open jar)
D. *Protect and Discriminate*[a] 　1. Detect moving and then constant light touch/deep pressure 　2. Protect: Differentiate between sharp/dull and hot/cold 　3. Kinesthesia; proprioception 　4. Localization of tactile stimuli finger identification and Two-point discrimination 　5. Stereognosis; graphesthesia	NOTE: *Hand Evaluations*, like the Jebsen Hand Function Test, are composite batteries that test prehension patterns, grip strength, hand ROM, writing, fastenings, etc.	D. *Oral Motor Coordination* 　1. Tongue Control 　2. Jaw Control 　3. Lip Control

[a]See perceptual-cognitive issues for related or overlapping concerns.

---

progression for regaining discriminative sensation, but there are general adjuncts to learning (22). Trombly suggests starting with a general sensory warm-up of vigorous rubbing. Cognitive strategies, such as trying to guess the characteristics of the stimulus (e.g., is it hard or round?) and opening the eyes after every attempt to confirm accuracy are recommended. It is also important to prevent fatigue. A few 5- to 10-minute sessions are better than a single 20- to 30-minute session. Sensory retraining is very draining, and the patient must be committed to make it work.

COORDINATION AS SMOOTHNESS

Ruling out Cerebellar Dysfunction

The definition of coordination as smooth movement came from the literature on cerebellar and basal ganglia disease. These diagnoses interfere with a person's ability to quickly start and stop a movement, to judge distance and speed accurately, and to move smoothly. Neurologists developed clinical tests for all of these functions

(see Table 16.1). Dysdiadochokinesis and the rebound phenomenon evaluate the ability to quickly start and stop a movement. Dysmetria evaluates the distance and speed of movement. Dyssynergia tests smoothness of movement. As Table 16.1 shows, other diseases like posterior column spinal cord lesions can produce signs of incoordination.

Smoothness Equals Speed

While few therapists see patients with cerebellar tumors, smoothness is still an issue we address with many patients who have motor impairment. Abnormal sensory input described at the beginning of this chapter can make patients appear clumsy.

Tests for smoothness are divided into screening tools and tests for manual dexterity. Screening tools like writing and fastenings on clothing require subjective clinical judgment for interpretation. Screening tools like the Nine-Hole Pegtest use speed as a normative measure.

Standardized test of manual dexterity also evaluate the smoothness of movement in the form of speed (see

Table 16.1.
Diseases That Affect Coordination

Basal Ganglia Lesions	*Unilateral Neocerebellar Lesions*

Basal Ganglia Lesions

1. *Athetosis*
   - Continuous, writhing motions that are too irregular to imitate accurately
   - Writhing becomes exaggerated with effort; not present during sleep
   - Lack of stability of neck, trunk, and proximal joints
   - Muscle tone can fluctuate from high to low

2. *Huntington's Chorea*
   - Continuous rapid jerky irregular movements of face and distal joints
   - Movements may occur during sleep
   - Muscles are hypotonic

3. *Parkinson's Disease*
   - Cog-wheel rigidity
   - Bradykinesia (e.g., difficulty initiating movement)
   - Resting tremor
   - Slow, shuffling gait with minimal arm swing that gradually accelerates out of control
   - Lack of facial expression
   - Monotone speech pattern

Unilateral Neocerebellar Lesions
- Ataxic gait[a] with a tendency to fall to same side as lesion
- Intention tremor
- Dysdiadochokineses (e.g., lacks rapidly alternating pronation and supination)
- Rebound phenomenon (e.g., resists elbow flexion and then lets go; patient's hand hits his chest)
- Dysmetria (e.g., past pointing during the finger-to-nose test)
- Dyssynergia (e.g., lack of smooth motion during heel-to-shin test)
- Nystagmus, especially when looking toward the side of the lesion
- Equilibrium: sways both with eyes closed and eyes open
- Ipsilateral hypotonia

Spinal Cord Posterior Column Lesion
- Loss of proprioception and discriminative tactile sensation
- Ataxic gait[a] due to loss of proprioception
- Dysmetria, especially with eyes closed due to loss of proprioception
- Equilibrium: sways ONLY with eyes closed due to loss of proprioception

[a]Ataxic gait = wide-based, staggering gait with irregular cadence.

Memory Aid 16.1). These tests include the Minnesota Rate of Manipulation Test, the Purdue Pegboard Test, the Crawford's Small Parts Dexterity Test, and the Jebsen Hand Function Test. The Jebsen Test requires the patient to write, turn cards, pick up small objects, stack checkers, estimate the weight of weighted cans, and perform simulated eating as quickly as possible.

COORDINATION OF TWO OR MORE BODY PARTS

When therapists talk about coordination, they are referring to more than smoothness. They are also concerned about the ability to coordinate two or more body parts at a time.

Basic Eye-Hand Coordination

The beauty of eyes and hands working together cannot be taken for granted. Children who are functioning at infant levels and adults who are emerging from coma frequently lack this basic skill. The primitive phase of eye-hand coordination is entitled Ocular-Manual Split (see Table 16.2). This stage is characterized by mutually exclusive visual regard and manipulation of objects. The subject can do one or the other, but not both together. The transitional stage, entitled Fleeting Eye-Hand Coordination, shows that looking and manipulation of objects fleetingly overlap in time. For example, the subject will look while reaching and then look away as soon as the object is in the hand only to be surprised later on when he/she sees the object in his/her hand. The mature phase is characterized by Prolonged Eye-Hand Coordination. The subject will finger and turn an object over in the hand while intently looking at it. Treatment consists of replicating the normal sequence of development.

Coordination of the Two Eyes

The two eyes must work together to produce a sharp image on the fovea of the retina. Convergence, ocular persistence, visual pursuits, quick localization, and saccades are discussed in the chapter on perceptual-cognitive issues. They are mentioned here to remind you to rule out poor ocular coordination. EYE-hand coordination may be impaired by poor ocular coordination as well as poor manual dexterity.

Bilateral Limb Coordination

Bilateral coordination is usually divided into several types, such as reciprocal movements (e.g., walking), symmetrical movements (e.g., clapping), and asymmetrical movements (e.g., holding a jar with one hand while turning the lid with the other hand). The NDT and biomechanical frames of reference assume that all three types of movements will return if underlying skills such as muscle tone and range of motion are rehabilitated.

Neurodevelopmental treatment does not require the patient to perform complex movements while being cognitively challenged (3). Yet, the patient must eventually initiate and coordinate movements of several extremities

Table 16.2.
Basic Eye-Hand Coordination

	Ocular-Manual Split	Fleeting Eye-Hand Coordination	Prolonged Eye-Hand Coordination
Essential Characteristics	1. Prolonged visual regard for one object held near face 2. Grasp reflex retains object placed in hand 3. Shakes/mouths objects with no visual regard of object	1. Glances around to inspect multiple objects 2. Visually directed reaching 3. Manipulation while looking away alternates with holding object still to look at it	1. Spontaneously looks at small visual details 2. Prolonged visual regard of object held in the hand while other hand manipulates small parts of the object
Visual Regard	Delayed focus on objects presented in midline 0–2 mo Prompt regard of objects presented in midline 3 mo Prolonged visual regard for objects 6 mo	Looks at own hands in mutual fingering 4 mo Glances from object to hand and back again 4 mo Pats and looks at object held in hand 5 mo	Spontaneously notices and fingers string attached to an object 8 mo Spontaneously notices pellet when it is dumped; then picks it up 9 mo
Ocular Pursuits	Follows object just past midline 2 mo Follows objects smoothly 180° in supine 2 mo Rapidly shifts glance between two objects 3 mo Demonstrates ocular convergence 4 mo	Alternately looks at, shakes, and mouths object 6 mo Visually directed reaching 6 mo Visually searches for dropped object and retrieves it 6 mo Holds object in each hand; looks back and forth between the two 7 mo	Spontaneously notices and pokes at clapper in bell with extended index finger 10 mo
Hand Function	Takes object placed in hand to mouth without looking at it 3 mo Shakes objects with NO visual regard 4–5 mo		

while interacting with an object. The patient needs to practice holding the toothbrush with the hemiplegic hand while the other hand squeezes the toothpaste tube. The patient must be able to walk down the street while watching other pedestrians instead of looking down to see what the hemiplegic leg is doing. It is safer to have the patient try activities that require simultaneous use of several extremities while being cognitively challenged with therapist supervision. We need to know the patient's real motor capabilities before we finalize the patient's discharge plans.

The biomechanical frame of reference also implies that once underlying deficits such as loss of range, strength, and endurance are remediated, the patient will automatically demonstrate good coordination. The therapist needs to watch the patient perform coordinated movements during a few functional activities to see if the patient is still using awkward, compensatory movements. The patient may not be aware that he/she is still lowering his/her head while eating or laterally flexing his/her trunk to reach for objects at chest height. Even well-educated, cognitively intact patients need to briefly practice coordination to assure us and themselves that they are generalizing the gains they achieved to functional tasks at home and work.

Oral Motor Coordination

Oral motor coordination is too complicated to discuss here. It includes treatment of medical conditions such as dental disease, normalization of oral sensation and reflexes, normalization of oral and axial muscle tone, and coordination of tongue, jaw, and lips. These three oral structures develop coordination at different rates for different eating tasks, such as spoon use and cup-drinking. As a general rule, tongue control emerges first, and lip control emerges last (see Table 16.3). Oral motor coordination is included here to remind you that most texts on adult physical disabilities ignore it. Extensive information is available in the pediatric literature.

MINI-CASE STUDY

Creating the Narrative Hypothesis

Sam is a 65-year-old male who was admitted with an infected right foot and bilateral foot deformities secondary

Table 16.3.
Occupational Therapy Feeding Checklist

MEDICAL PROBLEMS
  Dental disease _____ Malocclusion _____ Constipation/Diarrhea _____ Underweight _____ Habitual mouth breather _____
  Chronic ENT Problems _____ Poor appetite _____

POSITIONING PROBLEMS Circle: Extensor thrust/ ASTN reflex/ Foot reflexes/ Arm retraction/ Scoliosis/ Kyphosis/ Dislocated hip/ Narrow sitting base

TACTILE SENSITIVITY and REFLEXES
  Lips _____ Gums _____ Teeth _____ Palate _____ Tongue _____
  Response to textured foot _____ Toothbrushing _____
  Teething _____ Phasic bite reflex gone (3–5 mo) _____
  Gag reflex gone (7–9 mo) _____ Babkin gone (3 mo) _____ Rooting gone (3–5 mo) _____

MUSCLE TONE: Lips _____ Cheeks _____ Tongue _____

BOTTLE USE (age levels from Suzanne Morris)
  Tongue: Powerful true suck (0–1 mo) _____ Suckling (extensor thrust) (1–2 mo) _____
       ½ Suckling/½ true suck (4–6 mo) _____ True suck (up and down) (7 mo) _____
  Lips: Corners contact nipple (0–3 mo) _____ Firm closure w/no drips (4 mo) _____

SPOON USE
  Tongue: ½ Suckling/½ true suck (4–6 mo) _____ True suck (up and down) (7 mo) _____
       Stays in mouth as spoon is presented (6 mo) _____
       Can swallow independently of preceding suck (7–9 mo) _____
  Jaw: Jaw opening graded for size of spoon (6 mo) _____
  Lips: Firm closure on spoon using upper lip to clean off food (7–9 mo) _____
     Lips closed while swallowing pureed food (7–9 mo) _____

CUP DRINKING
  Tongue: Poor coordination for sucking, swallowing, and breathing (4–6 mo) _____
       Coordinate suck/swallow/breath by pulling away every 1–3 sips (7–9 mo) _____
       Can suck/swallow/breath in a long sequence without choking (13–15 mo) _____
  Jaw: Moves it up and down while drinking (7–9 mo) _____
     Inhibits up/down motion by biting on rim of cup (13–15 mo) _____
  Lips: Firm lip closure on cup without biting rim (16–18 mo) _____

CHEWING
  Tongue: Moves food from side of mouth with tongue (7–9 mo) _____
  Jaw: Munching (4–5 mo) _____ Vertical chew (6 mo) _____ Rotary chew (16–18 mo) _____
     Bites soft food w/poor grading & associated head movements (7–9 mo) _____
     Bites soft food w/graded opening/no associated head motion (10–12 mo) _____
     Bites hard food w/graded opening/no associated head motion (16–18 mo) _____
  Lips: Open but active during chew (7–9 mo) _____ Closed and active 16–18 mo) _____

---

to diabetes of 20 years. He had a B/K amputation of his RLE and an amputation of his left big toe. No LE prostheses were ordered at the time of discharge. He also has hypertension and atrial fibrillation. He will return to his two-story house with 6 steps at the front door. He has a wife but no children. He already has a commode and tub chair at home.

Based on the diagnosis of long-standing diabetes, I would expect peripheral neuropathy that would impair sensation and coordination (hypothesis #1) but not range of motion or strength (hypothesis #2). I would also expect poor healing and skin condition (hypothesis #3) based on the poor circulation that is associated with diabetes. The hypertension and atrial fibrillation make me wonder if his activities are currently restricted enough to impair endurance (hypothesis #4). The presence of a commode and tub chair at home make me even more suspicious about endurance. Is the bathroom on the second floor at home? Was

it too tiring for him to climb the stairs several times a day? Based on his discharge plans, I need to know about his daily routine (hypothesis #5). His age suggests that he is retired. Is his wife supportive (hypothesis #6)?

Designing an Evaluation Package

I would screen ROM and strength and do comprehensive testing for sensation, coordination, and endurance. I would carefully inspect his skin for deterioration. I would screen his level of independence in ADL and ask about his daily routine at home.

Test Results

Passive range of motion is mildly restricted for shoulder rotation and elbow extension due to arthritic involvement of these joints. Strength is WNL. Proprioception and localization of tactile stimuli are impaired in all four extremities. Stereognosis and sharp/dull are impaired in BUEs due to slow responses. His skin is dry, shiny, and hairless from midcalf down on the LLE. Coordination is −2.0 standard deviations for both hands on the Nine-Hole Pegtest. He repeatedly knocked pegs off the table with his ring and little fingers. His writing is illegible when signing his name with his dominant left hand. He is "slightly" deconditioned. All ADLs are done sitting. He can stand for 10 minutes in the standing box and walk 100 feet with the walker.

He requires constant supervision to sequence the use of the walker while walking and transferring and to sequence the use of crutches to climb 12 steps. He won't be given a LE prosthesis. He is independent in eating, bed mobility, dressing on the edge of the bed, and wheelchair maneuvers in his room.

Interpreting Test Result

Generating a Cue Interpretation List

1. *Impaired sensation/coordination*
   + Impaired kinesthesia and protective sensation
   + Impaired discrimination sensation
   + Manual dexterity is −2.0 S.D. bilaterally
   Confirmed as written
2. *Normal ROM and strength*
   + Strength is WNL
   + PROM is WNL except for mild loss of shoulder/elbow ROM
   Revision: Mild loss of shoulder/elbow ROM
3. *Poor healing/skin condition*
   + Poor circulation/healing
   + Poor skin condition BLEs
   Confirmed as written
4. *Poor endurance*
   + Only walking 100 feet with walker/no RLE prosthesis
   + two-story house with six front steps
   + Does ADLs sitting on edge of bed in hospital
   + Already has commode and tub chair at home
   + Hypertension/atrial fibrillation
   Confirmed as written
5. *What is his daily routine at home?* No information available.
6. *Is his wife supportive?* No information available.
New. Independent in ADLs only in sitting: not allowed to stand during ADLs such as shaving; needs constant supervision to handle ambulatory aids; independently maneuvers wheelchair in hospital room; won't be given LE prosthesis
   Evaluating the Narrative Hypotheses. Hypotheses #1, #3, and #4 were easily confirmed. Hypothesis #2

had to be revised. Arthritis was not part of his medical history or presenting problem. The medical chart gave no information about hypotheses #5 and #6. Interviews are recommended.

The new information about the need for supervision when using ambulatory aids is a surprise. Many diabetic patients have poor LE sensation and still learn how to safely manipulate these devices. Is the heart condition too severe to permit weightbearing on UEs? Are the foot deformities on his spared foot too severe for foot-flat gait? Is there a cognitive deficit that makes him unsafe? Does the family lack insurance to cover the cost of the prosthesis? More information is needed.

Deficits Ignored by the Biomechanical Frame of Reference

Poor circulation, poor healing ability, and impaired protective sensation are significant deficits because inadvertent bumps and scrapes can cause further damage. Further amputations may be necessary if he doesn't learn compensatory strategies to protect his LEs.

His loss of discriminative sensation in BUEs is significant enough to impair the manual dexterity of his dominant hand. Since his signature is illegible, did his wife sign his medical release forms? Will she have to sign the checks to pay the medical bills? How does he feel about this loss?

SUMMARY

It is vital that you recognize and address sensory motor issues that are ignored by the biomechanical and NDT frames of reference. The ability to tolerate being touched and moved are essential for implementing these frames of reference. If pain is unbearable, success of all other approaches will depend on reducing that pain. Whether a patient is safe when asked to move also depends on the return of somatosensation or on learning compensatory strategies that substitute for lost sensation.

Coordination must not be taken for granted either. It is especially poor in brain-damaged adults who lack smoothly graded movements that are independent of pathological synergies. Brain-damaged adults usually regress motorically when first exposed to cognitive and emotional challenges created by purposeful activities. These patients benefit from coordination training in a functional context. Even a cognitively intact patient may need to try one highly coordinated task before going home to see if he/she generalizes gains in ROM, strength, and endurance to complex activities.

STUDY QUESTIONS

1. For tactile defensiveness, what type of stimulus should you use for the most impaired patient, and who should apply it?
2. For vestibular hypersensitivity, what type of stimulus should you use for the most impaired patient, and when do you stop?
3. What is the difference between P1 and P2?
4. T or F: The purpose of the "pain kit" is to eliminate pain.
5. What is the first discriminative tactile sensation to be lost and the last to return?
6. What type of sensation is a good prognosticator for sensory and motor return?
7. How are proprioception and kinesthesia evaluated?
8. Coordination is divided into what two skills?
9. What are the characteristics of the transition stage of Basic Eye-Hand Coordination?
10. Oral motor coordination requires motion of what three structures?

References

1. Ayres AJ. Sensory integration and learning disabilities. Los Angeles: Western Psychological Services, 1972.
2. Pedretti LW, Pasquinelli S. A frame of reference for occupational therapy in physical dysfunction. In: Pedretti LW, Zoltan B, eds. Occupational therapy practice skills for physical dysfunction. 2nd ed. St. Louis: CV Mosby, 1990:1.
3. Dutton R. Guidelines for using both activity and exercise. Am J Occup Ther 1989;43:573.
4. Voss DE, Ionta MK, Myers BJ. Proprioceptive neuromuscular facilitation. 3rd ed. New York: Harper & Row, 1985.
5. Adam M. Bobath certification (8-week course). Memphis, 1982.
6. Ayres AJ. Sensory integration and the child. Los Angeles: Western Psychological Services, 1979.
7. Gatchel RJ, Mayer TG. Functional restoration for spinal disorders. Philadelphia: Lea & Febiger, 1988:218.
8. McCormack GL. Pain management by occupational therapists. Am J Occup Ther 1988;42:582.
9. Maitland GD. Vertebral manipulation. 2nd ed. London: Butterworths, 1977.
10. Wall P, Melzack R. The gate control theory of pain management. Brain 1978;101:971.
11. Bruening L. Reflex sympathetic dystrophy—therapist viewpoint. Paper presented at the Surgery and Rehabilitation of the Hand Symposium and Workshop, Philadelphia, 1987.
12. Myers B, Mukoyama S, Becker P. Proprioceptive neuromuscular facilitation. Two-week course at the Rehabilitation Institute of Chicago, 1985.
13. Mastrangelo R. RSD—still a baffling disorder. Advance for Occupational Therapy 1989;2:9.
14. Brown EJ. Misinformation and misdiagnosis hamper chronic pain treatment. Advance for Occupational Therapy 1989;6:1.
15. Neistadt ME. Stress management. In: Hopkins HL, Smith HD, eds. Willard and Spackman's occupational therapy. 7th ed. Philadelphia: JB Lippincott, 1980:321.
16. Carlton RS. The effects of body mechanics instruction on work performance. Am J Occup Ther 1987;41:16.
17. Zoltan B, Siev E, Freishtat B. Perceptual and cognitive dysfunction in the adult stroke patient. Revised ed. Thorofare, NJ: Slack, Inc., 1989:59.
18. Carpenter MB. Human neuroanatomy. 7th ed. Baltimore: Williams & Wilkins, 1976:137.
19. Powers W. Functional neuroanatomy. Graduate course offered at Boston University, 1978.
20. American Occupational Therapy Association. Uniform terminology. 2nd ed. Rockville, MD: AOTA, 1987.
21. Bell-Krotoski J. Components of sensibility assessment. Paper presented at the Surgery and Rehabilitation of the Hand Symposium and Workshop, Philadelphia, 1987.
22. Trombly CA, Scott AD. Evaluation and treatment of somatosensory sensation. In: Trombly CA, ed. Occupational therapy for physical dysfunction. 3rd ed. Baltimore: Williams & Wilkins, 1989:41.
23. Wynn-Parry CB. Rehabilitation of the hand. 4th ed. London: Buttersworths, 1981.
24. Schneider LH. A surgeon's approach to nerve repair. Paper presented at the Surgery and Rehabilitation of the Hand Symposium and Workshop, Philadelphia, 1987.

CHAPTER / 17

Homeostatic Issues

Until recently, therapists did not typically treat critically ill patients. Today, therapists routinely treat medically unstable patients in intensive care, on postsurgical wards, and in rehabilitation programs where patients may be transferred before they can tolerate daily therapy. This change in health care delivery creates a crisis of identity. The therapist is supposed to restore function, but is required to do no harm! This is difficult to accomplish with a medically unstable patient because **homeostatic issues** are life-threatening concerns. When there is a conflict between therapy goals and homeostasis, the homeostatic issues must always be given first priority.

Establishing measurable objectives and prescribing procedures to restore homeostasis are the sole purview of the physician. However, therapists spend more time with patients than doctors, so therapists have an important role to play in homeostasis. For example, how do you teach upper extremity dressing without dislodging the IV needle when the patient puts on a shirt? This is an example of the therapists's role in homeostasis, which is not usually discussed in print.

One responsibility therapists have always had for restoring homeostasis is to observe and report signs and symptoms. **Signs** are objective observations, while **symptoms** are subjective complaints. Physicians are rarely in the therapy department or at bedside during therapy to interpret signs and symptoms for therapists. Therapists must perform a form of triage. They must decide if signs and symptoms warrant: (*a*) a brief rest, (*b*) downgrading of treatment, (*c*) a return to the nursing floor, or (*d*) an immediate call to the physician. If a physician is called or paged, signs and symptoms must be as specific as possible so the doctor can give you specific instructions.

Therapists may even implement lifesaving procedures instead of calling the doctor or nurse. Therapists are not trained in school to perform lifesaving procedures, but expectations are changing as more hospitals provide in-service training to therapists. Today, it is not unthinkable for a therapist to suction a tracheotomy or change settings on a ventilator as directed by the physician. Little consensus exists about which lifesaving procedures a therapist should perform, so role delineation must be determined by each individual facility.

Homeostatic issues such as orthostatic hypotension are discussed in physical disability textbooks, but this information is fragmented. It is scattered across separate chapters on specific diagnoses. Homeostatic issues are purposefully not organized by diagnosis in this text. Many patients have multiple homeostatic deficits regardless of their "primary diagnosis." For example, a burn patient can have fractures from jumping out of a window. A patient with diabetes probably has high blood pressure, which is discussed only in cardiac chapters. Students should use the tables in this chapter to think beyond the primary diagnosis for the current admission as they read a medical chart. I have assumed that the reader has already taken a medical conditions course, so be prepared to look up medical terminology if necessary.

RESPIRATORY SYSTEM

One of the first priorities is to ensure adequate oxygen exchange. This can be achieved by using special equipment that keeps the patient's airway open and helps the patient breathe. Examples include a ventilator and tracheotomy (see Table 17.1). The physician will determine physiological readiness for independent breathing and select ventilator settings for Intermittent Mandatory Ventilation (IMV) (1). IMV alternately provides a preset volume of air and opportunities that let the patient breathe at whatever frequency and volume is demanded by an activity. IMV gives the patient both respiratory support and emotional reassurance that independent breathing is possible.

Therapists have an important role to play in weaning patients from this equipment (1). Weaning can still be

Table 17.1.
Homeostasis: Postulates

Goals: By System	Method/Rationale	Application: Examples
I. *Respiratory System*	*Observation*, which detects signs and symptoms	Monitor rate, rhythm, location
A. *Adequate oxygen exchange* will be maintained by using	*Equipment*, that maintains a patent airway or helps the patient breath	1. Ventilator 2. Tracheotomy
	Procedures, that remove accumulated secretions that block the airway	1. Suctioning 2. Assisted coughing
B. *Vital capacity* will be increased to 2,000+ cc by using	*Procedures*, that strengthen respiratory muscles	Triflow exercises
C. *Aspiration* will be prevented by using	*Equipment*, that removes excess fluid from the stomach	Track daily totals for nasogastric tube
D. *Pulmonary emboli* will be controlled by using	*Observation*, which detects signs and symptoms	Report sudden onset of chest pain, shoulder pain, and dyspnea
	Anticoagulants, which prevent clot formation	Check chart for heparin, etc.
	Thrombolytic drugs, which dissolve clots	Check chart for streptokinase, etc.

emotionally stressful. Weakened muscles and "air hunger" can create a sense of breathlessness. Occupational therapists can reduce anticipatory anxiety with relaxation techniques. Therapists can also improve respiratory conditioning by matching the demands of a purposeful activity to current respiratory capacity.

Adequate oxygen exchange can also be ensured by using procedures that remove accumulated secretions blocking the airway. Currently, patients are going to the therapy department with suctioning machines that therapists are expected to use until assisted coughing is possible. Suctioning is not a good long-term solution because it irritates the lining of the bronchial tubes (2). This stimulates more secretion and eventually causes scarring and stenosis. Therefore, assisted coughing is started by everyone on the team as soon as possible.

The inability to cough may be due to an absent cough reflex, the inability to take a deep breath, or the inability to forcefully exhale (2). Each deficit requires a separate solution. The therapist may have to stimulate the cough reflex by applying a few drops of sterile water in the tracheotomy to irritate the back of the throat to initiate coughing. The inability to take a deep breath is essential because you can't cough without sufficient air in your lungs. The therapist can use an Ambu bag if the patient isn't on a ventilator to force extra air into the lungs just before coughing. The inability to forcefully exhale can be facilitated with an "abdominal thrust" and "ptussive squeeze." Compression is applied on the abdomen and over the ribs a few seconds before the patient tries to cough. A video entitled "Towards Independence: Assisted Cough" clearly demonstrates all these techniques (2).

Adequate oxygen exchange is ensured by observing the rate, rhythm, and location of breathing. **Rate** is mea-

sured in breaths per minute. It is normal for a newborn to have a resting rate of 85 breaths per minute. A normal adult at rest breathes between 15 and 20 times per minute. **Rhythm** can be regular or irregular and deep or shallow. For example, Chene-Stokes breathing is characterized by shallow, then deep, then shallow breaths, and then finally no breathing. This is abnormal but not fatal. Hyperventilation creates a gasping rhythm that blows off excessive amounts of CO_2. This can lead to dizziness and, if severe enough, to tetany and cyanosis. Kuss-mal rhythm is constant heavy breathing associated with diabetic acidosis.

The **location** of breathing is reported by naming the body parts that are visibly moving during respiration. Movement of the belly is normal. When patients become anxious, the upper chest also begins to expand during inspiration. Most abnormal of all is "reverse breathing" or "sternal notching" while at rest. A visible notch appears at the top of the sternum every time the tendons of the sternocleidomastoid muscle bow out at their insertion. In normal individuals, the accessory muscles for inspiration, like the sternocleidomastoid, are recruited only during exertion. However, patients with a weak diaphragm and weak external intercostals have to recruit accessory muscles for inspiration, even at rest. A patient with "sternal notching" AT REST cannot be stressed aerobically until the primary inspiratory muscles are strengthened. Abnormal rates, rhythm, and location should be monitored and reported.

Eventually, the patient's vital capacity needs to be increased to at least 2,000 to 2,500 cc to support activity (1). **Vital capacity** is the total volume of gas exchanged between maximum inhalation and maximum exhalation. Increasing vital capacity is achieved by using procedures that gradually strengthen the respiratory muscles. For example, the physician may prescribe Triflow exercises. The patient must elevate the plastic ball inside the clear Triflow tube by taking a deep breath and then exhaling into the apparatus for as long as possible. The goals for this procedure are determined by the physician. These exercises are repeated every hour or so throughout the patient's daily routine. The therapist is expected to set time aside during therapy to do Triflow exercises.

Inhalation of fluid from the stomach into the lungs must be prevented by using an aspirator that removes this excess fluid. The aspirator applies suction through a nasogastric (NG) tube that goes into the stomach. An NG tube is used until internal bleeding can be brought under control or excess bile and stomach acid secretions are metabolized as gastrointestinal (GI) function returns. For example, 5% of spinal cord patients have GI bleeding and an absence of peristalsis for the first week post-injury (3). The NG tube is removed as soon as bowel sounds return. The nurse records the amount of fluid removed each day. The therapist needs to check daily totals to track the patient's progress, which determines how aggressive therapy can be.

Finally, the therapist and nurse are essential for control of pulmonary emboli. These blood clots have very serious consequences, but they can be dissolved by using medication and observation. The therapist should check the medical chart to see if the patient is taking an anticoagulant, like heparin, to prevent clots from forming, or a thrombolytic drug, like streptokinase, which promotes digestion of fibrin to dissolve the clot (4). These drugs are a warning that an embolus is a potential or continuing problem. The therapist should immediately call the nurse or doctor if he/she observes a sudden onset of chest pain, shoulder pain, or dyspnea in these high-risk patients.

CARDIOVASCULAR SYSTEM

Myocardial infarction (MI) and congestive heart failure (CHF) are two common ailments of the cardiovascular system. Both are life-threatening and require the use of observation to detects signs and symptoms. While both conditions produce dyspnea, angina, arrhythmias, and fatigue, other signs and symptoms help to differentiate these two conditions. An MI is characterized by diaphoresis and nausea or vomiting, while CHF is characterized by peripheral edema, audible lung congestion, and confusion or inattentiveness. Of the two conditions, CHF is more likely to be overlooked. This is a chronic condition that may be omitted in the medical chart because it is not the presenting diagnosis for the current admission to the hospital. Confusion or inattention can also be misinterpreted as senility or cognitive impairment. Immediate reporting of these signs and symptoms

guide the physician's plan of care so he/she can supervise the therapist.

Cardiac symptoms need to be described as concretely as possible. Chest pain can be described by location (e.g., at the incision site), intensity (on a scale of 1 to 4), duration (over 15 minutes is more serious), and type (e.g., burning). Dyspnea can be described by noting how many breaths it takes for the patient to count from 1 to 15 (i.e., three or more breaths is considered serious). It is also helpful for the therapist to note what activity the patient was performing when the symptoms occurred. A pattern may emerge that can be modified during the next treatment session.

Both an acute MI and chronic CHF require the use of procedures that enforce intermittent rest (see Table 17.2). Objective signs can provide guidelines that ensure rest. A normal adult has a resting heart rate (HR) of 60 to 100 beats per minute (BPM) and a resting blood pressure reading of 120/80. If a patient exceeds these norms while at rest, the therapist should talk to the physician before starting any treatment. The therapist should provide rest for acutely ill patients if the HR goes up more than 20 to 30 BPM during an activity, the HR does not return to baseline after resting for 5 minutes after an activity, or the systolic BP goes up more than 20 mm or doesn't go up at all. Some physicians set a target HR and BP that the therapist must not exceed. These signs are invaluable even for patients with cardiac telemetry. Artifacts in the printout can occur if the patient sneezes, coughs, moves, or starts to sweat. Therapists are not legally qualified to interpret EKG strips, but they can stop treatment and call the physician if the EKG readings suddenly change. Energy conservation procedures can also ensure rest and are explained in the chapter on rehabilitation.

Patients who don't have a heart condition can still have cardiovascular problems. **Orthostatic hypotension** is a sudden loss of blood pressure when sitting or standing up. It can occur in any patient who is deconditioned from extended bed rest. It is important to find out from the nurses when a patient on strict bed rest first receives orders to "dangle at bedside." This means letting the patient sit up on the side of the bed with legs dangling over the edge and constant supervision. While orthostatic hypotension is not life-threatening, it is frightening and dangerous for patients to pass out and fall down. The therapist can gradually reverse orthostatic hypotension by making sure the patient is wearing equipment during therapy that substitutes for loss of the calf muscle pump, such as elastic stockings, and by incorporating proper positioning, which gradually stresses the cardiovascular system in every treatment session.

Deep vein thromboses (DVTs) can be very dangerous if they break loose. Therapists must carefully watch

Table 17.2.
Homeostasis: Postulates

Goals: By System	Method/Rationale	Application: Examples
II. *Cardiovascular System* A. *Myocardial infarction* will be repaired by using	*Observation*, which detects signs and symptoms	1. Report dyspnea/fatigue/angina/arhythmias; diaphoresis/nausea 2. Monitor HR/BP telemetry
	Procedures, that enforce rest	1. Follow HR/BP guidelines 2. Use energy conservation
B. *Congestive heart failure* will be monitored by using	*Observation*, which detects signs and symptoms	1. Report dyspnea/fatigue/angina/arrhythmias; peripheral edema/lung congestion/confusion 2. Monitor HR/BP
	Procedures, that ensure rest	1. Follow HR/BP guidelines 2. Use energy conservation
C. *Orthostatic hypotension* will be reversed by using	*Equipment*, that substitutes for loss of vasoconstriction and calf muscle pump	1. Abdominal binders 2. TEDs stocking/Ace leg wraps
	Positioning, which gradually stresses the cardiovascular system	1. Raise head of bed gradually 2. Gradually raise reclining W/C
D. *Deep vein thrombosis* (DVTs) will be reversed by using	*Observation*, which detects signs	Report unilateral limb swelling and localized increase in body temperature
	Procedures, which prevent clots from being dislodged before they can be dissolved	1. D/C ROM of involved area 2. Limb compression and elevation
	Drugs, that prevent clot formation	Check chart for anticoagulants
	Drugs, that dissolve clots	Check chart for thrombolytics
E. *Severe peripheral edema* will be reduced by using	*Procedures*, that release dangerously high peripheral pressure that are compressing local structures	1. Escharotomy for circumferential burns 2. Fasciotomy

for unilateral swelling and localized increase in body temperature of a limb. If these signs are present, the therapist should stop treatment IMMEDIATELY and call the physician. Compression and elevation of the extremity while on bed rest are used to prevent clots from being dislodged. The therapist should look in the medical chart for prescription of anticoagulants and thrombolytic drugs just as he/she does for pulmonary emboli.

Limb-threatening peripheral edema produces compression of blood vessels and nerves that is severe enough to require amputation if left untreated. Escharotomies and fasciotomies are the procedures used to deal with these vascular problems. Readings on burns and hand injuries are good places to look if you need an explanation of this material. Less severe forms of peripheral edema are discussed in the biomechanical frame of reference because it restricts range of motion.

IMMUNE SYSTEM

Infections can be prevented by using drugs that kill infectious agents, procedures that remove exudates, and procedures that prevent transmission (see Table 17.3). Doctors often prescribe antibiotics to prevent infection in cases at high risk. To be forewarned about the poten-

tial for infection, check the chart for drugs such as antibiotics. The spread of infections can also be prevented by using procedures that remove exudates as a medium for germ growth. For example, therapists may teach outpatients how to clean the metal pins that are stabilizing a fracture. Before treating a patient, therapists should ask the nurse to change soiled dressings. This removes exudate and will prevent the wound from being abraded during movement by sticky or stiff dressings. Being present for dressing changes gives the therapist a chance to see the current state of the wound. For example, newly grafted skin that is purple with yellow spots is probably infected (5).

The spread of infections can be prevented by using universal precautions, which prevent the transmission of germs. Infections that can be transmitted include *Staphylococcus* and ringworm (skin), hepatitis and *Salmonella* (food and feces), tuberculosis (mucous), mononucleosis (saliva), and AIDS (blood and genital fluids) (6). Universal precautions are necessary to protect the therapist and to prevent the therapist from transmitting an infection from one patient to the next. Patients who get insulted when you put on gloves may not understand that you are considering their safety as you move from patient to patient.

Table 17.3.
Homeostasis: Postulates

Goals: By System	Method/Rationale	Application: Examples
III. *Immune System* *Infections* will be prevented by using	*Drugs*, which kill infectious agents	Check chart for antibiotics
	Procedures, that remove exudates as a medium for germ growth	1. Pin care for hand patient 2. Report soiled dressing to nurse
	Procedures, that prevent transmission	*Universal precautions:* 1. Wear gloves each and every time you expect to come in contact with body fluids, and remove them immediately 2. Promptly wash hands and surfaces that come in contact with body fluids 3. Handle sharp instruments and soiled linen carefully 4. Mask and gown with TB patients
IV. *Integumentary System* A. *Decubiti* will be prevented by using ALL of the following methods, if necessary	*Observation*, which detects early signs of skin breakdown	1. Pressure mark: Red but still blanches; redness disappears after 20–30 minutes 2. Pressure area: Red or red-blue; doesn't blanch well; feels mushy; redness disappears after several hours
	Procedures, that temporarily relieve pressure over bony prominences	1. Push-up on armrest of wheelchair 2. Lateral or forward weight-shift
	Equipment, that redistributes pressure across wider area	1. W/C seat cushion 2. Hardwood W/C seat insert
	Equipment, that eliminates pressure over bony prominences	1. Sacral cut-out in W/C 2. Foam donut 3. Lie prone or side-lie on gurney cart
B. Wound Healing	See Immune System: preventing infection and biomechanical frame of reference: maintaining ROM	

Universal precautions prevent contact with blood or any body fluids that contain blood, whether the blood is visible or not. This can include saliva, mucous, urine, vaginal fluids, spinal fluid, and synovial fluid (6, 7). Universal precautions are especially important whenever you have a break in your own skin, even something as small as a paper cut conner rash, or hangnail. Occupational therapists come in frequent contact with body fluids. Examples include making a splint for a limb with an open wound, suctioning a patient, providing oral motor facilitation, engaging in toilet, bathing, and dressing training, transferring a patient with a catheter, teaching skin and stump care, and changing soiled sheets on mat tables.

You must use physical barriers such as gloves EACH AND EVERY time you anticipate contact with body fluids. You must also remove the gloves before touching anything else, like a bed rail or nurse's call button (6, 7). Failure to immediately remove the gloves transfers infectious agents to environmental surfaces. If a lab coat has been exposed to body fluids, you should put on a clean lab coat before going to lunch or working with another patient. Your facility must provide gloves and launder lab coats for you (6, 7). Ask your supervisor to show you how to safely put on and take off gloves and lab coats.

If you experience unplanned contact with body fluids, you should immediately implement decontamination procedures (6). Promptly wash all exposed skin and eye wear. Think about what you may have on your hands before you eat, smoke, apply eye make-up, or put in contact lenses. Hand-washing is your best defense against infection. Washing is especially effective with the AIDS virus, which is easily killed by soap and water (6). It is also important to quickly clean environmental surfaces. Waiting for housekeeping to clean the floor or table top can result in body fluids being spread all over the OT department by people and by objects like wheelchairs and exercise equipment. Use an EPA-approved solution like water with 10% bleach (6). Finally, it is important to avoid shaking out soiled sheets. Roll the sheet in on itself and dispose of it immediately in the proper container.

Wet, dripping, or oozing materials are regulated waste (6). They must be put in closable containers that prevent leakage. These materials must be deposited into a color-coded receptacle (e.g., red basket liner in a metal can with a foot pedal). Regulated waste must be collected separately from other trash. Soiled linen must not be put in regular laundry carts.

One instance when wearing gloves is not sufficient is working with patients with tuberculosis. These patients will have a sign posted on their door indicating that everyone should put on a mask and gown in addition to gloves. Since the tuberculosis bacillus is quite large, it cannot pass through these simple physical barriers (8).

Universal precautions also include handling sharp instruments carefully (6, 7). For occupational therapists, this includes IV needles that pull out during exercise or ADLs, needles used during needlework, scissors used during splint-making, and woodworking tools. Report all sticks immediately by following the procedures of your facility's Post Exposure Plan.

INTEGUMENTARY SYSTEM

The skin is one of the most vital organs in the body. It protects against infection, controls body temperature, maintains proper fluid balance, and provides sensory input (5). After burns and other traumatic injuries, decubiti are the most common cause of skin loss. If the staff fail to prevent a decubitus, the patient will require surgery and several months of totally weight-free positioning to heal. This is an expensive and devastating process, which is why experienced therapists use all available methods to prevent decubiti (see Table 17.3).

High-risk patients include people who are bed-ridden, wheelchair-bound, wear splints, have poor sensation, or have poor circulation. Patients with many diagnoses are at high risk for decubiti. These include patients with advanced diabetes, burns, spinal cord injuries, and elderly patients with thin, frail skin.

The therapist should check the bony prominences of high-risk patients during every treatment session regardless of how many other people are checking the patient's skin. Patients should be begin skin self-inspection for pressure marks and pressure areas as soon as possible. The staff member designated to teach this procedure varies from facility to facility. The patient trainer may be the therapist, the nurse, or even the social worker.

The first line of defense against decubiti is observation of signs that detect skin damage in various stages (9). **Pressure marks** are characterized by reddened skin that still blanches when pressure is briefly applied with a finger. Once pressure is relieved, the redness usually disappears in 20 to 30 minutes. A **pressure area** is characterized by skin that is red or red-blue and does not blanch well. The flesh feels mushy. The redness requires several hours to disappear. A pressure area indicates that damage to underlying tissues has occurred, even though the skin looks intact. Once a hole in the skin appears, damage to underlying tissue may already be extensive, but it's hard to tell if muscle and bone necrosis have set in until the wound is debrided. As the *Merck Manual* describes, "The ulcer is like an iceberg, a small visible surface with an extensive unknown base" (10,

p. 2449). A hole in the skin is not a good method of early detection, which is why knowing about pressure marks and pressure areas is so important!

The second line of defense is procedures that temporarily relieve pressure from bony prominences. These procedures should be implemented as soon as a pressure MARK is found! Patients with spinal cord injuries are told to shift their weight off of their buttock for 30 seconds every 30 minutes. Pictures of weight shifts to relieve pressure are available in the spinal cord literature, but they can apply to any patient.

If pressure MARKS persist or turn into pressure AREAS, you must go to your third line of defense. This is equipment that can either redistribute pressure across a wider surface area, such as a seat cushion, or can eliminate pressure completely, such as a rubber donut for the heel. The patient may even have to come to therapy lying on a gurney cart. Examples of equipment are listed on Table 17.3. Discussions about this equipment are most prevalent in chapters on closed-head and spinal cord injury.

Therapists are often consulted as experts on seat cushions for wheelchairs. Specific seat cushions are good for different situations. For example, in one study, patients with spinal cord injury had more trochanter decubiti with the Jay cushion (11). The ROHO cushion provided better pressure relief, but the spinal cord-injured patients initially felt unstable on this cushion. The sides of the ROHO cushion are not sloped like the Jay cushion. Therapists have to take many issues into account when recommending seat cushions.

The therapist's concern for the integumentary system also includes wound healing. For example, open reduction of traumatic hand injuries is common today. Surgeons often elect to leave the skin open until the exudate is reduced. The therapist's role during wound healing focuses on control of infection and maintenance of ROM. See the chapter on the biomechanical frame of reference for an extensive discussion on maintenance of ROM during wound healing.

METABOLIC SYSTEM

Two problems commonly seen by therapists are patients with diabetes or electrolyte imbalance. Patients with diabetes often end up in therapy because it often leads to a stroke, heart attack, or amputation. The therapist's primary responsibility is to observe for signs and symptoms of diabetic coma and insulin shock, which can emerge as the therapeutic regime stresses the patient (see Table 17.4). It is especially practical for the therapist to monitor skin condition, pulse, and breathing patterns. In diabetic coma, the patient presents the paradox of dry, red skin with labored breathing and rapid pulse. In insulin shock, the patient presents the paradox of

Table 17.4.
Homeostasis: Postulates

Goals: By System	Method/Rationale	Application: Examples
V. *Metabolic System* 　A. *Diabetic coma* will be 　　reversed by using	*Observation*, which detects signs and symptoms	Report dry red skin with labored breathing and rapid pulse; headache; irritability; nausea; vomiting
	Drugs, which reverse imbalance	Call nurse to give insulin
	Procedures to prevent imbalance	Modulate level of exertion
B. *Insulin shock* will be 　　reversed by using	*Observation*, which detects sign and symptoms	Report sweaty pale skin with shallow respiration and normal pulse; abnormal behavior; double or blurred vision
	Food, which reverses imbalance	Call nurse to give orange juice
	Procedures to prevent imbalance	Modulate level of exertion
C. *Electrolyte imbalance/ 　　protein deficiency* will 　　be reversed by using	*Procedures*, that reverse protein and electrolyte imbalance	1. Track protein supplements 2. Handle IV tubing safely to prevent dislodgement
VI. *Urologic System* 　A. *Infections* will be 　　prevented by using	*Procedures*, that prevent return of waste products to bladder	Prevent catheter backflow and dislodgement
	Procedures that prevent stagnation of waste products	Force fluids per doctor's orders
B. *Bladder-emptying* will 　　be achieved by using	*Procedures* that substitute for voluntary initiation	Intermittent catheterization program
	Equipment that collects urine	1. Male external collection devices 2. Indwelling catheter

cold, sweaty, pale skin with shallow respiration and a normal pulse. A patient slipping into diabetic coma may also exhibit irritability and complain of nausea and headache. The patient slipping to insulin shock may exhibit abnormal behavior and complain about blurred or double vision.

While therapists don't administer insulin and orange juice to restore metabolic balance, they are expected to stop treatment and call the nurse if diabetic coma or insulin shock occur. The nurse may come down to the therapy department or have the patient transported back to the nursing floor. Therapists are definitely expected to modulate the patient's level of exertion. Every time the patient becomes more physically active, insulin levels have to be readjusted. Minor imbalances of insulin, food intake, and exertion are inevitable until the patient's activity level finally plateaus. This makes observation and modulation of exertion a daily necessity.

Electrolyte imbalance is a common metabolic problem in critically ill patients. For example, a patient with a massive burn has massive fluid loss, which results in low protein levels. If this protein deprivation is not corrected, the patient will begin to break down his/her own muscles for protein (5). While the therapist doesn't insert IVs or provide protein supplements, he/she should track these procedures on a daily basis. Tolerance for protein supplements and IVs cannot be assumed.

Protein supplements taste terrible; IVs become infiltrated or get pulled out. Since fluctuations in electrolyte balance can occur hourly, it is worthwhile to check the nurse's notes every day before treating such a patient. A nurse's observations can help the therapist predict the patient's tolerance for stress, tendency to pass out, and ability to attend and recall instructions.

Therapists use common sense when dealing with IVs. They should handle IV tubes safely and tell the nurses whenever an IV has been pulled out. When rolling, dressing, and transferring patients, the therapist should first make sure there is sufficient slack in the tubing. Move the IV pole close to the patient and trace the full length of the tube to make sure it is clear. The tubing can get caught under the patient or stuck in the bedrail. Once you take the IV bag down to move it, always make sure it is kept elevated above the heart to prevent backflow! When dressing a patient, pass the IV bag through the sleeve before having the patient put on the garment. These simple precautions are easy to remember once they become a habit.

UROLOGIC SYSTEM

Bladder infections can cause the patient to miss therapy sessions and eventually lead to kidney shutdown and death. The therapist must use correct procedures to prevent catheter backflow and dislodgement (see Table

17.4). Backflow can cause bladder infections by returning stagnant waste products in the collection bag to the dark, warm environment created by the bladder. Backflow is prevented by *always* holding and hooking the collection bag on a fixture that is *lower* than the patient's bladder. The bag and tube quickly become coated with solid wastes that will be dumped back into the bladder if the bag is raised high enough. For example, *don't* hook the bag on the head of the bed or the wheelchair armrest or backrest! Tube dislodgement can be prevented by carefully freeing the tube from sheets, bedrails, and other obstructions and by moving the collection bag *first* to make sure there is sufficient slack in the tube. If the tube will not reach to the new location, you need to know *before* you start to move the patient! Tube dislodgement can pull the catheter out while the balloon at the end of the tube is still inflated. This balloon can injure the lining of the urethra and make it prone to infection.

Another procedure to prevent bladder infections is to force fluids when prescribed by the physician. Large amounts of fluid create a high turnover rate of urine. This means the therapist must offer water or other fluid during every treatment session and report the number of cc's to the nurses. Forcing fluids is safe if the patient has voluntary control or has an indwelling catheter. Conversely, fluids should be restricted for patients on an intermittent catheterization program to prevent dangerous overdistension of the bladder.

An empty bladder prevents infections because it has no medium for germ growth. Bladder emptying will be achieved by equipment that collects urine, like cathethers, and by procedures that substitute for voluntary initiation. For example, a spinal cord patient with an upper motor neuron injury can learn to initiate bladder emptying by reflex action (3). Gentle suprapubic tapping or stroking of the inner thigh is done BEFORE catheterization to stimulate reflex emptying. The patient is then temporarily catheterized to remove and measure any residual urine. This procedure is repeated every 4 hours until the patient begins to consistently have postvoid residuals of 50 to 100 cc. The intervals between catheterizations can then be gradually lengthened. Eventually, the patient just keeps track of fluid intake, which enables him to predict when the bladder will become sufficiently distended to ensure reflex emptying. The daily routine is then scheduled around these predictable times. This program can succeed only if the therapist adjusts the therapy schedule to accommodate it.

SKELETAL SYSTEM

Three skeletal deficits that can interfere with accelerated treatment are osteoporosis, heterotopic ossification, and fractures. Osteoporosis can be prevented or retarded by using procedures that gradually stress the bones (see Table 17.5). Without weightbearing, the bone begins to dissolve. Progressively longer periods of weightbearing will be prescribed by the physician as early as possible. Weightbearing is prescribed even if a limb will not regain voluntary movement because eventually the slightest movement by an attendant can fracture a bone with severe osteoporosis. The occupational therapist usually incorporates weightbearing into other activities, such as working in a standing table, rather than letting the patient sit or stand idly.

The therapist must be alert for heterotopic ossification in patients with spinal cord injury, severe burns, traumatic head injuries, and some types of muscular dystrophy. Signs and symptoms include heat, swelling, loss of passive range of motion, and complaints of pain in a particular joint. The joints most commonly affected are the shoulders, hips, elbows, and knees. Ankylosis of the joint will occur if the ossification is not detected early and treated immediately. The procedure that retards the laying down of bony tissue in these joints is aggressive ROM. This procedure will be uncomfortable for the patient, but he/she needs to know that the alternative is complete loss of range of motion if this condition is not treated.

Fractures could be placed in either the homeostasis or biomechanical chapters. Since biomechanical techniques, such as partial range of motion, may be prescribed by the physician before fractures are completely healed, I am concerned about separating fracture considerations from biomechanical techniques. For this reason, I have placed fractures in the chapter on the biomechanical frame of reference, where the discussion can be simultaneous.

AUTONOMIC NERVOUS SYSTEM

Autonomic dysreflexia is a vasomotor response characterized by a sudden onset of a severe pounding headache, severely increased blood pressure, and flushing and diaphoresis above the level of the spinal cord lesion (3). It can be interrupted by procedures that decrease blood pressure (see Table 17.5). For example, sitting the patient upright helps the blood pool in the lower extremities and lowers the blood pressure. It can also be interrupted by procedures that remove the noxious stimulus that caused the reaction. Some of these procedures are implemented by the nurse, like catheterizing a patient with an overdistended bladder or loosening impacted bowels. Other procedures can be implemented by the therapist, including unkinking the catheter tubing and emptying an overfilled catheter bag.

Temperature control can be maintained by using simple procedures like putting on or taking off clothing.

Table 17.5.
Homeostasis: Postulates

Goals: By System	Method/Rationale	Application: Examples
VII. *Skeletal System* A. *Osteoporosis* will be prevented by using	*Procedures* that gradually stress the bone matrix through weightbearing	1. Standing table 2. Sitting in W/C
B. *Heterotopic ossification* will be prevented by using	*Observations,* which detect signs and symptoms	Heat, pain, swelling, and loss of ROM of a specific joint
	Procedures that retard the laying down of bony tissue in joint spaces	Aggressive passive ROM
C. *Fractures*	See biomechanical frame of reference: structural stability for treatment methods	
VIII. *Autonomic Nervous System*	*Observation,* which detects signs	Sudden severe pounding headache; severely increased BP; flushing and diaphoresis above level of SCI
A. *Autonomic dysreflexia* will be interrupted by using	*Procedures* that decrease blood pressure	1. Immediately sit patient *UP* 2. Monitor BP until stable
	Procedures that remove noxious stimuli	Unkink catheter tube, loosen impacted bowels, etc.
B. *Temperature* will be maintained using	*Procedures* that normalize body temperature	1. Cooling fan/turn up heat 2. Put on extra clothing
C. *Stress ulcers* will be eliminated by using	*Procedures* that reduce stress	1. Relaxation techniques 2. Counseling

Stress ulcers are a less easily remediated autonomic nervous system response. Procedures that reduce stress, such as relaxation techniques, may be implemented by the therapist, psychologist, nurse, or social worker.

SUMMARY

The therapist's role in homeostasis is highly variable. It varies from facility to facility, patient to patient, and even day to day. To meet this varying need, therapists must understand the homeostatic goals and procedures prescribed by the physician, observe their patients carefully and consistently, and communicate daily with physicians and nurses.

Yet, the therapist doesn't just observe and report. Recovery of homeostasis is also dependent on the therapist's actions. The therapist is responsible for implementing precautions, performing some lifesaving procedures, scheduling therapy time around homeostatic programs, being flexible when homeostatic issues disrupt therapy plans, and explaining homeostatic procedures to the patient. Therapists have a dozen small opportunities each day to hasten the patient's return to a stable medical state (see Memory Aid 17.1).

STUDY QUESTIONS

NOTE: Many of these study questions are not easy to answer by just skimming this chapter. Intensive reading is recommended!

1. Why must the therapist know how to assess signs and symptoms independently?

2. What equipment, procedures, and observations are therapists responsible for to ensure adequate oxygen exchange and increase vital capacity?
3. What are the signs and symptoms that differentiate between a pulmonary embolus and DVTs?
4. What are the signs and symptoms that differentiate between a myocardial infarction and congestive heart failure?
5. Where should you look for warnings that local or systemic infection control procedures have been ordered?
6. What is the difference between a pressure mark and a pressure area?
7. What procedures and equipment are used to prevent decubiti?
8. How do skin conditions and breathing patterns differ for diabetic coma and insulin shock?
9. What procedures does the therapist implement for electrolyte imbalance?
10. Do you lower or raise the IV bag? Do you lower or raise the catheter bag? Why?
11. When do you force fluids, and when do you restrict fluids?
12. What is the difference between treating osteoporosis and treating heterotopic ossification?
13. Why do you sit a patient up when he/she has autonomic dysreflexia but lie him/her down when he/she has orthostatic hypotension?
14. How do the procedures for orthostatic hypotension and autonomic dysreflexia differ?

Memory Aid 17.1.

Homeostatic Issues

I. Respiratory System

   A. Oxygen exchange
   B. Vital capacity
   C. Aspiration
   D. Pulmonary emboli

II. Cardiovascular System

   A. Myocardial infarction
   B. Congestive heart failure
   C. Orthostatic hypotension
   D. Deep vein thrombosis
   E. Peripheral edema, only if it is limb-threatening
      (See chapter on biomechanical frame of reference to learn
      how reduce edema that impairs ROM)

III. Immune System

   A. Infections

IV. Integumentary System

   A. Decubiti
   B. Wound healing

V. Metabolic System

   A. Diabetic coma
   B. Insulin shock
   C. Electrolyte imbalance
   D. Protein deficiency

VI. Urologic System

   A. Infections
   B. Emptying

VII. Skeletal System

   A. Osteoporosis
   B. Heterotopic ossification
      (Fractures discussed in "Structural Stability" section of
      chapter on biomechanical frame of reference)

VIII. Autonomic Nervous System

   A. Autonomic dysreflexia
   B. Temperature control
   C. Stress ulcers

References

1. Affleck A, Lieverman SL, Polon JP, Rohrkemper KR. Providing occupational therapy in an intensive care unit. Am J Occup Ther 1986;40:323.
2. Dallas Rehabilitation Foundation. Toward independence: Assisted cough (videocassette). Dallas, 1987.
3. Kraft C. Bladder and bowel management. In: Buchanan LE, Nawoczenski DA, eds. Spinal cord injury. Baltimore: Williams & Wilkins, 1987:81.
4. Poe TE. Pharmacology. In: Malone T. Physical and occupational therapy: drug implications for practice. Philadelphia: JB Lippincott, 1989:15.
5. Crouthammel R. Burn rehabilitation. Lecture presented at Temple University, 1990.
6. National Safety Council. Bloodborne pathogens. Boston: Jones and Bartlett, 1993.
7. Medcom, Inc. Universal Precautions: AIDS and hepatitis B (videocassette). Garden Grove, CA, 1991.
8. Silverman B. Controlling infectious diseases. Lecture presented at Temple University, 1992.
9. Dallas Rehabilitation Foundation. Toward independence: important considerations in wheelchair seating (videocassette). Dallas, 1987.
10. Berkow R, editor-in-chief. Merck manual. 16th ed. Rahway, NJ: Merck Research Laboratories, 1992:2449.
11. Garber SL, Dylerly LR. Wheelchair cushions for persons with spinal cord injury: an update. Am J Occup Ther 1991;45:550.

SECTION VI

COMBINING FRAMES OF REFERENCE

CHAPTER 18

Case Simulation: Burns

Therapists use more than one frame of reference to treat a single patient. As the "Deficits Not Addressed" sections in the case simulations show, a single frame of reference cannot address all the domains of concern that have an impact on a person's life. Therapists who combine frames of reference use an eclectic approach. This doesn't mean that they have abandoned frames of reference. It means that they go shopping for the best prescriptive mix that meets each individual's needs.

As this chapter will show, different approaches can intertwine so smoothly that it may be difficult to see where one frame of reference ends and the next begins. See Figure 18.1 for one example of how postulates regarding intervention from different frames of reference can be seamlessly combined in a single treatment session. Note that frames of reference are not stated explicitly; they are implied by the type of methods used.

One strategy for combining frames of reference is to use the procedural track to turn what we know about the different stages of recovery for a disease into a plan for action. A single frame of reference has to shift its procedural focus as stage-specific causes change. For example, sensory-motor concerns for a burn patient may shift from pain of the burn site during the pre-grafting stage to hypersensitivity of grafted skin during the post-grafting stage. The importance of one frame of reference can also diminish while another becomes more dominant as stage specific causes change. For example, during the grafting stage, homeostatic concerns like fluid loss may be significantly reduced, while psychosocial concerns, such as unrealistic expectations for the cosmetic appearance of skin grafts, may become paramount.

A second strategy for combining frames of reference is to use the interactive track to turn what we know about the person's life and what we can hypothesize about his/her reactions into a plan for action. Data that can be gathered quickly include information about roles and the presence of family members. Additional data like values, interests, environmental demands, and environmental resources can be obtained through subsequent conversations with the patient and family. This information will definitely affect the therapist's discharge goals.

A third strategy for combining frames of reference is to use the guidelines for prioritizing goals, as discussed in Chapter 2. These guidelines suggest that particular frames of reference take center stage when they address concerns that are too dangerous to leave untreated, are functionally significant, have the potential for short-term change, or must be treated directly. For example, during the pre-grafting stage, homeostatic issues like infection are paramount. However, biomechanical issues, like increasing strength, may be too dangerous to address in the same period.

The easiest way to show you how frames of reference are combined is to use the burn case study described in Chapter 2 as a model. This chapter has been divided into three sections for the pre-grafting, grafting, and post-grafting stages of recovery for burns. Each section contains procedural and interactive hypotheses, a list of concerns for this particular patient, and suggestions for prioritizing short-term goals. In addition, each section has been organized by the domains of concern listed in Memory Aid 2.2, so you may want to look at this memory aid as you read. The chapter ends with a brief visit to the interactive track.

PRE-GRAFTING STAGE

Procedural and Interactive Hypotheses

Homeostatic concerns during the pre-grafting stage are dominated by the respiratory, vascular, integumentary, immune, and metabolic systems. The shock phase usually lasts for 2 to 3 days after the injury (1). If there is an inhalation burn, oxygen exchange may be impaired. When blood vessels are burned on all sides of an extrem-

Deficit/Cause/Goal/FO	Methods/Rationales	Specific Activity
Deficit: Unable to move LUE	*Elevation,* which allows gravity to remove excess peripheral fluids	*W/C arm trough* will be attached to left side of W/C. Patient's forearm and hand are positioned in the center of the trough whenever his/her arm is at rest.
Cause: edema, flexor synergy, spasticity, and left unilateral neglect secondary to CVA	*Pressure,* which reduces filtration of fluids out of the capillaries	*Retrograde massage* is administered to left hand for 5 minutes with patient's elbow resting on the table and forearm held in a vertical position by therapist.
Short-term Goals: —left hand volume 650 ml —passive elongation with minimal resistance at beginning of scapular protraction and moderate resistance at mid-range of supination —active weight shift on protracted scapula in side-lie with moderate physical assistance —look to left side 4 out of 5 times with constant cuing	*Passive elongation,* which gives sensation of elongated LUE	*Handling.* Patient lies supine on a mat table with therapist's hands under the scapula and cupping the posterior forearm while facing the patient. Gradually passively elongate patient's arm into scapular protraction and supination. After patient relaxes, have him/her roll into left side while the therapist maintains the scapula in protraction and forearm in supination.
Functional Outcome: patient will use RIPs during LUE dressing with intermittent cuing and minimal physical assistance	*Limb weight shifts,* which let patient initiate while therapist maintains inhibition	*Sorting laundry.* Patient is in side-lie with therapist's hands placed as described above and with a pillow under patient's head. Patient uses sound hand to sort towels and washcloths that are placed on a small table positioned at mat table height just below patient's shoulder height. Linens will be dropped in boxes placed on near left and far right corners of table. Therapist waits for patient to initiate rolling slightly forward to reach for and drop linens.
	Transfer of training approach, which remediates underlying deficits	*Sorting laundry.* Patient will be given constant verbal cuing to place linens in box on near left corner.

Figure 18.1. Combining Frames of Reference in Activities

ity from a circumferential burn, severe fluid accumulation can create a tourniquet effect (2). This can lead to limb ischemia and amputation if escharatomy is not performed (1). Skin loss creates the potential for toxic infections. Bacteria that live on dead tissue may be present by the fourth day, so septic shock and death are very real concerns (1). Finally, the loss of skin can also lead to life-threatening fluid loss (2). Fluid loss can result in electrolyte imbalance, loss of protein as the body metabolizes its own muscles, kidney shut-down, and finally death. Electrolyte imbalance may make the patient pass out, so elevating the patient into the upright position may have to be gradual (2).

Sensory-motor concerns in the pre-grafting stage include pain and loss of sensation. Second-degree burns are painful, partial thickness burns that expose nerve endings (3). However, it is not easy to accurately assess the depth of a burn. The true depth of a burn is most accurately assessed by the amount of time needed for it to heal (2). Areas that heal before 3 weeks are likely to be painful second-degree burns. It is ideal if the therapist can treat the patient soon after pain medications

have been administered (3). On the other hand, a third-degree burn that lacks sensation takes at least 3 weeks to heal. Try to picture doing sensory testing on an open wound to determine if sensation is absent. Until sensory testing can be done, the therapist must use clinical observation to identify areas that potentially lack sensation and prevent further damage to these burned body parts.

Biomechanical concerns in the pre-grafting stage include structural instability and edema. If the burn is severe enough, it can burn through the skin and expose damaged tendons. Finger tendons are not protected by a thick muscle mass. The lymphatic system may not be able to absorb the excess interstitial fluid, so there may be peripheral edema, which will affect ROM for at least 6 days (1). Edema is especially likely if the lymph nodes in the armpit were affected.

The loss of ROM and endurance should not be an issue. Even patients with severe burns often have full ROM during the acute stage (2). Since patients are asked to do self-care as early as possible, early ROM exercises are usually not done until the medical crisis is over (2). Loss of endurance is also not likely. Sitting and walking endurance can be maintained by making the patient sit up and walk as much as possible. Bed rest, full nursing care, and wheelchairs are no longer prescribed during the early stages of burn (2). Patients who are immobilized and given full assistance during this acute stage become fearful about moving later on (2).

The primary psychosocial concern may be the patient's loss of internal control. Loss of control may become evident if the patient doesn't understand the medical emergency procedures, which can be frightening and painful. Fear of death and mutilation are understandable. Stress reactions, such as depression, may not set in during this early stage because the patient is still in mental and physical shock.

In the perceptual-cognitive domain, attention and abstract reasoning must be informally assessed in the pre-grafting stage. It may be temporarily impaired due to pain and pain medications. Patients may remember very little of these first few days or become confused about what was done and said. Abstract reasoning could be impaired by an undetected closed head injury resulting from a car accident. If clinical signs are subtle, a mild closed head injury might temporarily go undetected while urgent homeostatic issues are addressed.

Rehabilitation concerns should be minimized during pre-grafting if there is a unilateral burn. Most ADLs can be performed one-handed. However, ADLs that require two hands, such as cutting meat and tying hospital scrub pants, may be impaired.

The next section explains how to identify which concerns have been confirmed for this particular patient and how to turn information about the medical condition and the person into a plan for action.

Initial Concerns During Pre-grafting

Pre-grafting concerns for this patient have been listed in Table 18.1. Medical and psychosocial information should be used to create a holistic picture of what has to be addressed by the occupational therapist.

Patient data were sparse at the time of admission (1). He is an automobile worker with deep second- and third-degree burns over 10% of his left arm and hand from a car accident. The burned areas include his left shoulder and axilla, the anterior surface of his left arm, and the dorsum of his left hand. He has a wife and two teenage sons. He is their sole source of support.

Two homeostatic concerns have been ruled out for this patient. Inhalation burn and limb-threatening edema are not present. There was no report of inhalation burn, and the patient was able to do all his self-care with no report of fatigue (1), so depressed respiration is probably not a problem. There is no evidence of a circumferential burn, and life-threatening edema was not reported. These data illustrate how the reader has to read between the lines of a medical chart. Wellness is often implied by a lack of data.

Homeostatic concerns for this patient in the pre-grafting stage include the immune and metabolic systems. Even a superficial burn can be turned into a full-thickness injury from infection (3). Therefore, the potential for infection makes universal precautions mandatory. The therapist must also be prepared to schedule therapy around dressing changes, which are an important way to remove exudate to prevent bacterial growth. During this 2- to 3-day period of shock, the therapist should track nutrition and electrolyte status daily in the nursing notes. Is he eating all of his high-calorie, high-protein diet? Can he walk without feeling faint? What are his complaints and vital signs? Only 10% of his body was burned, so metabolic concerns should be at a minimum. Yet how well the patient feels in general will affect his participation in therapy.

The sensory-motor concern about pain was confirmed. The patient complained of pain, but sensory testing was not done (1). It is assumed that the therapist was cautious about preventing damage to areas with third-degree burns that lack sensation.

Biomechanical concerns about structural instability and edema were confirmed. Precautions against active fist-making were ordered, so structural instability of the extensor tendons is likely (1). The patient should be told to avoid using his burned hand to grab his bed bar for support or pushing himself upright with his burned hand (2). In this particular case, only finger flexion was impaired by edema. Hand elevation was started immediately (1).

The initial evaluation shows that the predictions for normal ROM and endurance were only partially confirmed. This patient's AROM is normal except for shoulder flexion and abduction, which are limited to 145° and severe restrictions of AROM for MP, PIP, and DIP flexion (1). To maintain ROM, splints may be worn over the dressings of third-degree burns whenever the patient is at rest (2). This patient wore an axillary splint to maintain the shoulder in 90° of abduction, an elbow conformer splint to hold the elbow in 5° of flexion, and a hand splint to maintain the fingers in complete extension while at rest (1). The only splint that might be worn continuously, except during exercises and dressing changes, is the hand splint that protects the extensor tendons (1). The normal strength of his sound right arm was maintained by one-handed self-care activities. Strength data imply that endurance was maintained by an active self-care program.

No data were reported on psychosocial concerns. Yet it is unwise to assume that a verbal but highly stressed patient understands unfamiliar medical procedures. Early patient and family education are essential. The

Table 18.1.
Concerns for This Patient Across Stages of Recovery

Domains	Pre-Grafting Stage	Grafting Stage	Post-Grafting Stage
HOMEOSTASIS	Possible infection Possible fluid loss Possible electrolyte imbalance Ruled out inhalation burn	Possible infection	Possible stress ulcers Possible heterotopic ossification
SENSORY-MOTOR	Pain from second-degree burn Sensory loss from third-degree burn	Pain of donor site/graft sites Sensory loss from third-degree burn	Impaired coordination of left hand Hypersensitivity of skin
BIOMECHANICAL	Loss of structural stability of extensor tendons Edema of burned left hand Loss of ROM of burned LUE Ruled out loss of strength of RUE Ruled out loss of endurance	Loss of structural stability of grafted skin & donor site Edema of left hand/LLE donor site Loss of ROM of burned LUE Ruled out loss of strength of RUE Possible loss of sitting endurance	Possible loss of structural stability of dry grafted skin Possible scar formation to further reduce ROM of burned LUE Loss of ROM of burned LUE Loss of strength of left hand Possible loss of walking endurance
MOHO	Possible loss of internal control	Implied loss of internal control Need data on roles and interests Need data on human resources	Need data on values and habits Need data on financial resources Need data on expectations of family and employer
PSYCHOSOCIAL	Possible lack of understanding of emergency procedures Possible fear of mutilation	Possible lack of understanding of grafting precautions Possible unrealistic expectations for cosmetic appearance of grafts Depression and social withdrawal	Possible lack of understanding of scar prevention procedures Ruled out unrealistic expectations about loss of function Decreased stress reactions Need data on impact of inability to relieve tension with golf
COGNITIVE	Ruled out poor cognition due to pain, pain meds, head injury secondary to MVA		
REHABILITATION	Independent except for hair care despite fist-making precautions	Independent in self-care except for hair care	Need data on necessity of modified work tasks

occupational therapist often explains and makes sure the patient truly understands what is being done to him/her and why. Patient education often comes up in an unplanned way as the conversation warrants. The therapist must listen carefully to the patient to make sure that he/she understands what the therapist has said. In this case, fear of death is not likely because the patient is burned only over 10% of his body. The medical staff will reassure him about his good chance for survival. However, the fear of mutilation may cross his mind early because a deep second- or third-degree burn can look charred. More information is needed about the patient's fear of mutilation and his understanding of medical procedures.

The therapist reported that no cognitive deficits were observed (1). Potential cognitive deficits due to pain, pain medication, and a closed head injury have been ruled out.

Negligible self-care concerns were confirmed. Performing ADLs one-handed should be especially easy for this patient since his dominant hand was spared. Yet fist-making precautions created a problem with two-handed ADLs. He independently performed all self-care activities with one hand except for washing and combing his hair (1). The therapist probably provided adaptive devices, such as a rocker knife, to make the patient independent. Yet the nurse must make sure that the patient doesn't receive unnecessary assistance during self-care.

Priorities During the Pre-Grafting Stage

Refer to Table 18.2 to see a summary of pre-grafting priorities. The number 1 indicates the top priority in the short-term treatment plan for this patient.

Homeostatic concerns take top priority. For example, the therapist must do nothing to infect the wound or

Table 18.2.
Prioritizing Goals for This Patient

Pre-Grafting Stage	Grafting Stage	Post-Grafting Stage
#1 Prevent infection Track fluid loss and electrolyte imbalance Prevent structural damage of extensor tendons/third-degree burns that lack sensation Keep pain manageable	#1 Prevent infection Prevent structural damage of grafted skin/ donor site/third-degree burns that lack sensation	#1 Investigate understanding of scar prevention procedures Prevent scar formation of grafted skin
#2 Reduce edema of left hand Maintain ROM in burned LUE	#2 Reduce edema of left hand Prevent edema of LLE donor site Maintain ROM in burned LUE	#2 Prevent structural damage of dry grafted skin Reduce hypersensitivity of grafted skin Increase ROM of burned LUE Increase left hand strength Increase hand coordination
#3 Investigate locus of control and fear of mutilation Investigate understanding of emergency procedures	#3 Keep pain manageable Investigate locus of control/roles/interests/ human resources Investigate understanding of grafting procedures Investigate expectations for appearance of skin grafts Reduce stress reactions	#3 Investigate values/habits/financial resources Investigate expectations of family and employer
#4 Maintain strength in RUE Maintain endurance Independence in two-handed self-care except for hair care	#4 Maintain strength in RUE Maintain sitting endurance Independence in two-handed self-care except for hair care	#4 Explore importance of golf Increase walking endurance Investigate modified work Track stress ulcers/heterotopic ossification

rupture the extensor tendons. Therapy may have to be curtailed because of lightheadedness from electrolyte imbalance. It takes only a few minutes to do a chart review and talk to the nurse before treatment begins to address this highest priority.

Note the use of service goals for homeostatic concerns. Since only physicians are licensed to write homeostatic outcome goals, therapists don't write homeostatic goals in the medical record. Therefore, occupational therapy students don't learn about the therapist's role regarding homeostatic concerns from the chart.

Another top priority is prevention of further structural damage to extensor tendons and any areas that lack sensation due to a third-degree burn. Until sensory testing can be done and the true burn depth can be determined, the therapist must follow fist-making precautions and use ongoing clinical observation to do no harm and to keep pain manageable.

The following goals have first priority during pre-grafting. Note the use of chunking to make the short-term plan more manageable:

1a. Prevent infection and track daily fluid loss and electrolyte imbalance;

1b. Prevent all further structural damage to extensor tendons and areas with third-degree burns that lack sensation; and

1c. Keep pain manageable based on subjective patient report.

The second priority in the pre-grafting stage is to reduce edema and maintain ROM. Treatment of these biomechanical concerns creates little interference with medical procedures, so it is safe and easy to put them in the pre-grafting treatment plan. To control edema and maintain ROM, the patient's left arm and hand simply need to be elevated and splinted whenever he is at rest. The therapist makes the proper orthotics and comes to the patient's room to make final adjustments. Note the need to do baseline testing to make some of the following goals measurable:

2a. Reduce peripheral edema of hand based on finger AROM; and

2b. Maintain AROM of burned RUE based on initial evaluation.

Psychosocial concerns are the third most important priority during pre-grafting. The following concerns may make him noncompliant with lifesaving procedures. If he doesn't cooperate with medical procedures, he will impede his entire plan of care.

3a. Investigate loss of internal control/fears of mutilation; and

3b. Investigate whether he understands medical procedures.

Remediation of strength and endurance are the last priority as long as homeostatic concerns are still stressed. Excessive resistance and prolonged duration are not safe at this time. However, independence in self-care tasks should be sufficient to maintain these assets without direct therapist intervention.

4a. Maintain strength of uninvolved RUE per initial evaluation;

4b. Maintain sitting/walking endurance per initial evaluation; and

4c. Perform all self-care activities except for hair care.

GRAFTING STAGE

Procedural and Interactive Hypotheses

This stage lasts about 5 days for each graft. Temporary grafts, such as cadaver, pig, or family member's skin may be used to temporarily cover the wounds, but only an autograft (from the patient himself) will survive permanently (2). Infection continues to be a major concern.

Sensory-motor concerns shift focus during the grafting stage. The donor site may hurt more the burned area. Patients have compared the pain from the donor site to a really bad paper cut (2). Pain from the burn site is probably less of an issue now because the patient has been reassured by the liberal use of pain medications (1). Potential damage due to loss of sensation should be easier to prevent now. As burn depth is confirmed by the time needed to heal, precautions can focus on those areas that have finally been confirmed as third-degree burns.

Grafting creates new biomechanical problems. Newly grafted skin lives on plasma until it becomes connected with the capillary bed (3). Excessive movement can destroy this capillary linkage and cause the graft to die. Therefore, new grafts are kept totally immobilized for 24 hours a day for the first 4 to 5 days (2, 3).

A lower extremity donor site also requires edema prevention during the grafting stage. The already stressed capillary bed of the LE donor site will be overloaded as blood rushes to the legs when the patient stands up (1). Elastic bandages should be worn on the LEs and static standing, and dangling the legs should be avoided to prevent LE edema. No active exercise of

the LE donor site is done for 2 to 3 days postoperatively (1), and no ambulation should be done for 6 days (3).

The number of psychosocial concerns multiply in the grafting stage. The continued loss of internal control and lack of understanding of medical procedures are now compounded by other factors. First, many patients have unrealistic expectations about the cosmetic appearance of skin grafts (2). Grafting is "reconstructive surgery" that tries to reestablish normal function. Patients may begin to build unrealistic expectations of regaining a normal appearance once grafting begins.

Second, shock has passed, and normal stress reactions are likely to appear. This is a good time to listen for and validate the patient's normal emotional reactions to physical trauma. Mobility restrictions during grafting and the continued loss of privacy due to hospitalization may now make the patient more aware of his inability to relieve tension with strategies such as leisure activities, exercise, sex, and socializing.

Shift in Concerns During Grafting

Refer to Table 18.1 to see how the domains of concern change from the pre-grafting to the grafting stages of recovery. There is a subtle shift in the therapist's plan for action.

The number of homeostatic concerns decline during the grafting stage. Fluid loss is gradually being corrected by a series of grafts. Yet the therapist continues to be concerned with infection. Universal precautions are still in effect. It is especially helpful for the therapist to see the grafts during dressing changes. Infected grafts may appear purple with yellow spots. These findings should be reported immediately (2).

No data regarding loss of sensation from the third-degree burn or pain of the grafted skin and the donor site were reported. This suggests that these are ongoing concerns that are being addressed by routine precautions.

The grafting stage produces a dramatic shift in focus for the biomechanical concerns of structural instability and edema. Concerns about structural instability have shifted from the burned areas to the grafted skin and donor site as split-thickness grafts were applied to the left arm (1). Concern about edema has expanded to include the LLE donor site. The LE donor site should be wrapped with an elastic bandage to support the fragile capillary bed (1). Finger flexion was still impaired by edema.

Concerns about ROM also shift dramatically. Range of motion data were obtained prior to grafting because UE movement was restricted for 5 days post-grafting (1). Pre-grafting test results show that this patient's active ROM was normal except for shoulder flexion and abduction, which were limited to 145° and severe restrictions of active ROM for MP, PIP, and DIP flexion. Despite these restrictions, AROM was discontinued for 5 days to maintain structural stability of his newly grafted skin (1). To maintain ROM, he wore the axillary, elbow, and hand splints on the LUE 24 hours a day for 5 days (1).

Biomechanical concerns about maintaining strength in the RUE and sitting endurance are unchanged. Active and resistive ROM was done to maintain Good strength of the RUE (1). Good strength of his sound RUE was also maintained by performing one-handed self-care activities. Sitting endurance can be maintained by making the patient sit up as much as possible.

However, the biomechanical concern about maintaining walking endurance has been dropped during the grafting stage. Active LE exercise cannot be started until 2 to 3 days post-grafting (1), and walking must be discontinued for 6 days post-grafting for LE donor sites (3).

Since the therapist must discontinue exercise of the grafted body parts, the grafting stage is a good time to explore psychosocial issues. This patient became depressed and withdrawn during the grafting stage (1). This suggests that he is experiencing a loss of internal control. Yet more information is needed about his locus of control, his understanding of grafting procedures, his expectations for the cosmetic appearance of grafts, and his roles, interests, and human resources, like his family. Interviewing the patient and his family about these issues will make it easier for the therapist to choose meaningful activities for the patient during the post-grafting stage.

Rehabilitation concerns remain the same during the grafting stage. The patient is still independent in self-care except for hair care (1).

Priorities During the Grafting Stage

See Table 18.2 to compare the pre-grafting and grafting stage priorities. Except for pain and loss of sensation, which drop in importance, short-term concerns expand rather than change priorities from the pre-grafting stage.

Prevention of infection is still primary. Nevertheless, homeostatic issues are still service goals and would not be documented by the therapist. Prevention of all further structural damage to the extensor tendons and areas with third-degree burns that lack sensation is also still primary. Structural stability concerns have been expanded to include the grafted skin and donor site. Structural stability concerns are so obvious to experienced therapists that they often don't write them in the chart. Here's how to proceed:

1a. Track medical records and report all evidence of infection; and

1b. Prevent all further structural damage to grafted skin/donor site areas with third-degree burns that have no sensation.

Reduction of edema and maintenance of ROM in the LUE remain the second most important set of goals because the patient needs the therapist's assistance to counteract the effects of 5 days of inactivity until the graft takes. Biomechanical and sensory-motor goals would definitely be charted. Note the continued use of chunking to make short-term plans more manageable. Here's how to proceed:

2a. Reduce edema of fingers/prevent edema of LLE donor site; and

2b. Maintain AROM of RUE at:
- 150° of shoulder flexion and abduction;
- 60° of MP flexion;
- 45° of PIP flexion;
- 10° of DIP flexion; and
- fingertips 1 inch away from distal palmar crease.

Psychosocial concerns remain the third priority, even though they have expanded in number. Psychosocial concerns are still a part of the underground practice of many occupational therapists working in physical dysfunction settings. These therapists address psychosocial concerns every day, but they don't necessarily document them. Concerns about pain and loss of sensation drop to a third-level priority. They are ongoing concerns that are being addressed by routine procedures. Note the continued need for testing to make goals measurable even this far into the patient's recovery. Here's how to proceed:

3a. Keep pain manageable based on clinical observation;

3b. Assess locus of control/roles/interests/human resources;

3c. Investigate whether he understands grafting procedures and his expectations for the cosmetic appearance of grafts; and

3d. Reduce stress reactions based on clinical observation.

Maintaining strength and sitting endurance still remain the therapist's last priority. They can often be maintained by self-care activities without direct therapist supervision. Here's how to proceed:

4a. Maintain Good muscle strength in sound RUE;

4b. Maintain sitting endurance based on initial evaluation;

4c. Encourage independence in self-care except for hair care.

POST-GRAFTING STAGE

Procedural and Interactive Hypotheses

Once the skin grafts take, homeostatic issues become secondary to the potential for heterotopic ossification and stress ulcers.

Grafted skin creates new sensory-motor concerns. It is likely to have hypersensitivity or dull sensation (1, 2). Grafted skin also needs to be protected from prolonged sunlight because it is more prone to sunburn and hyperpigmentation (1). Poor hand coordination secondary to poor sensation and disuse becomes an issue that can be explored since fist-making precautions have been lifted.

Structural instability is less of an issue now. Grafted skin lacks sweat and oil glands, so it is very dry and prone to structural damage (2).

Loss of ROM is the major biomechanical concern during the post-grafting stage. Grafted skin continues to develop scar tissue for up to 18 months (2). This scar tissue becomes contracted and can fill in spaces, like the space between the chin and the chest. These contractures can affect ROM both above and below the graft site (2). Therefore, active assistive ROM of grafted areas is usually ordered by the doctor on day 4 or 5 post-grafting. This is done with the dressings off to eliminate abrasions (2, 3). Since grafted skin can tighten in 20 to 30 minutes after stretching if prolonged stretch pressure is not provided, splinting, positioning, and pressure garments must be implemented consistently (2).

The need for scar prevention emerges during the post-grafting stage. However, many patients do not understand the need for aggressive scar prevention until after the scars form (2). One therapist who has many years of experience at a burn hospital motivates post-grafted patients by promising to delay the use of splints (2). She tells her patients that they won't have to wear splints if they maintain their ROM with scar massage, proper sleeping positioning, and consistent wearing of pressure garments.

Psychosocial concerns are still present, but they shift focus. Hopefully, the therapist has been able to investigate roles, interest, and human resources during the physically inactive grafting period and can now investigate more sensitive topics, such as his life-long values and habits, financial resources, and the expectations of his family and his employer. These issues can provoke a fear of losing function.

Leisure and work concerns can be addressed now that fist-making is permitted. The need to modify leisure and work activities should be evaluated at this point.

Shift in Concerns During Post-grafting

Refer to Table 18.1 to see how the concerns change from the pre-grafting to the grafting stages of recovery. There is a major shift in the therapist's plan for action. Considerable patient data were obtained during the post-grafting stage because many precautions were lifted (1).

Homeostatic concerns for the post-grafting stage are reduced to the potential for stress ulcers and heterotopic ossification.

Sensory-motor concerns also show a major shift in focus. The patient's skin was hypersensitive to light touch and temperature. His left hand score on the Jebsen-Taylor Hand Function Test was below the 10th percentile. This test measures speed while writing, turning cards, picking up small objects, stacking checkers, and eating.

Biomechanical concerns represent another major shift in the therapist's focus during the post-grafting stage. Structural stability of the grafted skin continues to be a concern, but for a different reason. Grafted skin is very dry, so cocoa butter has to be applied daily to keep the skin soft and supple (2).

Loss of ROM due to scar formation is highly likely, so his understanding of scar prevention procedures must be investigated immediately.

The therapist is cleared for the first time to aggressively increase ROM, strength, and walking endurance. Following treatment, AROM was WNL except for 150° of shoulder flexion and abduction and finger flexion of 60° for MP, 45° for IP, and 10° for DIP joints. During fist-making, the fingertips were 1 inch away from the distal palmar crease. LUE strength was Good except for the left hand. Left lateral and palmar pinch were 3 and 2 pounds respectively (below the 10th percentile). He had no gross grasp. Regaining walking endurance was not reported because it probably didn't need to be addressed with regard to therapist intervention.

This patient's stress reactions seem to be abating as seen by his increased motivation to resume his former roles and to actively participate in therapy (1). The inability to relieve tension using normal activities is less of a problem since he can still play cards and engage in light gardening and woodworking activities (1). However, his left hand fatigued easily when holding cards, so he used a card holder. He was unable to play golf because grafted skin could not accommodate sudden stretch. Whether the loss of golfing is serious to him has to be explored. Is golfing a strong or a weak interest? Is it a social or a physical interest? Fortunately, he appears to have a realistic understanding of his injury and vocational potential (1). The expectations of his family and employer, his values, habits, and financial resources still need to be investigated.

The therapist was able to evaluate self-care and leisure skills that require both hands (1). He was independent in all self-care and light home management tasks, such as raking and handling woodworking tools.

Priorities During the Post-Grafting Stage

Refer to Table 18.2 to help you see the dramatic shift in priorities from the grafting to post-grafting stage.

The first priority during the post-grafting stage is the patient's ability to understand and willingness to carry out scar prevention procedures. It is more difficult and expensive to reduce scars than to prevent them, yet many patients don't learn this until after they develop scar tissue. Proceed as follows:

1a. Investigate whether he understands scar prevention procedures; and
1b. Prevent all scar formation of the grafted skin.

Sensory-motor and biomechanical concerns shift from maintenance to regaining assets now that the therapist can aggressively evaluate and treat these areas. Structural instability, skin hypersensitivity, ROM, strength, and hand coordination are functionally significant because they are intimately related to leisure and work skills.

Note the mini-treatment sequence that begins with the application of cocoa butter to soften the dry skin and then desensitization to enable the patient to tolerate manual contact while being stretched to increase ROM. Strengthening immediately follows stretching to encourage the patient to use the gains achieved by the therapist's stretching. Strengthening should help the patient hold onto objects while manipulating them during fine motor coordination activities. At this point, strive to:

2a. Prevent all structural damage to dry grafted skin;
2b. Reduce hypersensitivity to tactile stimuli from baseline;
2c. Increase AROM of burned RUE to:
  ● 165° of shoulder flexion and abduction;
  ● 65° of MP flexion;
  ● 45° of PIP flexion;
  ● 10° of DIP flexion; and
  ● fingertips ½-inch away from distal palmar crease.
2d. Increase strength of burned left hand:
  ● 6 lbs for lateral pinch; and
  ● 4 lbs for tip pinch.
2e. Increase Jebsen-Hand Function Test score to 25th percentile.

Psychosocial concerns remain the third priority since this patient seems to be making a good adjustment. This psychosocial information will help the therapist select appropriate evaluation procedures listed in the fourth set of priorities. Next, you should:

3a. Investigate the expectations of his family and employer; and
3b. Investigate values, habits, and financial resources.

Endurance remains the lowest priority because it can probably be remediated without direct therapist intervention. The inability to relieve tension with familiar activities has dropped down to the last priority since he is going home and will be able to resume all leisure activities except for golf. Evaluation of work skills is also a low priority because it will probably be done on an outpatient basis. Homeostatic issues have dropped to the last priority because only the potential for stress ulcers and heterotopic ossification remain. At this stage:

4a. Increase walking endurance based on environmental demands;
4b. Explore the importance of losing the ability to play golf;
4c. Investigate need for modified work activities; and
4d. Track potential stress ulcers and heterotopic ossification.

INTERACTIVE TRACK

As you look at the previous lengthy list of short-term goals, you may wonder how experienced therapists implement so many goals at once. Exploring and empathizing with the personal life of a patient is achieved by using the interactive track (4). Two excerpts from a study of patient-therapist interactions will illustrate how multiple goals can be implemented simultaneously. Here is an example of how an experienced therapist (ET) seamlessly wove the interactive and procedural tracks together (5). A physical therapist carried on the following conversation while doing an Ultrasound treatment with patient X. This therapist was able to gather data about the patient's life-style and create an atmosphere of empathy.

ET: "Now I'm going to get started here (with the Ultrasound) and then gradually I'm going to have you bring that right knee up to your chest, but gradually. Now I'm going to do this with a little stretch. Did you do a lot of walking this morning?"

X: "Yes. I usually walk in the morning, about three blocks."

ET: "How did you feel?"

X: "OK when I first put my leg out. Initially, getting up in the morning; that is when it pulls. When I walk to the bus, it eases."

ET: "How is it during the course of the day?"

X: "It is better during the day but worse at night."

Another example shows how an experienced therapist

(ET) built her questions on the patient's responses (X) while a novice (NV) ignored the patient's comments in order to focus on the procedural track (5).

ET: "Do you live on the first floor or second floor?"
X: "The first floor. I'm very careful of going up the stairs."
ET: "Is there a railing on the steps? Do you use it?"
X: "Yes. I put both hands on the railing to come down."

versus

NV: "How are you feeling today? Any changes in your symptoms?"
X: "It has been acting up."
NV: "Feeling any better with traction?"
X: "I had traction before."
NV: "You made the full 15 minutes, right? Any problems with that?"

Goals such as "explore the expectations of the family and employer" can be implemented with informal conversation similar to the ones just given. Rather than planning when to address such a goal, it is best to let it come up spontaneously or to guide the conversation in this direction. When conversation flows naturally, patients feel that the therapist is really listening to their concerns and cares about them.

CONCLUSIONS

Students who practice using frames of reference one at a time are well equipped to combine frames of reference in the clinic. Starting with one frame of reference ensures a successful experience and a detailed understanding of the clinical reasoning process. This gives students the confidence and experience they need to generalize what they have learned on their first frame of reference to new frames of reference. Finally, an assignment that combines frames of reference enables students to be aware of how experienced therapists treat the total patient.

References

1. Chan SW, Pedretti LW. Burns. In: Pedretti LW, Zoltan B, eds. Occupational therapy practice skills for physical dysfunction. 2nd ed. St. Louis: CV Mosby, 1985: 279.
2. Crouthammel R. Burns. Lecture presented at Temple University, Philadelphia, 1989.
3. Alvarado MI. Burns. In: Trombly CA, ed. Occupational therapy for physical dysfunction. 4th ed. Baltimore: Williams & Wilkins, Chapter 41, 1995.
4. Fleming MH. The therapist with the three track mind. Am J Occup Ther 1991;45:1007.
5. Jensen GM, Shepard KF, Hack LM. The novice versus the experienced clinician: insights into the work of the physical therapist. Phys Ther 1990;70:314.

APPENDIX:
Reliability, Test Validity, and Sensitivity

I. RELIABILITY

Reliability is defined as how consistently you can get the same test results over and over. There are many kinds of reliability, but three important ones are discussed below.

A. *Reliability coefficients vs. standard deviation scores.* A **correlation coefficient** ranges from $+1.0$ to -1.0. A correlation of 0.0 indicates that no correlation exists. A correlation of $+1.0$ indicates a perfect positive correlation (i.e., if one test score is high, the other is also high). A correlation of -1.0 indicates a perfect negative correlation (i.e., if one score test is high, the other test score is low). This is different from a **standard deviation score** that varies from -4.0 to $+4.0$. A standard deviation score of 0.0 indicates average performance, and all scores from $+1.0$ to -1.0 are considered to be within normal limits.

B. *Inter-rater Reliability* is how well TWO OR MORE OBSERVERS agree on how to score the SAME SUBJECT taking a test one time. Because simultaneous observation by several people can be disconcerting to many subjects, researchers often videotape a subject and then ask the observers to score the behavior they see. Good inter-rater reliability means that administrative and scoring protocols are very clearly written and that observers are using these protocols in a very similar way. Inter-rater reliability is typically reported as percentage of agreement or the strength of correlation between the raters' scores.

C. *Intra-rater Reliability* is how well two or more consecutive measurements on the SAME SUBJECT taken by the SAME OBSERVER on the same day agree. The time interval between measurements is usually a few minutes to a couple of hours to reduce the number of intervening variables that can change the patient performance. Good intra-rater reliability means that the observer is consis-

tently using the same test procedures. It does not necessarily mean that the observer is using standardized procedures! He/she may be using his own consistent method of evaluation.

D. *Test-Retest Reliability* is how well a SUBJECT'S TWO SCORES on the SAME TEST agree when the test is administered on TWO DIFFERENT DAYS. The interval between the two administrations varies from 1 day to 2 weeks. Good test-retest reliability means that the patient's performance is consistent. Good test-retest reliability is not always possible when subjects are inherently variable. For example, volatile medical conditions, like a patient coming out of a coma, can cause a patient's behavior to change hourly. Test-retest reliability is typically reported as the strength of correlation between the two sets of scores.

E. *Size of Correlation Coefficient* is a guide for interpreting reliability. These coefficients have to be higher for clinic use because the consequences of any decision based on a test score can have severe consequences for your patient (e.g., denied a driver's license or sent to a nursing home). Subjects in research studies are protected from severe consequences by human subjects committees.

In the clinic	In research
.90 + is a high correlation	
.80 to .89 is moderate	
.70 to .79 is low	.70+ is a high correlation
.69 and below is unacceptable	.50 to .69 is moderate
	.30 to .49 is low
	.29 and below = no correlation

F. *Standard Error of Measurement* (SE meas) = how much a subject's score varies from his/her own "true" score. If a subject takes a test several times, his/her score would vary slightly depending on whether the subject was having a "good" or a "bad" day. Even well-standardized tests cannot control this slight individual variance. SE meas is usually reported as a range of raw scores. For example, the Stanford-Binet I.Q. test has an SE meas of ±4.5 points. So an I.Q. score of 100 means your true score is between 95.5 and 104.5.

SE meas is particularly important when a subject has a borderline score (e.g., is close to −1.0, like −1.3 or −0.7). If this subject had a bad day, which slightly depressed his/her "true score," you don't want to make major decisions based on this borderline score. You should add the SE meas spread to the subject's raw score and look up the new standard deviation score. For example, Susie's Space Visualization raw score was 6, which is a borderline standard deviation score. After adding 3.2 points to her raw score, her revised standard deviation score is still −1.1, so you can safely conclude that her Space Visualization skills are not within normal limits.

G. *Characteristics of Formal Assessments That Produce High Reliability*
   1. *Standardized test materials*
   2. *Administrative protocols* establish how to set up the test environment, how to use test materials, what order to give the test items, exact wording of verbal instructions, whether prompts can be given, when to stop the test, etc.
   3. *Scoring protocols* establish specific directions and rating keys that allow as little room as possible for disagreement among raters.
   4. *Guidelines for interpreting test results* make a test more reliable.
      a. *Standard Deviation Score* permits you to compare a subject to a normative group. Within normal limits is considered to be −1.0 to +1.0. Unfortunately, very few human behaviors have standard deviation scores. There are no standard scores for unusual behaviors like doorknob sucking. Even commonly observed behaviors like blood pressure have no standard deviation scores. Therefore, health care professionals often turn to less statistically sophisticated scoring guidelines.
      b. *Percentile Scores* are less desirable because the intervals between ranks change (see Fig. A.1). For example, the interval between 95 and 99 is much larger than the interval between 50 and 55. It takes a large change in raw score to produce a change in rank near the extremes of the distribution, but only a small change in raw score to produce a change in rank near the middle of the distribution.
      c. *Age-Equivalent Scores* tell us that a raw score is typical for a specific age level (e.g., Denver Developmental Screening Test)
      d. *Cut-off Scores* provide some agreed upon criteria for passing behavior (e.g., blood pressure cut-offs for hypertension)
      e. *Ranks on an ordinal scale* (e.g., the Manual Muscle Test with grades from Poor to Normal; the COTE with scores from 0 to 4)
      f. *Frequency counts* (e.g., number of times a patient exhibits a behavior during the initial evaluation)
      g. *Qualitative descriptions* (e.g., description of how asymmetrically a patient sits before treatment begins)
      h. *Present/Absent* (e.g., ASTN Reflex)
   5. *Longer tests.* Reliability is usually higher when a test is longer. If an I.Q. test has only one question and it happens to be something you don't know, I would falsely conclude that you are retarded. If I use many test items, then special knowledge and early test anxiety should have less impact on your final test score. For example, test-retest reliability for the full-scale Wechsler Intelligence Scale for Children (WISC) is .95, but it is .65 to .88 for the shorter WISC subtests.

II. *TEST VALIDITY*
   Validity is defined as how well a test measures what it claims to measure. Just because an author puts a name, like visual figure-ground, in a test title doesn't mean it tests that skill. There are several kinds of validity, but three important ones are listed below.
   A. *Face Validity* asks if you intuitively believe that the test measures what it says it measures on "face value."
   B. *Content Validity* asks if the test measures the content that was taught. Test items are drawn from a specific course of instruction (e.g., anatomy course) or a uniform set of experiences (e.g., FW II). However, learning experiences can change over time and from one situation to the next. Therefore, content validity is useful ONLY when you are trying to decide if a test covers the exact same content that you have taught. One method for establishing content validity is to ask a panel of experts if they agree about what items should be on a test. Another method is to show differentiation among subjects. For example, item #6 on the California Reading Achievement Test was able to discriminate between 7th and 10th graders:

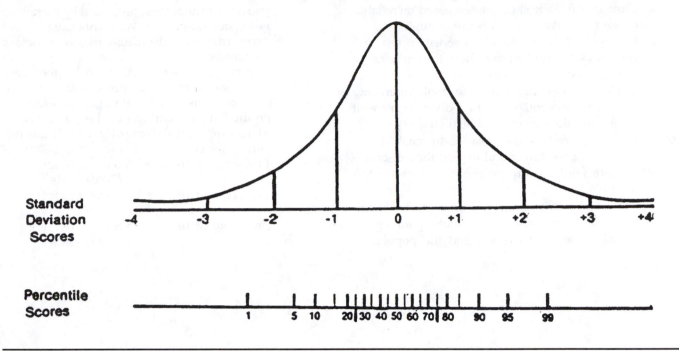

Standard Deviation Scores

-4   -3   -2   -1   0   +1   +2   +3   +4

Percentile Scores

1   5   10   20 30 40 50 60 70 80   90   95   99

Figure A.1.

Grade 7	Grade 8	Grade 9	Grade 10
77% pass the item	83% pass	88% pass	95% pass

C. *Construct Validity* asks if the test measures a construct (e.g., a fundamental human trait) that exists in the general population. This trait is inborn, like intelligence. No special experience, like Head Start is required. You must know how this innate skill is distributed across the normal population before you can compare a subject's score against what you think is "normal." This type of validity is **norm-referenced** because a person is compared to a population norm.

1. *Methods for proving construct validity include:*
   a. *Differentiation among subjects* (e.g., number of cubes in a tower should increase with age)
   b. *Contrasted groups* (e.g., normal subjects and paranoid schizophrenics should get significantly different scores on a test of paranoid ideation)
   c. *Correlation with similar tests*. If two tests measure similar skills, a subject should get similar scores on the two tests.
   d. *Factor analysis* is the clustering of scores on tests that measure similar skills. Since few people are superior in every way, most subjects' scores on a battery of tests will cluster into "factors." See the example below of how one subject's strengths and weak-

nesses clustered into two innate factors.
Language test scores = 88, 86, and 82
Fine motor test scores = 75, 76, and 80

III. *SENSITIVITY*

A. *Definition.* Sensitivity is the ability to detect small changes. A sensitive test can award different scores for only slightly different behaviors. The example below shows that sensitivity doesn't mean a test has to have more test items; it just has to have sophisticated scoring criteria.

1. The Sewall Developmental Test is VERY sensitive
   6 months = sits briefly propped forward on extended arms
   7 months = sits unsteadily without propping on arms
   8 months = sits steady for 10 minutes after placed in sitting position
   9 months = sits up from supine by rolling onto side and then pushing up with hands

2. The Denver Developmental Screening Test is NOT sensitive
   6 months = sits without support for 5 seconds
   9 months = gets up to sit

B. *Need for Sensitivity.* Sensitivity is especially important to therapists who often do not completely "cure" a patient. To document the effectiveness of our treatment, we need tests that detect small changes over a short period of time.

Clinicians usually choose a test based on reliability and validity, but this is not enough!

C. *Ceilings and Basements*. Even sensitive tests are not usually sensitive throughout the entire range the test is designed to measure.

1. *Good ceilings* are sensitive to small differences at the upper end of test; they discriminate well among older or more skilled subjects.

2. *Good basements* are sensitive to small differences at the lower end of test; they discriminate well among younger or less skilled subjects.

3. *Matching*. When you are assessing a test's ceiling and basement, you are looking for a good match between the test and the population you are treating. Most tests used by therapists need good basements. We do not usually treat extraordinary individuals like world-class weightlifters.

4. *Plateauing*. Some tests do not have good ceilings because they measure a skill that naturally plateaus at a certain age. For example, on the Finger Identification Test, a raw score of 16 does not differentiate well among older subjects.

raw score of 16 = +1.6 S.D. score for
7 1/2-year-olds

raw score of 16 = +1.5 S.D. score for
8-year-olds

raw score of 16 = +1.5 S.D. score for
8 1/2-year-olds

FIGURE AND TABLE CREDITS

Figures

Figure 6.1. Redrawn from Jankowska E, Lundberg A. Interneurons in the spinal cord. TINS 1981;4:320.

Figure 7.2. From Norkin C, Levangie P. Joint structure and function. Philadelphia: FA Davis, 1983:275.

Figure 8.1. From Eggers O. Occupational therapy in the treatment of adult hemiplegia, Rockville, MD: Aspen Publications, 1984:24, 25.

Figure 8.2A. From Pedretti LW, Zoltan B, eds. Occupational therapy practice skills for physical dysfunction. 3rd ed. St. Louis: CV Mosby, 1990:222.

Figure 8.2B. From Bobath B. Adult hemiplegia: evaluation and treatment. 2nd ed. London: William Heinemann Medical Books Limited, 1978:76.

Figure 8.2C. From Eggers O. Occupational therapy in the treatment of adult hemiplegia. Rockville, MD: Aspen Publications, 1984:45.

Figure 8.3. From Pedretti LW, Zoltan B, eds. Occupational therapy practice skills for physical dysfunction. 3rd ed. St. Louis: CV Mosby, 1990:222.

Figure 8.4. From Pedretti LW, Zoltan B, eds. Occupational therapy practice skills for physical dysfunction. 3rd ed. St. Louis: CV Mosby, 1990:220.

Figure 9.2. From Eggers O. Occupational therapy in the treatment of adult hemiplegia. Rockville, MD: Aspen Publications, 1984.

Figure 9.3. From Eggers O. Occupational therapy in the treatment of adult hemiplegia. Rockville, MD: Aspen Publications, 1984:27.

Figure 9.4. From Eggers O. Occupational therapy in the treatment of adult hemiplegia. Rockville, MD: Aspen Publications, 1984:55.

Figure 9.5. From Eggers O. Occupational therapy in the treatment of adult hemiplegia. Rockville, MD: Aspen Publications, 1984.

Figure 15.1. From Allen CA. Occupational therapy for psychiatric diseases. Boston: Little, Brown & Co., p. 47.

Figure 15.2. From Allen CA. Occupational therapy for psychiatric diseases. Boston: Little, Brown & Co., p. 88.

Figure 16.1. From Hopkins and Smith. Willard and Spackman's occupational therapy. 7th ed. Philadelphia: JB Lippincott, p. 22.

Tables

Table 7.3A. From Brunnstrom S. Movement therapy in hemiplegia. Philadelphia: Harper & Row, 1970:38.

Table 7.3B. From Brunnstrom S. Movement therapy in hemiplegia. Philadelphia: Harper & Row, 1970:39.

Table 7.3C. From Brunnstrom S. Movement therapy in hemiplegia. Philadelphia: Harper & Row, 1970:39.

Table 7.10. From Erhardt RP. Developmental hand dysfunction. Laurel, MD: Remsco Publishing, 1982.

Table 15.4. From Brayman SJ. Comprehensive occupational therapy evaluation scale. Am J Occup Ther 1976;30:94.

Table 15.6. From Allen CK. Occupational therapy for psychiatric disease. Boston: Little, Brown & Co., 1985:65.

Table 15.7. From Allen CA, Earhart CA. Cognitive disabilities: expanded activity analysis. Workbook introduced at the Institute on Cognitive Disabilities. Phoenix, AZ, 1988.

Table 16.3. From: The normal acquisition of normal feeding skills. New York: Therapeutic Media, 1982.

INDEX

Page numbers in *italics* denote figures and Memory Aids; those followed by "t" denote tables.

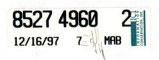

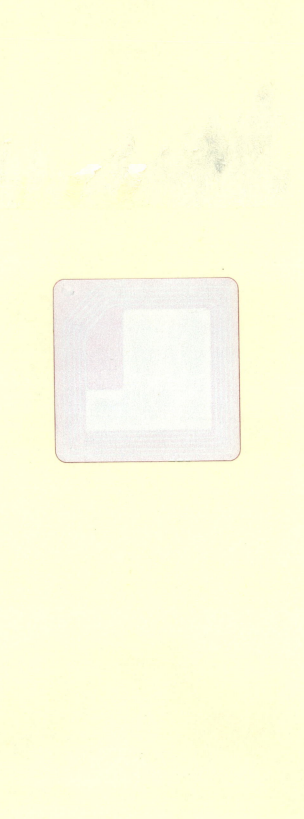